Advances in Treatment of Bipolar Disorders

Advances in Treatment of Bipolar Disorders

Edited by

Terence A. Ketter, M.D.

Professor of Psychiatry and Behavioral Sciences
and Chief, Bipolar Disorders Clinic
Stanford University, Stanford, California

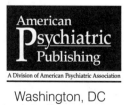

American Psychiatric Publishing
A Division of American Psychiatric Association

Washington, DC
London, England

Copyright © 2015 American Psychiatric Association
ALL RIGHTS RESERVED

Manufactured in the United States of America on acid-free paper
19 18 17 16 15   5 4 3 2 1
First Edition

Typeset in Palatino LT Std and Helvetica Lt Std

American Psychiatric Publishing

A Division of American Psychiatric Association
1000 Wilson Boulevard
Arlington, VA 22209-3901
www.appi.org

Library of Congress Cataloging-in-Publication Data
Ketter, Terence A., author, editor.
    Advances in treatment of bipolar disorders / edited by Terence A. Ketter. — First edition.
        p. ; cm.
    Includes bibliographical references and index.
    ISBN 978-1-58562-417-1 (pbk. : alk. paper)
    I. American Psychiatric Association. II. Title.
    [DNLM: 1. Bipolar Disorder—therapy. WM 207]
    RC516
    616.89′5—dc23
                                                                        2015006550

British Library Cataloguing in Publication Data
A CIP record is available from the British Library.

CONTENTS

Terence A. Ketter, M.D.
Shefali Miller, M.D.
Po W. Wang, M.D.

Terence A. Ketter, M.D.
Shefali Miller, M.D.
Po W. Wang, M.D.
Jenifer Culver, Ph.D.

Terence A. Ketter, M.D.
Shefali Miller, M.D.

Terence A. Ketter, M.D.
Shefali Miller, M.D.
Jenifer Culver, Ph.D.

Contributors

John O. Brooks III, Ph.D., M.D.
Associate Professor, Semel Institute for Neuroscience and Human Behavior, University of California Los Angeles, Los Angeles, California

Kiki D. Chang, M.D.
Professor, Department of Psychiatry and Behavioral Sciences, Stanford University School of Medicine, Stanford, California

Jenifer Culver, Ph.D.
Clinical Assistant Professor, Department of Psychiatry and Behavioral Sciences, Stanford University School of Medicine, Stanford, California

Terence A. Ketter, M.D.
Professor of Psychiatry and Behavioral Sciences; Chief, Bipolar Disorders Clinic, Stanford University, Stanford, California

Shefali Miller, M.D.
Clinical Assistant Professor, Department of Psychiatry and Behavioral Sciences, Stanford University School of Medicine, Stanford, California

Natalie L. Rasgon, M.D., Ph.D.
Professor, Department of Psychiatry and Behavioral Sciences, Stanford University School of Medicine, Stanford, California

Manpreet K. Singh, M.D., M.S.
Assistant Professor, Department of Psychiatry and Behavioral Sciences, Stanford University School of Medicine, Stanford, California

Mytilee Vemuri, M.D., M.B.A.
Clinical Assistant Professor, Department of Psychiatry and Behavioral Sciences, Stanford University School of Medicine, Stanford, California

Po W. Wang, M.D.
Clinical Professor, Department of Psychiatry and Behavioral Sciences, Stanford University School of Medicine, Stanford, California

Disclosures of Competing Interests

The following contributors to this book have indicated a financial interest in or other affiliation with a commercial supporter, a manufacturer of a commercial product, a provider of a commercial service, a nongovernmental organization, and /or a government agency, as listed below:

Terence A. Ketter, M.D.—*Grant/research support:* Agency for Healthcare Research and Quality, AstraZeneca, Cephalon (now Teva), Eli Lilly, Pfizer, Sunovion; *Consultant:* Allergan, Avanir, Depotmed, Forest, Genentech, Janssen, Merck, Sunovion, Teva; *Lecture honoraria:* Abbott, GlaxoSmithKline, Otsuka, Pfizer; *Royalties:* American Psychiatric Publishing; *Employee (spouse):* Janssen; *Stock (spouse):* Janssen.

Natalie L. Rasgon, M.D., Ph.D.—Current: Magceutics; *Research support:* American Diabetes Association, Corcept; *Consultant:* Shire, Sunovion, Takeda; Past: *PI of multi-site study:* Bayer; *Research support:* Forest, Glaxo-SmithKline, Pfizer, Wyeth; *Grant support:* Abbott; *Consultant:* Wyeth; *Speaker:* Bristol-Myers Squibb, Forest, Pfizer.

The following contributors to this book have indicated no competing interests to disclose during the year preceding manuscript submission:

Jenifer Culver, Ph.D.
Shefali Miller, M.D.
Manpreet K. Singh, M.D., M.S.
Po W. Wang, M.D.

Preface

Advances in Treatment of Bipolar Disorders is intended to be a concise, readable, timely guide to the most recent advances in the treatment of patients with bipolar disorder. Readers interested in older or more detailed information are referred to the earlier volume, *Handbook of Diagnosis and Treatment of Bipolar Disorders,* published by American Psychiatric Publishing in 2010. Although the pace of therapeutic advances has attenuated somewhat since the publication of the 2010 book, important new developments have continued, challenging clinicians to keep abreast of the most recent research and integrate it into their practice.

The ongoing movement toward providing evidence-based care continues to make appreciating the quality of data supporting interventions increasingly important. Thus, we emphasize in this book recent controlled studies and U.S. Food and Drug Administration (FDA) approvals. We strive to present the information needed for clinicians to balance the likelihood of benefit (using *number needed to treat* analyses) versus harm (using *number needed to harm* analyses) and then to provide individualized, state-of-the-art, evidence-based care. In this regard, plentiful figures and summary tables are provided to make the content clinician-friendly.

The information in this volume is based not only on controlled trials and FDA approvals but also on almost two decades of clinical research and clinical treatment experience by clinicians at Stanford University. Therefore, it offers an intermingling of evidence-based medicine and extensive personal clinical experiences to reflect our most up-to-date thinking about the diagnosis and management of bipolar disorder. Because this field is rapidly advancing, readers are encouraged to cross-reference our recommendations with other sources, in particular with the latest edition of the *Physicians' Desk Reference* for medication information.

I have many individuals to thank for their assistance in the preparation of this book: My wife Nzeera has been patient and understanding regarding my need to spend time on this volume. The chapter coauthors— John Brooks, Kiki Chang, Jenifer Culver, Shefali Miller, Natalie Rasgon,

Manpreet Singh, Mytilee Vemuri, and Po Wang—deserve particular appreciation. The editorial staff at American Psychiatric Publishing (APP)—in particular John McDuffie—have earned credit for their support, critical reading, and technical skill. The APP leadership—in particular Robert Hales—receive thanks for their confidence. Our colleagues and trainees at Stanford University deserve appreciation for their insights. Finally, but by no means least, a great debt is owed to patients and their families who consistently prove that each of them can teach us about bipolar disorder and its treatment on a daily basis.

We hope readers will find this volume helpful, and look forward to their feedback.

Terence A. Ketter, M.D.
January 2015

1 Diagnosis and Treatment of Bipolar Disorder

Terence A. Ketter, M.D.
Shefali Miller, M.D.
Po W. Wang, M.D.

Multiple important, clinically relevant developments regarding the diagnosis and treatment of bipolar disorder have occurred since the publication of *Handbook of Diagnosis and Treatment of Bipolar Disorders* in 2010 (Ketter 2010), challenging clinicians to keep abreast of the most recent research and integrate it into their practice. Arguably, the most important recent diagnostic development is the publication, in 2013, of DSM-5 (American Psychiatric Association 2013), which has superseded DSM-IV-TR (American Psychiatric Association 2000).

One review of bipolar disorder treatments opined that recent pharmacotherapy advances have remained modest (Geddes and Miklowitz 2013). Although the pace of pharmacotherapy advances did slow somewhat in the late 2000s and early 2010s compared with the early to mid-2000s, important new pharmacotherapeutic developments have continued. Indeed, between 2009 and 2013, the U.S. Food and Drug Administration (FDA) approved asenapine monotherapy (McIntyre et al. 2009, 2010) and adjunctive (added to lithium or valproate) therapy (Szegedi et al. 2012) for acute (DSM-IV-TR) manic and mixed episodes; risperidone long-acting injectable (LAI) formulation monotherapy (Quiroz et al. 2010) and adjunctive (added to lithium or valproate) therapy (Macfadden et al. 2009), ziprasidone adjunctive (added to lithium or valproate) therapy (Bowden et al. 2010), and aripiprazole adjunctive (added to lithium or valproate) therapy (Marcus et al. 2011) for bipolar disorder preventive treatment; and lurasidone monotherapy (Loebel et al. 2014b) and adjunctive therapy (Loebel et al. 2014a) for acute bipolar I depression. Also, in 2014, the olanzapine plus fluoxetine combination approval for adults with bipolar I depression was extended to include children and adolescents ages 10–17 years (Detke et al. 2015). In addition, in 2012, the FDA approved inhaled loxapine for agitation associated with bipolar I disorder (Kwentus et al. 2012). Table 1–1 lists the drugs approved by the FDA for bipolar disorder treatments.

Also in recent years, multicenter, randomized, double-blind, placebo-controlled trials have assessed the utility of ziprasidone monotherapy (Lombardo et al. 2012) and adjunctive (added to lithium, valproate, or lamotrigine) therapy (Sachs et al. 2011), olanzapine monotherapy (Tohen et al. 2012), and armodafinil adjunctive (added to lithium, valproate, lamotrigine, and/or olanzapine, risperidone, aripiprazole, ziprasidone [only with lithium and/or valproate] in three of three studies, or quetiapine, in the third study only) therapy (Ketter et al. 2013) in acute bipolar depression; cariprazine monotherapy (Citrome 2013; Starace et al. 2012), ziprasidone adjunctive (added to lithium or valproate) therapy (Sachs et al. 2012a, 2012b), and paliperidone monotherapy (Berwaerts et al. 2012b; Vieta et al. 2010) and adjunctive (added to lithium or valproate) therapy (Berwaerts et al. 2011) in acute mania; and paliperidone monotherapy (Berwaerts et al. 2012a) and aripiprazole adjunctive (added to lamotrigine) therapy (Carlson et al. 2012) for bipolar disorder preventive treatment.

Moreover, the International Society for Bipolar Disorders Antidepressant Use in Bipolar Disorders Task Force published its report on this controversial topic in 2013 (Pacchiarotti et al. 2013). Also, there has been increasing appreciation of the potential for rapid relief of depression with interventions that affect glutamatergic neurotransmission, such as adjunctive ketamine (Diazgranados et al. 2010; Zarate et al. 2012), and the utility of adjunctive deep brain stimulation in treatment-resistant depression (Berlim et al. 2014), although as of early 2015, such interventions remained only research (as opposed to clinical) tools. Finally, a recent review of bipolar disorder treatments noted that adjunctive psychosocial treatments have continued to advance (Geddes and Miklowitz 2013), and this important topic is discussed in Chapter 2, "Treatment of Acute Bipolar Depression"; Chapter 4, "Bipolar Disorder Preventive Treatment"; Chapter 5, "Treatment of Pediatric Bipolar Disorder"; and Chapter 7, "Treatment of Older Adults With Bipolar Disorder." Selected other important developments mentioned above are discussed in more detail in the remainder of this chapter.

■ Important Changes to Bipolar Disorder in DSM-5

In our opinion, the three most important changes for bipolar and related disorders in DSM-5 are, in rank order: 1) adding a "with mixed features"

TABLE 1–1. U.S. Food and Drug Administration–approved bipolar disorder treatments, with years of initial approval

Acute mania	Bipolar depression	Bipolar maintenance
1970, Lithium[P]	2003, Olanzapine+fluoxetine[*P]	1974, Lithium[P]
1973, Chlorpromazine	2006, Quetiapine XR (2008)	2003, Lamotrigine
1994, Divalproex ER (2005)	2013, Lurasidone[*]	2004, Olanzapine
2000, Olanzapine[*P]		2005, Aripiprazole[*P]
2003, Risperidone[*P]		2008, Quetiapine XR (adjunct)
2004, Quetiapine XR (2008)[*P]		2009, Risperidone LAI[*]
2004, Ziprasidone		2009, Ziprasidone (adjunct)
2004, Aripiprazole[*P]		
2004, Carbamazepine ERC		
2009, Asenapine[*]		

Note. ER, XR=extended-release formulation (FDA approval year in parentheses); ERC=extended-release capsule formulation; LAI=long-acting injectable formulation.
[P]Pediatric as well as adult (see Table 5–1 for pediatric bipolar disorder approval years).
[*]Adjunctive therapy (added to lithium or valproate) and monotherapy.

specifier for manic, hypomanic, and major depressive episodes; 2) permitting a full manic or hypomanic episode that emerges during antidepressant treatment and persists beyond the physiological effect of that treatment to be sufficient evidence for a manic or hypomanic episode; and 3) adding a "with anxious distress" specifier for manic, hypomanic, and major depressive episodes. These three changes all merit further discussion.

More Inclusive Approach to Mixed Symptoms

DSM-5 includes a new "with mixed features" specifier for manic, hypomanic, and major depressive episodes. Therefore, the mixed episodes of DSM-IV-TR have been eliminated in favor of manic episodes with mixed features in DSM-5. The DSM-5 Mood Disorders Work Group determined that permissible opposite pole symptoms for mixed features ought to be restricted to those not considered to be coincident in both (mood elevation and depression) poles, so that "overlapping" symptoms such as distractibility, irritability, and psychomotor agitation ought not be counted as mixed symptoms (Akiskal and Benazzi 2003; American Psychiatric Association 2013; Angst et al. 2011; Fiedorowicz et al. 2011; Goldberg et al. 2009; Maj et al. 2006; Sato et al. 2003, 2004; Swann et al. 2007, 2013; Zimmermann et al. 2009). In DSM-5, only "nonoverlapping" opposite pole symptoms have been permitted to count toward the "with mixed features" specifier, although this decision has been challenged (Koukopoulos and Sani 2014).

The DSM-5 "with mixed features" specifier requires at least three nonoverlapping opposite pole symptoms. Even though it has been acknowledged that the presence of as few as two mood elevation symptoms during major depressive episodes entails important properties associated with bipolar disorder and mixed states (Benazzi and Akiskal 2001; Zimmermann et al. 2009), it has also been suggested that a threshold of three opposite pole symptoms is a parsimonious approach to mixed states (Swann et al. 2009). However, requiring at least three "nonoverlapping" mood elevation symptoms may be insufficiently inclusive, because features distinguishing mixed from pure depressive episodes can emerge at even very low mood elevation symptom thresholds (Frye et al. 2009; Goldberg et al. 2009; Mazza et al. 2011; Shim et al. 2014; Swann et al. 2007, 2009). Thus, some investigators have found the DSM-5 approach to "with mixed features," although considerably more inclusive than the DSM-IV-TR approach to mixed symptoms, still overly exclusive, and have advocated even more inclusive approaches afforded by

1) permitting "overlapping" opposite pole symptoms to count toward mixed symptoms and/or 2) decreasing the number of necessary opposite pole symptoms from three to two, or even one (Koukopoulos et al. 2013).

Nevertheless, DSM-5 entails a considerably more inclusive approach to mixed symptom phenomenology compared with the overly exclusive, restricted approach of DSM-IV-TR, which had only full mixed episodes (syndromal manic episode concurrent with syndromal major depressive episode). Thus, DSM-5 includes the following patterns of mixed symptoms not included in DSM-IV-TR: 1) syndromal manic episode with subsyndromal depressive symptoms (as manic episode with mixed features); 2) syndromal hypomanic episode with syndromal or subsyndromal depressive symptoms (as hypomanic episode with mixed features); and 3) syndromal major depressive episode with subsyndromal mood elevation symptoms (as major depressive episode with mixed features). The last of these constructs, which in non–DSM-5 terms has been commonly referred to as "mixed depression," can occur not only in bipolar disorder but also in unipolar major depressive disorder.

DSM-5 stipulates that concurrent syndromal manic and major depressive symptoms (i.e., a DSM-IV-TR mixed episode) be considered as a manic episode with mixed features (rather than a major depressive episode with mixed features) because mania is considered to be generally more severe than depression. In contrast, DSM-5 does not stipulate whether a syndromal hypomanic episode concurrent with a syndromal major depressive episode ought to be considered a hypomanic episode with mixed features (as stated above, and as preferred by us) or a major depressive episode with mixed features (which may be preferred by some investigators and clinicians). In our view, calling such episodes hypomanic episodes with mixed features has the potential merit of drawing attention to the importance of being aware that standard antidepressants may provide inadequate efficacy (i.e., leaving the patient depressed) and/or tolerability (i.e., exacerbating mood elevation symptoms). Nevertheless, the complementary approach of calling such episodes major depressive episodes with mixed features may have the potential merit of drawing attention to the importance of addressing syndromal major depressive symptoms, which can be more severe than syndromal hypomanic symptoms (which by definition are not severe).

The silence in DSM-5 regarding how to characterize syndromal hypomanic symptoms accompanied by concurrent syndromal major depressive symptoms has the advantage of providing clinicians the flexibility of calling such presentations either hypomanic episodes with mixed features or major depressive episodes with mixed features, depending on individual presentations. For example, a bipolar I disorder patient with moderate syndromal hypomanic symptoms, mild (but syndromal) major depressive symptoms, and a history of antidepressant treatment–emergent psychotic mania might be better served by such a presentation being interpreted as a hypomanic episode with mixed features, consistent with the high priority of antimanic treatment and the need to avoid antidepressants. In contrast, a bipolar II disorder patient with severe syndromal major depressive symptoms, mild (but syndromal) hypomanic symptoms, and a history of adequate efficacy and tolerability with standard antidepressants might be better served by such a presentation being interpreted as a major depressive episode with mixed features, consistent with the potential utility of cautiously administering standard antidepressant medication along with antimanic treatment.

Arguably, DSM-5's inclusion of mixed depression (i.e., major depressive episode with mixed features) may be a more impactful innovation than inclusion of mixed mania or hypomania (i.e., manic or hypomanic episode with mixed features) for several reasons. First, mixed depression may involve a larger number of patients with unipolar major depressive disorder and bipolar disorder, whereas mixed mania or hypomania may involve only a smaller number of patients with bipolar disorder (but not unipolar major depressive disorder). Second, permitting mixed depressions in patients with unipolar major depressive disorder is consistent with the bipolar spectrum concept—that is, a continuum of mood disorders ranging from bipolar I disorder, to bipolar II disorder, to other specified or unspecified bipolar disorders (called "bipolar disorder not otherwise specified" in DSM-IV-TR), to mixed unipolar depression, to pure unipolar depression. Third, mixed compared with pure depressions may have different therapeutic implications, with antidepressants having poorer efficacy and/or tolerability in mixed compared with pure depression, independent of overall illness polarity (i.e., whether in the context of bipolar disorder or unipolar major depressive disorder).

More Inclusive Approach to Antidepressant Treatment– Emergent Mood Elevation

DSM-5 considers full hypomanic or manic episodes emerging during antidepressant treatment and persisting beyond the physiological effects of that treatment to be sufficient evidence for hypomanic or manic episodes, and thus sufficient evidence for a diagnosis of bipolar II disorder (provided the patient also has major depressive episodes) or bipolar I disorder, respectively. This is in contrast to the approach in DSM-IV-TR, which considered antidepressant treatment–emergent mood elevations as secondary to antidepressants and thus as not counting toward a primary bipolar disorder. DSM-5 (which avoids primary-secondary terminology) considers such episodes sufficient evidence for a true bipolar disorder, rather than merely indicating a substance/medication-induced phenomenon. Thus, bipolar disorder in DSM-5 (which considers persistent antidepressant treatment–emergent mania or hypomania to be bipolar disorder) is more inclusive than in DSM-IV-TR (which considers antidepressant treatment–emergent mania or hypomania to be a medication-induced disorder). The DSM-5 approach is consistent with data indicating that treatment-induced mania is within the bipolar spectrum, rather than merely representing a coincidental treatment complication (Dumlu et al. 2011), but has been criticized because there is likely only limited reliability when one is deciding whether or not mood elevation symptoms persist beyond antidepressant physiological effects in individual patients (Terao and Tanaka 2014). This reliability limitation could be avoided by dropping the "persisting beyond the physiological effects of that treatment" requirement, although making this change might serve to modestly further increase bipolar disorder inclusivity.

Acknowledgment of the Importance of Anxiety

For manic or hypomanic episodes as well as major depressive episodes, DSM-5 has added the specifier "with anxious distress," which is defined as the presence of at least two of the following symptoms: 1) feeling keyed up or tense, 2) feeling unusually restless, 3) difficulty concentrating due to worry, 4) fearing that something awful may happen, and 5) fearing loss of self-control. This innovation is noteworthy because anxiety disorder comorbidity is very common in patients with bipolar disorder and is often associated with important unfavorable illness characteristics, such as poorer mood (including more suicidality) and more substance use disorder comorbidity (McIntyre et al. 2006). Moreover, pharmacotherapy of anxiety in patients with bipolar disorder can be particularly challenging because of efficacy and tolerability limitations of antidepressants and the abuse potential of anxiolytics. Although older agents approved for the treatment of acute bipolar depression may also relieve anxiety (Hirschfeld et al. 2006; Tohen et al. 2007), the older second-generation antipsychotics can have substantive tolerability limitations (i.e., sedation and weight gain) (Calabrese et al. 2005; Thase et al. 2006; Tohen et al. 2003). Lurasidone, a second-generation antipsychotic that was more recently approved for acute bipolar depression, may also relieve anxiety but with fewer tolerability limitations than older approved agents (Loebel et al. 2014a, 2014b).

■ Important Potential Changes in Bipolar Disorder Missing From DSM-5

In our opinion, the three most important potential changes for bipolar and related disorders that are *missing* from DSM-5 include, in rank order: 1) underemphasis of a unitary dimensional approach to mood disorders, 2) underemphasis of inclusion of other clinical markers of bipolar disorder risk, and 3) lack of biomarkers for the diagnosis and treatment of bipolar disorder. These three missing potential changes merit further consideration.

Underemphasis of a Unitary Dimensional Approach to Mood Disorders

Arguably, DSM-5—by creating separate chapters for bipolar and related disorders and (unipolar) depressive disorders rather than combining bipolar and unipolar disorders in a single mood disorders chapter (as in DSM-IV-TR)—has taken at least a partial step backward in emphasizing the increasing evidence of a spectrum of mood disorders ranging from unipolar to bipolar disorder that has been supported by both American and European authors (Akiskal 2007; Akiskal et al. 1989; Angst et al. 2011). This bipolar spectrum controversy is but a manifestation of a long-standing dialogue regarding unitary versus segmented approaches to mood disorders, with the unitary (Kraepelinian) approach advocating the integration of unipolar and bipolar mood disorders based on the common feature of recurrence (Kraepelin 1921), and the segmented (Leonhardian) approach advocating the segregation of unipolar and bipolar mood disorders based on differential polarities (Leonhard 1957). Indeed, it could be argued that positioning the DSM-5 chapter on bipolar and related disorders between those of schizophrenia spectrum and other psychotic disorders and (unipolar) depressive disorders serves to emphasize a schizophrenia-bipolar-unipolar spectrum at the expense of a more specific bipolar-unipolar spectrum.

Some authors consider the DSM-5 definition of hypomania to be overly narrow or exclusive—because it requires either a longer-than-optimal minimum duration or a higher-than-optimal mood elevation symptom count—and opine that it ought to be made more broad or inclusive by decreasing symptom duration and count thresholds (the duration threshold has received more attention). DSM-5 has only partially acknowledged this position by including among the other specified bipolar and related disorders a list of presentations that do not meet criteria for specific bipolar and related disorders, including, among others, 1) major depressive episodes and short-duration (2- to 3-day) hypomanic episodes (i.e., of insufficient duration for full hypomanic episodes) (Benazzi 2001) and 2) major depressive episodes and hypomanic episodes with insufficient symptom count for full hypomanic episodes. Thus, the approach of DSM-5 may be interpreted as a less-than-complete acknowledgment of the potential utility of decreasing the minimum duration threshold for hypomanic episodes from 4 to 2–3 days.

Although it could also be argued that DSM-5 has taken a partial step forward with respect to acknowledging the mood disorders spectrum by permitting major depressive episodes with mixed features not only in bipolar and related disorders but also in (unipolar) depressive disorders, some authors contend that by using a relatively narrow and exclusive (as opposed to broad and inclusive) definition of mixed depression, DSM-5 has not gone far enough in acknowledging the bipolar-unipolar spectrum (Koukopoulos and Sani 2014).

Importantly, DSM-5 does not address the issue of degree of diagnostic uncertainty regarding (especially younger) patients with major depressive episodes who have not yet had a hypomanic or manic episode and therefore to date merit only a diagnosis of (unipolar) major depressive disorder. In the following subsection, we describe the several nonacute symptom clinical markers of risk for bipolar disorder outcome that could be used to develop a probabilistic model of risk of bipolar outcome among patients with major depressive episodes who have not yet had a hypomanic or manic episode.

Underemphasis of Inclusion of Other Clinical Markers of Bipolar Disorder Risk

As mentioned in *Handbook of Diagnosis and Treatment of Bipolar Disorders* (Ketter 2010), the risk of bipolar outcome among depressed individuals increases in the presence of several other (non-DSM) clinical markers, such as early age at onset of depression (i.e., before age 25), history of psychosis, family history of bipolar disorder, and atypical vegetative depressive symptoms (i.e., hypersomnia, hyperphagia, and psychomotor retardation). Indeed, 5 years prior to the publication of DSM-5, the International Society for Bipolar Disorders Diagnostic Guidelines Task Force published a proposed probabilistic approach to the risk of bipolar outcome in depressed individuals (Mitchell et al. 2008). For several years, investigators have advocated use of such non-DSM information in efforts to enhance the diagnosis and treatment of depressed individuals at high risk of bipolar outcome (Phelps and Ghaemi 2012; Sachs 2004).

It could be argued that DSM-5 took a partial step forward with respect to inclusion of other clinical markers of bipolar disorder risk by permitting a full manic or hypomanic episode that emerges during antidepressant treatment and persists beyond the physiological effect of that treatment to be sufficient evidence for a manic or hypomanic episode. Nevertheless, some investigators contend that DSM-5 has underemphasized the importance of multiple other bipolar outcome risk factors for depressed individuals.

Lack of Biomarkers for the Diagnosis and Treatment of Bipolar Disorder

Biomarkers have demonstrated diagnostic and treatment response monitoring utility in multiple branches of medicine. Unfortunately, to date, genetic studies in bipolar disorder have indicated complex polygenic inheritance related to multiple small-effect alleles (Craddock and Jones 1999; Craddock and Sklar 2009, 2013), so that in spite of compelling evidence of the heritability of bipolar disorder, genetic studies have not yet yielded clinically relevant biomarkers of bipolar illness risk or treatment response and have noted substantial bipolar-unipolar and bipolar-schizophrenia genetic overlap. Similarly, although neuroimaging studies have consistently demonstrated the neuroanatomical substrates of affective processing, they have also thus far failed to yield clinically relevant biomarkers of bipolar illness risk or treatment response (Cardoso de Almeida and Phillips 2013; Delvecchio et al. 2013; Redpath et al. 2013). Accordingly, it is not surprising that DSM-5 lacks biomarkers for the diagnosis and treatment of bipolar disorder. Nevertheless, investigators remain optimistic that research will eventually yield clinically relevant biomarkers for bipolar disorder (Goldstein and Young 2013; Phillips 2013; Teixeira et al. 2013).

Because mechanisms and phenotypes for adverse effects may be less complex and variable than those for bipolar disorder pathophysiology and therapeutic effects, it may be the case that clinically relevant biomarkers will emerge for adverse effects before they are identified for diagnosis or treatment response. Indeed, the current U.S. prescribing information for carbamazepine already includes a recommendation that Asians ought to be genetically tested and, if positive for the human leukocyte antigen (HLA) allele HLA-B*1502 (which indicates a marked increase in risk of serious rash), should not be treated with carbamazepine unless the benefit clearly outweighs the risk (Physicians' Desk Reference 2014).

■ References

Akiskal HS: The emergence of the bipolar spectrum: validation along clinical-epidemiologic and familial-genetic lines. Psychopharmacol Bull 40(4):99–115, 2007 18227781

Akiskal HS, Benazzi F: Family history validation of the bipolar nature of depressive mixed states. J Affect Disord 73(1–2):113–122, 2003 12507744

Akiskal HS, Cassano GB, Musetti L, et al: Psychopathology, temperament, and past course in primary major depressions, 1: review of evidence for a bipolar spectrum. Psychopathology 22(5):268–277, 1989 2690170

American Psychiatric Association: Diagnostic and Statistical Manual of Mental Disorders, 4th Edition, Text Revision. Washington, DC, American Psychiatric Association, 2000

American Psychiatric Association: Diagnostic and Statistical Manual of Mental Disorders, 5th Edition. Washington, DC, American Psychiatric Association, 2013

Angst J, Azorin JM, Bowden CL, et al; BRIDGE Study Group: Prevalence and characteristics of undiagnosed bipolar disorders in patients with a major depressive episode: the BRIDGE study. Arch Gen Psychiatry 68(8):791–798, 2011 21810644

Benazzi F: Is 4 days the minimum duration of hypomania in bipolar II disorder? Eur Arch Psychiatry Clin Neurosci 251(1):32–34, 2001 11315516

Benazzi F, Akiskal HS: Delineating bipolar II mixed states in the Ravenna-San Diego Collaborative Study: the relative prevalence and diagnostic significance of hypomanic features during major depressive episodes. J Affect Disord 67(1–3):115–122, 2001 11869758

Berlim MT, McGirr A, Van den Eynde F, et al: Effectiveness and acceptability of deep brain stimulation (DBS) of the subgenual cingulate cortex for treatment-resistant depression: a systematic review and exploratory meta-analysis. J Affect Disord 159:31–38, 2014 24679386

Berwaerts J, Lane R, Nuamah IF, et al: Paliperidone extended-release as adjunctive therapy to lithium or valproate in the treatment of acute mania: a randomized, placebo-controlled study. J Affect Disord 129(1–3):252–260, 2011 20947174

Berwaerts J, Melkote R, Nuamah I, Lim P: A randomized, placebo- and active-controlled study of paliperidone extended-release as maintenance treatment in patients with bipolar I disorder after an acute manic or mixed episode. J Affect Disord 138(3):247–258, 2012a 22377512

Berwaerts J, Xu H, Nuamah I, et al: Evaluation of the efficacy and safety of paliperidone extended-release in the treatment of acute mania: a randomized, double-blind, dose-response study. J Affect Disord 136(1–2):e51–e60, 2012b 20624657

Bowden CL, Vieta E, Ice KS, et al: Ziprasidone plus a mood stabilizer in subjects with bipolar I disorder: a 6-month, randomized, placebo-controlled, double-blind trial. J Clin Psychiatry 71(2):130–137, 2010 20122373

Calabrese JR, Keck PE Jr, Macfadden W, et al: A randomized, double-blind, placebo-controlled trial of quetiapine in the treatment of bipolar I or II depression. Am J Psychiatry 162(7):1351–1360, 2005 15994719

Cardoso de Almeida JR, Phillips ML: Distinguishing between unipolar depression and bipolar depression: current and future clinical and neuroimaging perspectives. Biol Psychiatry 73(2):111–118, 2013 22784485

Carlson BX, Ketter TA, Sun W, et al: Aripiprazole in combination with lamotrigine for the long-term treatment of patients with bipolar I disorder (manic or mixed): a randomized, multicenter, double-blind study (CN138–392). Bipolar Disord 14(1):41–53, 2012 22329471

Citrome L: Cariprazine in bipolar disorder: clinical efficacy, tolerability, and place in therapy. Adv Ther 30(2):102–113, 2013 23361832

Craddock N, Jones I: Genetics of bipolar disorder. J Med Genet 36(8):585–594, 1999 10465107

Craddock N, Sklar P: Genetics of bipolar disorder: successful start to a long journey. Trends Genet 25(2):99–105, 2009 19144440

Craddock N, Sklar P: Genetics of bipolar disorder. Lancet 381(9878):1654–1662, 2013 23663951

Delvecchio G, Sugranyes G, Frangou S: Evidence of diagnostic specificity in the neural correlates of facial affect processing in bipolar disorder and schizophrenia: a meta-analysis of functional imaging studies. Psychol Med 43(3):553–569, 2013 22874625

Detke HC, DelBello MP, Landry J, et al: Olanzapine/fluoxetine combination in children and adolescents with bipolar I depression: a randomized, double-blind, placebo-controlled trial. J Am Acad Child Adol Psychiatry 54(3):217–224, 2015 25721187

Diazgranados N, Ibrahim L, Brutsche NE, et al: A randomized add-on trial of an N-methyl-D-aspartate antagonist in treatment-resistant bipolar depression. Arch Gen Psychiatry 67(8):793–802, 2010 20679587

Dumlu K, Orhon Z, Özerdem A, et al: Treatment-induced manic switch in the course of unipolar depression can predict bipolarity: cluster analysis based evidence. J Affect Disord 134(1–3):91–101, 2011 21742381

Fiedorowicz JG, Endicott J, Leon AC, et al: Subthreshold hypomanic symptoms in progression from unipolar major depression to bipolar disorder. Am J Psychiatry 168(1):40–48, 2011 21078709

Frye MA, Helleman G, McElroy SL, et al: Correlates of treatment-emergent mania associated with antidepressant treatment in bipolar depression. Am J Psychiatry 166(2):164–172, 2009 19015231

Geddes JR, Miklowitz DJ: Treatment of bipolar disorder. Lancet 381(9878):1672–1682, 2013 23663953

Goldberg JF, Perlis RH, Bowden CL, et al: Manic symptoms during depressive episodes in 1,380 patients with bipolar disorder: findings from the STEP-BD. Am J Psychiatry 166(2):173–181, 2009 19122008

Goldstein BI, Young LT: Toward clinically applicable biomarkers in bipolar disorder: focus on BDNF, inflammatory markers, and endothelial function. Curr Psychiatry Rep 15(12):425, 2013 24243532

Hirschfeld RM, Weisler RH, Raines SR, et al; BOLDER Study Group: Quetiapine in the treatment of anxiety in patients with bipolar I or II depression: a secondary analysis from a randomized, double-blind, placebo-controlled study. J Clin Psychiatry 67(3):355–362, 2006 16649820

Ketter TA: Handbook of Diagnosis and Treatment of Bipolar Disorders. Washington, DC, American Psychiatric Publishing, 2010

Ketter TA, Calabrese JR, Yang R, et al: A double-blind, placebo-controlled, multicenter trial of adjunctive armodafinil for the treatment of major depression associated with bipolar I disorder. Paper presented at the 10th International Conference on Bipolar Disorder, Miami Beach, FL, June 13–16, 2013

Koukopoulos A, Sani G: DSM-5 criteria for depression with mixed features: a farewell to mixed depression. Acta Psychiatr Scand 129(1):4–16, 2014 23600771

Koukopoulos A, Sani G, Ghaemi SN: Mixed features of depression: why DSM-5 is wrong (and so was DSM-IV). Br J Psychiatry 203(1):3–5, 2013 23818531

Kraepelin E: Manic-Depressive Insanity and Paranoia. Edinburgh, ES Livingstone, 1921

Kwentus J, Riesenberg RA, Marandi M, et al: Rapid acute treatment of agitation in patients with bipolar I disorder: a multicenter, randomized, placebo-controlled clinical trial with inhaled loxapine. Bipolar Disord 14(1):31–40, 2012 22329470

Leonhard K: [Classification of Endogenous Psychoses]. Berlin, Akademie Verlag, 1957

Loebel A, Cucchiaro J, Silva R, et al: Lurasidone as adjunctive therapy with lithium or valproate for the treatment of bipolar I depression: a randomized, double-blind, placebo-controlled study. Am J Psychiatry 171(2):169–177, 2014a

Loebel A, Cucchiaro J, Silva R, et al: Lurasidone monotherapy in the treatment of bipolar I depression: a randomized, double-blind, placebo-controlled study. Am J Psychiatry 171(2):160–168, 2014b

Lombardo I, Sachs G, Kolluri S, et al: Two 6-week, randomized, double-blind, placebo-controlled studies of ziprasidone in outpatients with bipolar I depression: did baseline characteristics impact trial outcome? J Clin Psychopharmacol 32(4):470–478, 2012 22722504

Macfadden W, Alphs L, Haskins JT, et al: A randomized, double-blind, placebo-controlled study of maintenance treatment with adjunctive risperidone long-acting therapy in patients with bipolar I disorder who relapse frequently. Bipolar Disord 11(8):827–839, 2009 19922552

Maj M, Pirozzi R, Magliano L, et al: Agitated "unipolar" major depression: prevalence, phenomenology, and outcome. J Clin Psychiatry 67(5):712–719, 2006 16841620

Marcus R, Khan A, Rollin L, et al: Efficacy of aripiprazole adjunctive to lithium or valproate in the long-term treatment of patients with bipolar I disorder with an inadequate response to lithium or valproate monotherapy: a multicenter, double-blind, randomized study. Bipolar Disord 13(2):133–144, 2011 21443567

Mazza M, Mandelli L, Zaninotto L, et al: Factors associated with the course of symptoms in bipolar disorder during a 1-year follow-up: depression vs. sub-threshold mixed state. Nord J Psychiatry 65(6):419–426, 2011 21728783

McIntyre RS, Soczynska JK, Bottas A, et al: Anxiety disorders and bipolar disorder: a review. Bipolar Disord 8(6):665–676, 2006 17156153

McIntyre RS, Cohen M, Zhao J, et al: A 3-week, randomized, placebo-controlled trial of asenapine in the treatment of acute mania in bipolar mania and mixed states. Bipolar Disord 11(7):673–686, 2009 19839993

McIntyre RS, Cohen M, Zhao J, et al: Asenapine in the treatment of acute mania in bipolar I disorder: a randomized, double-blind, placebo-controlled trial. J Affect Disord 122(1–2):27–38, 2010 20096936

Mitchell PB, Goodwin GM, Johnson GF, et al: Diagnostic guidelines for bipolar depression: a probabilistic approach. Bipolar Disord 10(1 pt 2):144–152, 2008 18199233

Pacchiarotti I, Bond DJ, Baldessarini RJ, et al: The International Society for Bipolar Disorders (ISBD) task force report on antidepressant use in bipolar disorders. Am J Psychiatry 170(11):1249–1262, 2013 24030475

Phelps J, Ghaemi SN: The mistaken claim of bipolar 'overdiagnosis': solving the false positives problem for DSM-5/ICD-11. Acta Psychiatr Scand 126(6):395–401, 2012 22900986

Phillips ML: Brain-behavior biomarkers of illness and illness risk in bipolar disorder: present findings and next steps. Biol Psychiatry 74(12):870–871, 2013 24246363

Physicians' Desk Reference 2015, 69th Edition. Montvale, NJ, PDR Network, 2014

Quiroz JA, Yatham LN, Palumbo JM, et al: Risperidone long-acting injectable monotherapy in the maintenance treatment of bipolar I disorder. Biol Psychiatry 68(2):156–162, 2010 20227682

Redpath HL, Cooper D, Lawrie SM: Imaging symptoms and syndromes: similarities and differences between schizophrenia and bipolar disorder. Biol Psychiatry 73(6):495–496, 2013 23438631

Sachs GS: Strategies for improving treatment of bipolar disorder: integration of measurement and management. Acta Psychiatr Scand Suppl (422):7–17, 2004 15330934

Sachs GS, Ice KS, Chappell PB, et al: Efficacy and safety of adjunctive oral ziprasidone for acute treatment of depression in patients with bipolar I disorder: a randomized, double-blind, placebo-controlled trial. J Clin Psychiatry 72(10):1413–1422, 2011 21672493

Sachs GS, Vanderburg DG, Edman S, et al: Adjunctive oral ziprasidone in patients with acute mania treated with lithium or divalproex, part 2: influence of protocol-specific eligibility criteria on signal detection. J Clin Psychiatry 73(11):1420–1425, 2012a 23218158

Sachs GS, Vanderburg DG, Karayal ON, et al: Adjunctive oral ziprasidone in patients with acute mania treated with lithium or divalproex, part 1: results of a randomized, double-blind, placebo-controlled trial. J Clin Psychiatry 73(11):1412–1419, 2012b 23218157

Sato T, Bottlender R, Schröter A, et al: Frequency of manic symptoms during a depressive episode and unipolar 'depressive mixed state' as bipolar spectrum. Acta Psychiatr Scand 107(4):268–274, 2003 12662249

Sato T, Bottlender R, Sievers M, et al: Evaluating the inter-episode stability of depressive mixed states. J Affect Disord 81(2):103–113, 2004 15306135

Shim IH, Woo YS, Jun TY, et al: Mixed-state bipolar I and II depression: time to remission and clinical characteristics. J Affect Disord 152–154:340–346, 2014 24144581

Starace A, Bose A, Wang Q, et al: Cariprazine in the treatment of acute mania in bipolar disorder: a double-blind, placebo-controlled, phase III trial. Paper presented at the 165th Annual Meeting of the American Psychiatric Association, Philadelphia, PA, May 5–9, 2012

Swann AC, Moeller FG, Steinberg JL, et al: Manic symptoms and impulsivity during bipolar depressive episodes. Bipolar Disord 9(3):206–212, 2007 17430294

Swann AC, Steinberg JL, Lijffijt M, et al: Continuum of depressive and manic mixed states in patients with bipolar disorder: quantitative measurement and clinical features. World Psychiatry 8(3):166–172, 2009 19812754

Swann AC, Lafer B, Perugi G, et al: Bipolar mixed states: an international society for bipolar disorders task force report of symptom structure, course of illness, and diagnosis. Am J Psychiatry 170(1):31–42, 2013 23223893

Szegedi A, Calabrese JR, Stet L, et al; Apollo Study Group: Asenapine as adjunctive treatment for acute mania associated with bipolar disorder: results of a 12-week core study and 40-week extension. J Clin Psychopharmacol 32(1):46–55, 2012 22198448

Teixeira AL, Barbosa IG, Machado-Vieira R, et al: Novel biomarkers for bipolar disorder. Expert Opin Med Diagn 7(2):147–159, 2013 23530885

Terao T, Tanaka T: Antidepressant-induced mania or hypomania in DSM-5. Psychopharmacology (Berl) 231(1):315, 2014 24247478

Thase ME, Macfadden W, Weisler RH, et al; BOLDER II Study Group: Efficacy of quetiapine monotherapy in bipolar I and II depression: a double-blind, placebo-controlled study (the BOLDER II study). J Clin Psychopharmacol 26(6):600–609, 2006 17110817

Tohen M, Vieta E, Calabrese J, et al: Efficacy of olanzapine and olanzapine-fluoxetine combination in the treatment of bipolar I depression. Arch Gen Psychiatry 60(11):1079–1088, 2003 14609883

Tohen M, Calabrese J, Vieta E, et al: Effect of comorbid anxiety on treatment response in bipolar depression. J Affect Disord 104(1–3):137–146, 2007 17512607

Tohen M, McDonnell DP, Case M, et al: Randomised, double-blind, placebo-controlled study of olanzapine in patients with bipolar I depression. Br J Psychiatry 201(5):376–382, 2012 22918966

Vieta E, Nuamah IF, Lim P, et al: A randomized, placebo- and active-controlled study of paliperidone extended release for the treatment of acute manic and mixed episodes of bipolar I disorder. Bipolar Disord 12(3):230–243, 2010 20565430

Zarate CA Jr, Brutsche NE, Ibrahim L, et al: Replication of ketamine's antidepressant efficacy in bipolar depression: a randomized controlled add-on trial. Biol Psychiatry 71(11):939–946, 2012 22297150

Zimmermann P, Brückl T, Nocon A, et al: Heterogeneity of DSM-IV major depressive disorder as a consequence of subthreshold bipolarity. Arch Gen Psychiatry 66(12):1341–1352, 2009 19996039

2 Treatment of Acute Bipolar Depression

Terence A. Ketter, M.D.
Shefali Miller, M.D.
Po W. Wang, M.D.
Jenifer Culver, Ph.D.

Depression continues to be the most pervasive mood challenge for patients with bipolar disorder. Arguably, the most important recent diagnostic advances in bipolar depression are changes in DSM-5 (American Psychiatric Association 2013), which has added a "with mixed features" specifier for depressive (and manic or hypomanic) episodes and now permits a full manic or hypomanic episode that emerges during antidepressant treatment and persists beyond the physiological effect of that treatment to be sufficient evidence for a manic or hypomanic episode (i.e., this episode can be given a bipolar disorder diagnosis rather than merely being considered a medication reaction). In spite of these advances, diagnosis of bipolar depression remains challenging, with the greatest unmet diagnostic need in bipolar depression remaining the need for early, accurate differentiation from unipolar major depressive disorder.

The most important recent evidence-based therapeutic advance for bipolar depression occurred in the summer of 2013, when the U.S. Food and Drug Administration (FDA) approved lurasidone monotherapy (Loebel et al. 2014b) and adjunctive therapy (Loebel et al. 2014a) for acute bipolar depression. However, this approval only brought the total number of FDA-approved acute bipolar depression treatments to three, all of which have a second-generation antipsychotic (SGA) medication component and hence greater side-effect challenges than mood stabilizers or antidepressants. Consequently, the greatest unmet therapeutic need in bipolar disorder remains the need for effective, well-tolerated treatments for bipolar depression. This need appears to be fueling ongoing clinical efforts to find treatments for bipolar depression that can provide adequate tolerability. In that regard, the role(s) for antidepressants in bipolar depression remains controversial, as demonstrated in an important recent review by the International Society for Bipolar Disorders (ISBD) Antidepressant Use in Bipolar Disorders Task Force (Pacchiarotti et al. 2013), which indicated that for many clinical scenarios, antidepressant use in bipolar depression should be limited or avoided.

■ Evolving Trends in Treatment of Acute Bipolar Depression

The optimal approach to acute bipolar depression continues to be a topic of spirited debate. The historical influence of older approaches such as antidepressants plus antimanic agents, combined with the limited number of FDA-approved agents for acute bipolar depression and their associated side-effect burdens, likely contributes importantly to this controversy. Hence, although systematic data support only a very limited number of acute bipolar depression treatments, clinical practice has historically involved very different approaches. Indeed, a European study found that between 1994 and 2009, among 2,246 inpatients with acute bipolar depression, 85% took more than one class of psychotropic, with 74% taking antidepressants (commonly combined with lithium or valproate), 55% taking antipsychotics, 48% taking anticonvulsants, and only 33% taking lithium (Haeberle et al. 2012).

However, approaches to acute bipolar depression may be beginning to change. For example, by 2010, among 221 European inpatients with acute bipolar depression, quetiapine (alone and combined) was the most frequently prescribed drug (in 39% of the patients) (Haeberle et al. 2012). Among 597 primarily euthymic or depressed outpatients referred to an American bipolar disorder clinic between 2000 and 2011, combination therapies were very common, with patients taking on average 2.6 psychotropic medications, and between 2000–2005 and 2006–2011 lamotrigine, quetiapine, and aripiprazole usage more than doubled (Hooshmand et al. 2014).

In this chapter, we describe advances in evidence-based treatment of acute bipolar depression, starting with interventions with the most evidence to support their use and endeavoring to reconcile these with divergent contemporary clinical practices, such as the use of antidepressants and other adjunctive treatments.

■ Treatment of Acute Bipolar Depression: Balancing the Likelihood of Benefit and Harm

The potential benefits (therapeutic effects) of treatments for bipolar disorder must be considered in the context of potential harms (side effects). Although the existence of a medication's potential benefits and the possibility of being worthwhile, in spite of risks of potential harms, can be imputed via the existence of FDA indications, clinicians and patients commonly seek more detailed assessments of benefit versus harm.

Studies have increasingly reported potential benefits and harms by analyzing the *number needed to treat* (NNT) and the *number needed to harm* (NNH), respectively. The NNT is the expected number of subjects who would need to be treated to yield one additional good outcome compared with a control intervention (Laupacis et al. 1988). In this chapter, we consider NNTs for response (i.e., at least a 50% decrease in depressive symptoms) in acute bipolar depression. For example, the NNT for response is calculated by assessing the reciprocal of the difference in the response rates for a treatment and a control intervention. There is a convention to round up the NNT to the next higher integer, although some have advocated that NNTs from 1 to 100 ought to be reported to at least one decimal place (Stang et al. 2010). Thus, if a medication and placebo had response rates of 48% and 25%, respectively, then the NNT for response would be $100\% / (48\% - 25\%) = 100\% / 23\% = 4.3$, which would be rounded up to 5. Lower NNTs represent better outcomes, with single digits (preferably low single digits) generally representing adequate outcomes in acute bipolar depression. Most FDA-approved treatments for bipolar disorder have single-digit NNTs (Ketter et al. 2011). Alternative treatments may have NNTs as high as the low teens with good tolerability, in the setting of few other well-tolerated agents having lower NNTs.

All FDA-approved bipolar disorder treatments have at least one boxed warning regarding the risk of serious adverse effects (Ketter et al. 2011). Although important, such boxed warnings do not generally represent the most common side effects that cause treatment discontinuation (e.g., sedation/somnolence, weight gain, and akathisia) (Ketter et al. 2011). Harms (i.e., side effects) can be quantified using NNH, which is the number of patients who would have to be treated before one additional patient would be expected to experience an adverse effect, compared with a control intervention (Ketter et al. 2011). The NNH for an adverse effect is calculated by assessing the reciprocal of the difference in the adverse-effect rates for a treatment and a control intervention, so that if a medication and placebo had sedation/somnolence rates of 40% and 20%, respectively, the NNH for sedation/somnolence would be 100%/(40%–20%)=100%/20%=5. That is, five patients would need to be treated to expect to encounter one more patient with sedation/somnolence compared with placebo. As with NNT, there is a convention to round up NNH to the next higher integer. Higher NNHs represent better outcomes, with double digits generally representing adequate outcomes, depending on the severity of the harm (Ketter et al. 2011).

Because treatments should be more likely to help than to harm, we seek interventions with lower NNTs than NNHs, commonly with a goal of having no more than a single-digit NNT (i.e., at least approximately 10% more efficacy than placebo) and at least a double-digit NNH (i.e., no more than approximately 10% excess risk of adverse effects over placebo) (Ketter et al. 2011). Striving for an NNH higher than twice the NNT can further increase the likelihood of good versus bad outcomes, with help being more than twice as likely as harm compared with placebo.

In this chapter, we report NNHs for the clinically relevant adverse effects resulting in the greatest increases in harm over placebo (i.e., the adverse effects yielding the lowest NNH, based on available published data) for each acute bipolar depression treatment. For instance, although clinicians are commonly appropriately concerned about the potential for serious rash as an adverse effect of lamotrigine, the prevalence of serious rash in lamotrigine-treated patients is low (1 in 1,000–2,000) (Calabrese et al. 2002), and placebo-controlled lamotrigine studies in acute bipolar depression yielded an NNH for benign rash of 44 for lamotrigine compared with placebo (Calabrese et al. 2008; Ketter et al. 2011). However, the NNH for somnolence with lamotrigine compared with placebo in such studies was 37 (Calabrese et al. 2008). We therefore report the NNH for somnolence as the most clinically relevant harm to consider when evaluating potential benefits and harms of lamotrigine treatment for acute bipolar depression, although this will vary according to individual patient and provider characteristics and preferences.

The benefit:harm ratio is called the *likelihood to help or harm* (LHH) and is defined as NNH/NNT (Akobeng 2008; Straus 2002). An LHH greater than 1 is advantageous, demonstrating that compared with placebo, a treatment is more likely to help than to harm. In this volume, to make such calculations more clear, NNTs, NNHs, and LHHs are provided as one-decimal numbers rather than whole numbers. For example, if an intervention had an advantageous combination of NNT=4.8 and NNH=24.8, the LHH would be 24.8/4.8=5.2, meaning that compared with placebo, the intervention was more than five times as likely to yield benefit versus harm. An LHH of less than 1 is disadvantageous, because compared with placebo, the treatment is more likely to harm than to help. As an example, if an intervention had a disadvantageous combination of NNT=18.3 and NNH=6.1, the LHH would be 6.1 / 18.3=0.3, meaning that compared with placebo, the intervention was only one-third as likely to yield benefit versus harm (or was three times as likely to yield harm vs. benefit). NNTs, NNHs, LHHs, and selected blind medication side-effect rates for selected treatments for acute bipolar depression are provided in Table 2–1.

Alternative measures of potential harms not reported in this volume include NNH for all-cause discontinuation compared with placebo and NNH for adverse-effect-related discontinuation of drug compared with placebo. Although such metrics may yield more comprehensive information about medication tolerability than NNHs for individual spontaneously reported adverse effects, discontinuation rates in clinical trials may be confounded by variable degrees of patient and investigator motivation to have patients complete the study. As a result, NNHs for all-cause and adverse-effect-related discontinuation may underestimate clinically relevant harms associated with a drug compared with placebo that are likely to be encountered in routine practice. Indeed, such NNHs are commonly higher than those for spontaneously reported specific adverse effects, and occasionally are even negative (reflecting lower rates than with placebo).

Risk management strategies vary markedly among patients and clinicians, so it is crucial to personalize assessments of benefits versus harms. Investigators and clinicians commonly opine that treatments that are more potent with respect to therapeutic effects (i.e., have lower NNTs) also tend to be more potent with respect to adverse effects (i.e., also have lower NNHs), whereas treatments that are more tolerable (i.e., have lower risk of adverse effects and higher NNHs) also tend to be less potent with respect to therapeutic effects (i.e., also have higher NNTs). However, systematic data supporting such opinions are limited. Investigators and clinicians also commonly consider the potencies for therapeutic and adverse effects of interventions to be broadly similar within drug classes, and potency ranks (for both therapeutic and adverse effects) across classes from highest to lowest to be 1) SGAs, 2) mood stabilizers (other than lamotrigine), and 3) lamotrigine and antidepressants, although within medication classes, newer compared with older treatment options commonly represent tolerability enhancements (Figure 2–1). Once again, however, systematic data supporting this notion are limited. Thus, in the treatment of acute bipolar depression, antidepressants may entail

TABLE 2–1. Numbers needed to treat, numbers needed to harm, likelihood to help or harm, and selected blind medication harm (side-effect) rates for selected acute bipolar depression treatments

Medication	NNT	NNH	LHH	Harm	BMH (%)
Second-generation antipsychotics					
Olanzapine+fluoxetine[1]	3.9	5.2	1.3	Weight gain[a]	19.5
Quetiapine (monotherapy)[2,3]	5.5	4.0	0.7	Sed/som[b]	30.4
Lurasidone (monotherapy)[4]	4.6	14.3	3.1	Akathisia[c]	9.4
Lurasidone (adjunctive therapy*)[5]	6.7	15.5	2.3	Nausea[d]	17.5
Olanzapine (monotherapy)[1,6,u]	9.0	4.9	0.5	Weight gain[e]	20.9
Aripiprazole (monotherapy)[7,u]	44.0	4.8	0.1	Akathisia	24.4
Ziprasidone (monotherapy)[8,u]	887.0	83.3	0.1	Somnolence	16.4
Ziprasidone (adjunctive therapy†)[9,u]	NR	5.7	NR	Somnolence	22.4
Mood stabilizers					
Lithium (monotherapy)[10,u]	14.9	10.8	0.7	Nausea[f]	16.9
Lamotrigine (monotherapy)[11,12,u]	11.9	36.4	3.1	Somnolence	9.5
Antidepressants					
Antidepressants (adjunctive therapy‡)[13,u]	28.6	208.7	7.3	TEAS	7.7
Paroxetine (monotherapy)[14,u]	45.5	14.8	0.3	Nausea	12.4
Other					
Armodafinil (adjunctive therapy§)[15-18,u]	14.9	30.4	2.0	Headache[g]	13.7

TABLE 2–1. **Numbers needed to treat, numbers needed to harm, likelihood to help or harm, and selected blind medication harm (side-effect) rates for selected acute bipolar depression treatments** *(continued)*

Note. **Boldface** indicates drug names for U.S. Food and Drug Administration (FDA)–approved acute bipolar depression treatments. BMH = blind medication harm rate; LHH (NNH/NNT) = likelihood to help or harm compared with placebo; NNH = number needed to harm compared with placebo (for clinically relevant side effect with lowest NNH); NNT = number needed to treat compared with placebo (for antidepressant response); NR = not reported; TEAS = treatment-emergent affective switch. NNTs, NNHs, and LHHs are rounded up to the next higher first decimal place (in contrast to being rounded up to the next higher integer in the text and figures). Weight gain indicates ≥7% weight gain.

*Added to lithium or valproate.

[+] Added to lithium, valproate, or lamotrigine.

[‡] Added to lithium, valproate, carbamazepine, or second-generation antipsychotic.

[§] Added to lithium, valproate, lamotrigine, and/or olanzapine, risperidone, aripiprazole, or ziprasidone (only with lithium/valproate) in three of three studies, or quetiapine, in third study only.

[a] Somnolence with olanzapine+fluoxetine: NNH = 11.9, LHH = 1.0, BMH = 20.9%.

[b] Sed/som indicates sedation (Calabrese et al. 2005) or somnolence (Thase et al. 2006); ≥7% weight gain with quetiapine: NNH = 19.0, LHH = 3.5, BMH = 7.5%.

[c] Nausea with lurasidone: NNH = 16.2, LHH = 3.5, BMH = 13.9%.

[d] Akathisia with adjunctive lurasidone: NNH = 29.8, LHH = 4.5, BMH = 7.7%.

[e] Somnolence with olanzapine: NNH = 8.2, LHH = 0.9, BMH = 22.7%.

[f] Somnolence with lithium: NNH = 20.0, LHH = 1.3, BMH = 8.8%.

[g] Anxiety with armodafinil in first study: NNT = 8.3, NNH = 28.3, LHH = 3.4, BMH = 3.5%.

[u] Interventions lacking FDA approval for acute bipolar depression.

Source. Data from [1]Tohen et al. 2003; [2]Calabrese et al. 2005; [3]Thase et al. 2006; [4]Loebel et al. 2014b; [5]Loebel et al. 2014a; [6]Tohen et al. 2012; [7]Thase et al. 2008; [8]Lombardo et al. 2012; [9]Sachs et al. 2011; [10]Young et al. 2010; [11]Geddes et al. 2009; [12]Calabrese et al. 2008; [13]Sidor and Macqueen 2011; [14]McElroy et al. 2011; [15]Ketter et al. 2013; [16]Frye et al. 2013; [17]Adler et al. 2014; [18]Frye et al. 2014.

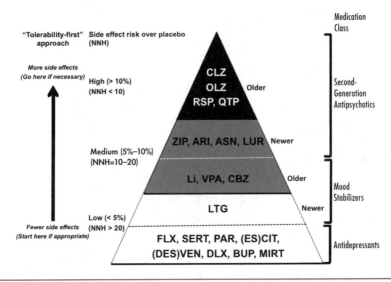

FIGURE 2–1.   Schematic for adverse effects of psychotropic medications.
Note.   Pharmacological potency may entail covarying benefits (therapeutic) and harms (adverse effects). ARI=aripiprazole; ASN=asenapine; BUP = bupropion; CBZ=carbamazepine; CLZ=clozapine; (ES)CIT= (es)citalopram; (DES)VEN = (desmethyl)venlafaxine; DLX=duloxetine; FLX=fluoxetine; Li=lithium; LTG = lamotrigine; LUR=lurasidone; MIRT=mirtazapine; NNH=number needed to harm; OLZ = olanzapine; PAR=paroxetine; QTP=quetiapine; RSP=risperidone; SERT = sertraline; VPA=valproate; ZIP=ziprasidone.

fewer adverse-effect risks than mood stabilizers or SGAs but at the cost of diminished efficacy. Clinicians and patients commonly utilize a "tolerability-first" approach, starting (if appropriate) with agents with better tolerability at the potential expense of poorer efficacy before moving on (if necessary) to agents with more robust efficacy at the potential expense of poorer tolerability.

In certain instances, patients may be characterized as having currently urgent illness, such as severe, acute bipolar depression, with substantial acute risk of suicide attempt, psychiatric hospitalization, or severe financial (e.g., bankruptcy), occupational (e.g., job loss/disability), or psychosocial (e.g., relationship loss) consequences. In contrast, in other instances, patients may be considered to have currently nonurgent illness, such as mild to moderate chronic bipolar depression, without substantial current risk of suicide attempt, psychiatric hospitalization, or severe financial, occupational, or psychosocial consequences. The compelling and immediate need for efficacy in patients with currently urgent illness may warrant consideration of more effective treatments with more favorable single-digit NNTs, which may mitigate safety/tolerability limitations of having less favorable single-digit NNHs, such as SGAs (Ketter et al. 2011). In contrast, a compelling need for safety/tolerability in patients with currently nonurgent illness may warrant consideration of better-tolerated treatments with more favorable double-digit NNHs, which may mitigate efficacy limitations of having less favorable double-digit NNTs, such as lamotrigine or antidepressants. In fact, it is common to encounter a clinical approach to acute bipolar depression of starting, in less urgent situations, with better-tolerated treatments (e.g., lamotrigine or antidepressants, if appropriate) in spite of less robust therapeutic effects, before proceeding to treatments with greater potential therapeutic effects (such as mood stabilizers and SGAs, if necessary) but also with potentially greater risks of adverse effects.

Treatment selection in evidence-based medicine requires not only considering controlled and observational data regarding treatment efficacy/effectiveness and safety/tolerability, but also integrating individual patient characteristics, such as bipolar illness history, efficacy history, safety/tolerability history, and patient preferences, as described in Table 2–2.

■ Updated Five-Tier Approach to Acute Bipolar Depression

Optimal treatment of acute bipolar depression entails finding the intervention(s) with the best combination of efficacy and safety/tolerability for individual patients. Recent advances in treatments for acute bipolar depression are reviewed in this section, using a five-tier system presented in Table 2–3, which is an update of that published in *Handbook of Diagnosis and Treatment of Bipolar Disorders* (Ketter 2010). This system is a hybrid approach, combining evidence-based medical information of efficacy and tolerability with more empirical constructs, such as familiarity and patient acceptability, to prioritize treatments in a fashion broadly consistent with American clinical practice and treatment guidelines for currently available treatments, and to highlight promising new research that may ultimately translate into new clinical treatments.

As of early 2015, three Tier I treatment options had FDA approval for the treatment of acute bipolar depression, and were thus supported by the most compelling evidence of efficacy, and hence were important candidates for patients with urgent bipolar depression. Lurasidone, which

TABLE 2–2. Current and prior individual patient characteristics influencing treatment selection

Bipolar illness history	Prioritize treatments with best match to current or most recent episode polarity and severity or urgency (e.g., presence or absence of mixed, psychotic, and suicidal symptoms), illness polarity predominance, episode sequence (e.g., mania then depression then well interval, *vs.* depression then mania then well interval, *vs.* continuous cycling), illness course (e.g., rapid cycling), and other illness characteristics predicting treatment responses (e.g., "classical" bipolar I disorder without mood-incongruent delusions and without comorbidity, which predicts potential lithium response), taking into account psychiatric and medical comorbidities, as well as illness characteristics of first-degree relatives.
Efficacy history	Prioritize treatments with current and prior acute and preventive efficacy, taking into account psychiatric comorbidity. Integrate efficacy data from first-degree relatives.
Safety/tolerability history	Prioritize treatments with current and prior acute and preventive safety/tolerability, and best-matching other characteristics predicting safety/tolerability (e.g., avoiding use of carbamazepine in Asians with the human leukocyte antigen (HLA) allele HLA-B*1502, which is a biomarker for risk of serious rash), taking into account medical comorbidity. Integrate safety/tolerability data from first-degree relatives.
Patient preferences	Consider patient preferences because they can impact positive and negative placebo responses as well as adherence. Integrate preferences of significant others.

received FDA approval for monotherapy and adjunctive treatment of acute bipolar depression in 2013, was the only addition to Tier I since publication of *Handbook of Diagnosis and Treatment of Bipolar Disorders* (Ketter 2010). Although lurasidone appears better tolerated (less weight gain and somnolence) than the two older Tier I treatments (olanzapine plus fluoxetine combination and quetiapine monotherapy), tolerability limitations of Tier I treatments may still lead clinicians and patients, after comparing the benefits and harms, to consider treatments in other tiers, particularly Tier II or Tier III. Indeed, in clinical practice and in some treatment guidelines, some Tier I treatments continued to be considered to have equal or even lower priority than better-tolerated alternatives such as lithium and lamotrigine in Tier II, or even adjunctive antidepressants in Tier III.

Tier II treatment options, as of early 2015, had not changed since publication of *Handbook of Diagnosis and Treatment of Bipolar Disorders* (Ketter 2010). Tier II treatments lacked FDA approval for the treatment of acute bipolar depression (and hence had less compelling evidence of efficacy than Tier I options) but had mitigating advantages such as bipolar maintenance indications, enhanced safety/tolerability (relative to Tier I options), or familiarity of use that made them attractive for a substantial number of patients. Hence, Tier II options were important candidates for patients with currently nonurgent bipolar depression. Indeed, in clinical practice and in some treatment guidelines, these medications continued to be considered first-line interventions in spite of absence of an FDA indication for acute bipolar depression.

Tier III treatment options, as of early 2015, lacked FDA approval for the treatment of acute bipolar depression and generally had less compelling evidence of efficacy than Tier I or II options. Although adjunctive antidepressants were ranked highly by some, but not all, experts, treatment guidelines generally continued to not consider Tier III agents to be first-line interventions, but cited at least some of them as intermediate-priority options. Nevertheless, some Tier III options had mitigating advantages, such as bipolar maintenance indications, enhanced safety/tolerability (especially relative to Tier I options), or familiarity of use that could make them attractive for selected patients; also, in certain circumstances, some of these interventions could be considered early on (e.g., psychotherapy or electroconvulsive therapy [ECT] in pregnant women with acute bipolar depression). In view of recent multicenter randomized controlled trials (RCTs) indicating some promise for adjunctive armodafinil, and older more limited data supporting adjunctive modafinil in acute bipolar depression, in this update these agents have been moved up from Tier IV to Tier III. Although there is a substantial and growing evidence

TABLE 2–3. An updated five-tier approach to the management of acute bipolar depression

Tier	Priority	Description	Treatment options
I	High	FDA approved	SGAs
			Olanzapine plus fluoxetine, quetiapine monotherapy, **lurasidone monotherapy and adjunctive therapy**
II	High	High priority unapproved	Mood stabilizers
			Lithium, lamotrigine
			Adjunctive antidepressants
			Adjunctive modafinil, armodafinil
			Other mood stabilizers
			Divalproex, carbamazepine
			Other SGAs
			Olanzapine monotherapy, aripiprazole,[a] risperidone, **ziprasidone,**[a] asenapine, clozapine
III	Intermediate	Other clinical options	Electroconvulsive therapy
			Adjunctive psychotherapy
			Family-focused therapy, cognitive-behavioral therapy, interpersonal and social rhythm therapy, group psychoeducation, **dialectical behavior therapy**

TABLE 2–3. An updated five-tier approach to the management of acute bipolar depression *(continued)*

Tier	Priority	Description	Treatment options
IV	Low	Novel adjunctive options	Thyroid hormones
			Pramipexole
			Topiramate
			Stimulants
			Sleep deprivation
			Light therapy
			Ramelteon
			Nutriceuticals
			Vagus nerve stimulation
			Transcranial magnetic stimulation
V	None[b]	Research treatments	**Adjunctive ketamine**
			Adjunctive deep brain stimulation

Note. **Boldface** indicates treatments with important new developments. FDA=U.S. Food and Drug Administration; SGA=second-generation antipsychotic.
[a]Ineffective in controlled acute bipolar depression trials, as of early 2015.
[b]Not yet clinical options.
Source. Adapted from Ketter TA: *Handbook of Diagnosis and Treatment of Bipolar Disorders.* Washington, DC, American Psychiatric Publishing, 2010. Copyright 2010, American Psychiatric Publishing. Used with permission.

base to support the use of adjunctive psychotherapy in acute bipolar depression, it remains in Tier III due to availability/feasibility limitations. For adjunctive psychotherapy and some other Tier III treatments, advances in research, familiarity, and/or availability/feasibility may ultimately be sufficient to merit their consideration for placement in even higher tiers.

Tier IV treatment options, as of early 2015, lacked FDA approval for the treatment of acute bipolar depression and generally had even more limited evidence of efficacy than Tier I, II, or III options. Treatment guidelines have uniformly considered these modalities to be low-priority interventions, if mentioning them at all. Nevertheless, some Tier IV options could prove attractive for carefully selected patients, after consideration of Tier I–III treatments (e.g., for patients who are treatment resistant or intolerant to Tier I–III treatments). For some of these treatments, advances in research may ultimately provide sufficient evidence to merit their consideration for placement in higher tiers. For example, ramelteon, which has been added at the Tier IV level because of limited evidence of efficacy in acute bipolar depression, could be promoted to a higher tier should data from current clinical research prove positive.

The new Tier V is reserved for innovative treatments that research suggests could have promise but are thus far too novel and carry too substantive safety/tolerability risks to be considered clinical (as opposed to research) tools. As of early 2015, only adjunctive ketamine and adjunctive deep brain stimulation (DBS) have been included in this tier.

Tier I: FDA-Approved Acute Bipolar Depression Treatments

As of early 2015, the FDA-approved treatments for acute bipolar depression were the olanzapine plus fluoxetine combination, quetiapine monotherapy, and lurasidone as monotherapy or adjunctive therapy. Because all of these treatments have an SGA component, they have more substantive side-effect challenges than do mood stabilizers, antidepressants, and most other novel agents used in the management of acute bipolar depression. As described in greater detail in the SGA subsection below, the recently approved newer SGA lurasidone appears to provide adequate efficacy yet better tolerability than the older approved SGAs. However, even with the improved side-effect profile of lurasidone, tolerability limitations of Tier I treatments may lead clinicians and patients, after comparing the benefits and harms, to consider treatments in other tiers, particularly those in Tier II or adjunctive antidepressants, which are in Tier III. Indeed, in clinical practice and in some treatment guidelines, some Tier I treatments have been considered to have priority that is equal to or even lower than some Tier II options or even adjunctive antidepressants, which are in Tier III (Goodwin and Consensus Group of the British Association for Psychopharmacology 2009; Grunze et al. 2010; Kasper et al. 2008; National Institute for Health and Clinical Excellence 2006; Yatham et al. 2013). Finally, because lurasidone was only recently approved, it is only noted as a second-line option in the 2013 Canadian Network for Mood and Anxiety Treatments (CANMAT) and ISBD collaborative update of CANMAT guidelines for the management of patients with bipolar disorder (Yatham et al. 2013).

Second-Generation Antipsychotics

SGAs have been increasingly used in bipolar disorder treatment, challenging the older view that antipsychotics were mere adjuncts for acute mania that needed to be minimized or discontinued during other phases of bipolar disorder management. Emerging data indicate that although SGAs have overlapping efficacy profiles for acute mania, they appear to have distinctive efficacy profiles for acute bipolar depression (De Fruyt et al. 2012; Geddes and Miklowitz 2013). Thus, although the olanzapine plus fluoxetine combination, quetiapine monotherapy, and lurasidone as monotherapy and adjunctive therapy have FDA approval for the treatment of acute bipolar depression (and are thus in Tier I), other SGAs such as olanzapine (as monotherapy), risperidone, aripiprazole, ziprasidone, asenapine, and clozapine lack sufficient evidence of efficacy and safety/tolerability to receive FDA approval for the treatment of acute bipolar depression.

Olanzapine plus fluoxetine combination and quetiapine monotherapy. As noted in *Handbook of Diagnosis and Treatment of Bipolar Disorders* (Ketter 2010) and illustrated in Figure 2–2 and listed in Table 2–1, for the two older FDA-approved treatments for acute bipolar depression, double-blind, placebo-controlled studies yielded similar favorable (single-digit) NNTs for Montgomery-Åsberg Depression Rating Scale (MADRS) response (≥50% improvement) compared with placebo (4 for the olanzapine plus fluoxetine combination and 6 for quetiapine monotherapy) (Calabrese et al. 2005; Thase et al. 2006; Tohen et al. 2003). However, these treatments also had unfavorable (single-digit) NNHs compared with placebo (6 for ≥7% weight gain with the olanzapine plus fluoxetine combination, and 5 for sedation/somnolence with quetiapine). Thus, although these two older FDA-approved treatments had adequate efficacy,

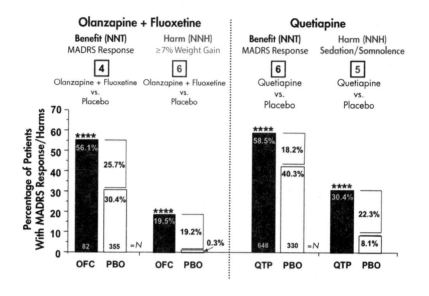

FIGURE 2–2.   Benefits and harms of older second-generation antipsychotics approved by the U.S. Food and Drug Administration (FDA) for acute bipolar depression: olanzapine+fluoxetine combination and quetiapine monotherapy.

Note.   Older second-generation antipsychotics with FDA approval for acute bipolar depression were similarly likely to yield benefit and harm compared with placebo (i.e., numbers needed to treat were similar to numbers needed to harm). MADRS=Montgomery-Åsberg Depression Rating Scale; NNH=number needed to harm (for adverse effects vs. placebo); NNT=number needed to treat (for MADRS response vs. placebo); OFC=olanzapine+fluoxetine combination; PBO=placebo; QTP=quetiapine.

****$P<0.001$ vs. placebo.

Source.   Adapted from Ketter TA: *Handbook of Diagnosis and Treatment of Bipolar Disorders.* Washington, DC, American Psychiatric Publishing, 2010. Copyright 2010, American Psychiatric Publishing. Used with permission. Olanzapine plus fluoxetine combination data (*left*) from Tohen et al. 2003; quetiapine monotherapy data (*right*) pooled from Calabrese et al. 2005 and Thase et al. 2006.

their clinical utility was substantially limited by being similarly likely to yield benefit (response) and harm (side effects) compared with placebo (i.e., they had LHHs of 1.3 and 0.7, respectively; Table 2–1).

Lurasidone as monotherapy and as adjunctive therapy.   In 2013, lurasidone received FDA approval for acute bipolar depression in patients with bipolar I disorder, not only as monotherapy but also as adjunctive therapy (added to lithium or valproate), based on multicenter, randomized, double-blind, placebo-controlled trials. Lurasidone monotherapy had a favorable (single-digit) NNT for response compared with placebo of 5, as well as a favorable (double-digit) NNH for akathisia compared with placebo of 15 (Figure 2–3, left; Table 2–1) (Loebel et al. 2014b). Therefore, lurasidone monotherapy compared with placebo not only was efficacious but was more than three times as likely to yield benefit (response) as harm (akathisia) (i.e., LHH=3.1; Table 2–1). Additionally, lurasidone adjunctive therapy (added to lithium or valproate) compared with placebo had a favorable (single-digit) NNT for response compared with placebo of 7 as well as a favorable (double-digit) NNH for nausea compared with placebo of 16 (Figure 2–3, right; Table 2–1) (Loebel et al. 2014a). Thus, lurasidone adjunctive therapy compared with placebo was also more than twice as likely to yield benefit (response) as harm (nausea) (i.e., LHH = 2.3; Table 2–1). Taken together, these data indicated that lurasidone, as monotherapy or adjunctive therapy, had a favorable benefit: harm ratio that was not offset by reduction in efficacy, making it an important new treatment option for bipolar I depression.

Tier II: High-Priority Unapproved Treatment Options for Acute Bipolar Depression

As noted in the introduction to this section, safety/tolerability limitations of the three Tier I FDA-approved treatments for acute bipolar depression may lead clinicians and patients to consider other options. In assessing alternative acute bipolar depression treatments that lack FDA approval for acute bipolar depression, one approach is to first consider medications that are approved for bipolar disorder preventive treatment. As of early 2015, such agents included the mood stabilizers lithium and lamotrigine, as well as the SGAs olanzapine, aripiprazole, risperidone, and ziprasidone (quetiapine has FDA approval for acute bipolar depression and therefore is in Tier I). Among these agents, the mood stabilizers lithium and lamotrigine have familiarity and/or safety/tolerability advantages accompanied by at least some systematic data supporting their utility in the acute and/or preventive management of bipolar depression. These qualities have contributed to lithium and/or lamotrigine alone or in combination with antidepressants being considered high-priority options for acute bipolar depression in multiple treat-

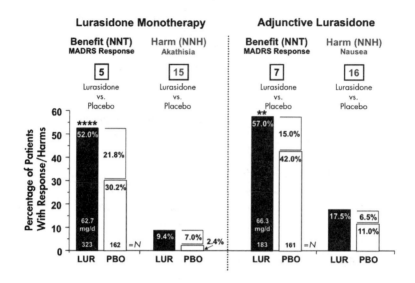

FIGURE 2–3.   Benefits and harms of the newer second-generation antipsychotic lurasidone, which was approved by the U.S. Food and Drug Administration (FDA) in 2013 for acute bipolar I depression treatment as monotherapy and as adjunctive (added to lithium or valproate) therapy. *Note.*   For both monotherapy and adjunctive (added to lithium or valproate) therapy, lurasidone, was more than twice as likely to yield benefit as harm compared with placebo (i.e., had NNH >2×NNT), with adequate efficacy (i.e., single-digit NNT). LUR=lurasidone; MADRS=Montgomery-Åsberg Depression Rating Scale; NNH=number needed to harm (for adverse effects vs. placebo); NNT=number needed to treat (for response vs. placebo); PBO=placebo. $^{**}P<0.01$, $^{****}P<0.001$ vs. placebo. *Source.*   Lurasidone monotherapy data (*left*) from Loebel et al. 2014b; lurasidone adjunctive therapy data (*right*) from Loebel et al. 2014a.

ment guidelines (Goodwin and Consensus Group of the British Association for Psychopharmacology 2009; Grunze et al. 2010; Hirschfeld 2007; Kasper et al. 2008; National Institute for Health and Clinical Excellence 2006; Suppes et al. 2005; Yatham et al. 2013). In contrast, the SGAs olanzapine, aripiprazole, ziprasidone, and risperidone, which are approved for bipolar disorder preventive treatment (but not for acute bipolar depression), have safety/tolerability and/or efficacy limitations that make them lower-priority options, as discussed in the later section on Tier III treatment options for acute bipolar depression.

Mood Stabilizers

Mood stabilizers are considered foundational treatments for bipolar disorder. Lithium and lamotrigine compared with divalproex and carbamazepine continue to have more evidence supporting their efficacy in acute bipolar depression.

Lithium. Lithium has long been considered the gold-standard treatment for bipolar disorder. As monotherapy or in combination with an antidepressant, lithium has been considered a first-line treatment for acute bipolar depression in multiple practice guidelines (Goodwin and Consensus Group of the British Association for Psychopharmacology 2009; Grunze et al. 2010; Hirschfeld 2007; Kasper et al. 2008; National Institute for Health and Clinical Excellence 2006; Suppes et al. 2005; Yatham et al. 2013).

Lithium, although commonly better tolerated than SGAs (Figure 2–1, Table 2–1), appears to have only modest acute antidepressant effects. This was demonstrated in an 8-week multicenter, randomized, double-blind, placebo-controlled trial in depressed patients (62% with bipolar I disorder and 38% with bipolar II disorder) described in the text (although not illustrated) in *Handbook of Diagnosis and Treatment of Bipolar Disorders* (Ketter 2010), and now illustrated in Figure 2–4 (Young et al. 2010). In that quetiapine manufacturer–sponsored study, lithium (mean dose and serum concentration were 981 mg/day and 0.61 mEq/L, respectively—conservative lithium dosing was a limitation) had double-digit NNHs for nausea of 11 (Table 2–1) and for somnolence of 20 (Figure 2–4, right; Table 2–1, legend footnote *f*); however, this was in the context of an unfavorable (double-digit) NNT for response of 15 (Figure 2–4, left; Table 2–1). Thus, lithium was similarly likely to yield benefit (response) and harm (nausea or somnolence) compared with placebo, in the setting of only modest efficacy (not significantly different from placebo); these findings are consistent with lithium being a Tier II (rather than Tier I) option for acute bipolar depression. In contrast, in this study quetiapine had an unfavorable (single-digit) NNH for somnolence of 8, although this was in the context of a favorable (single-digit) NNT for response of 8. Thus, quetiapine, like lithium, was similarly likely to yield benefit (response) and harm (somnolence) compared with placebo, although quetiapine had adequate efficacy (significantly superior to placebo), consistent with it being a Tier I (rather than a Tier II) option for acute bipolar depression. In this study, treatment-emergent affective switch (TEAS) rates were low with both lithium (2.2%) and quetiapine (3.2%), and were only nonsignificantly higher than with placebo (0.8%).

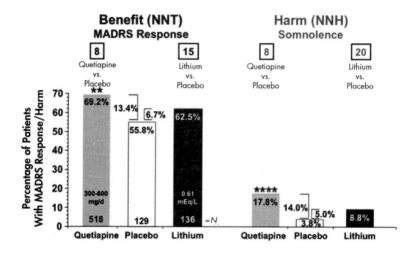

FIGURE 2–4.   Benefits and harms of lithium (and quetiapine) in acute bipolar depression.

Note.   Lithium (double-digit NNT and NNH) and quetiapine (single-digit NNT and NNH) were both similarly likely to yield benefit and harm (i.e., had NNTs that were comparable to their NNHs). However, quetiapine (but not lithium) had adequate efficacy and thus was approved by the U.S. Food and Drug Administration for acute bipolar depression (also see Figure 2–2, *right*). MADRS = Montgomery-Åsberg Depression Rating Scale; NNH=number needed to harm (for somnolence vs. placebo); NNT=number needed to treat (for response vs. placebo).

**P<0.01, ****P<0.001 vs. placebo.

Source.   Data from Young et al. 2010.

Figure 2–4 includes assessment of the risk of somnolence with lithium versus quetiapine. Although somnolence was the harm with the lowest positive NNH for quetiapine, it was not so for lithium. Indeed, the harm with the lowest positive NNH for lithium was nausea, which occurred in 16.9% of patients taking lithium versus 7.6% taking placebo (NNH=10.8; Table 2–1) and yielded an unfavorable LHH of 0.7 (Table 2–1), indicating that for lithium compared with placebo, nausea was more likely than response. This example demonstrates how findings of NNH and LHH analyses vary, depending on the harm selected, emphasizing the importance of individualizing such assessments.

Lamotrigine.   Lamotrigine, which received FDA approval for bipolar I disorder preventive treatment in 2003, has greater ability to delay depressive (as opposed to manic) episodes (Goodwin et al. 2004). Aside from serious rash, which may occur in 1 of every 1,000 patients with bipolar disorder (Calabrese et al. 2002; Physicians' Desk Reference 2014), lamotrigine has a tolerability profile similar to that of antidepressants and superior to that of SGAs and the other mood stabilizers lithium, divalproex, and carbamazepine (Figure 2–1, Table 2–1). Despite early hopes for this agent based on an encouraging large, controlled study suggesting some antidepressant efficacy in acute bipolar I depression (Calabrese et al. 1999), four subsequent acute bipolar depression RCTs failed to demonstrate efficacy superior to that with placebo, so that lamotrigine did not receive FDA approval for acute bipolar depression. In spite of the medication's efficacy limitations in acute bipolar depression, lamotrigine's ability to delay depressive episodes and good tolerability have led it to be considered a first-line treatment for acute bipolar depression in multiple treatment guidelines (Goodwin and Consensus Group of the British Association for Psychopharmacology 2009; Hirschfeld 2007; Kasper et al. 2008; Malhi et al. 2009; Suppes et al. 2005; Yatham et al. 2013).

In a pooled analysis of five double-blind, placebo-controlled studies in acute bipolar depression, lamotrigine compared with placebo had a favorable (double-digit) NNH for somnolence of 37 (Figure 2–5, right; Table 2–1); however, this was in the context of an unfavorable (double-digit) NNT for response of 12 (Figure 2–5, Table 2–1) (Calabrese et al. 2008; Geddes et al. 2009). Thus, although lamotrigine was more than three times as likely to yield benefit (response) as harm (somnolence) compared with placebo (LHH=3.1; Table 2–1), this favorable benefit:harm ratio was offset by inadequate efficacy, consistent with lamotrigine being a Tier II (rather than Tier I) option for acute bipolar depression.

Tier III: Other Treatment Options for Acute Bipolar Depression

Treatment of bipolar depression is sufficiently challenging that clinical need commonly exceeds the evidence-based treatment options discussed thus far in this chapter. In this subsection we consider other treatment options with even more limited evidence of efficacy than the abovementioned Tier I and Tier II treatments.

An important but controversial approach to acute bipolar depression is to combine standard antidepressants (which have FDA approval for unipolar major depressive disorder but not for acute bipolar depression) with antimanic agents. This strategy has been considered first line in multiple European guidelines (Goodwin and Consensus Group of the Brit-

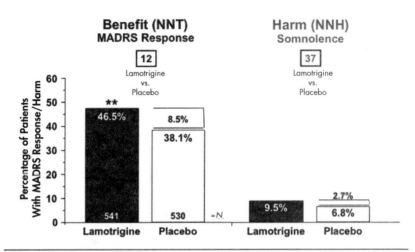

FIGURE 2–5.   Benefits and harms of lamotrigine in acute bipolar depression.

Note. Lamotrigine was more than three times as likely to yield benefit (MADRS response) as harm (somnolence) compared with placebo (i.e., had NNH > 3 × NNT), but at the cost of inadequate efficacy. Thus, lamotrigine was not approved by the U.S. Food and Drug Administration for acute bipolar depression. MADRS=Montgomery-Åsberg Depression Rating Scale; NNH= number needed to harm (for somnolence vs. placebo); NNT=number needed to treat (for MADRS response vs. placebo).

**$P<0.01 vs. placebo.

Source. Adapted from Ketter TA: *Handbook of Diagnosis and Treatment of Bipolar Disorders.* Washington, DC, American Psychiatric Publishing, 2010. Copyright 2010, American Psychiatric Publishing. Used with permission. Lamotrigine benefit data (*left*) from Geddes et al. 2009; lamotrigine harm data (*right*) from Calabrese et al. 2008.

ish Association for Psychopharmacology 2009; Grunze et al. 2010; National Institute for Health and Clinical Excellence 2006) as well as a Canadian guideline (Yatham et al. 2013) but has received lower priority in American guidelines (Calabrese et al. 2004; Hirschfeld 2007; Keck et al. 2004; Suppes et al. 2005). The data supporting the efficacy of such practice are limited, and increasingly results of RCTs are challenging perceptions that this strategy ought to be a high priority. Thus, in the current updated hierarchy, adjunctive antidepressants remain in Tier III.

In view of recent multicenter RCTs indicating some promise for adjunctive armodafinil in acute bipolar depression, and older more limited data supporting adjunctive modafinil in acute bipolar depression, in this update these agents have been moved up from Tier IV to Tier III.

Other Tier III alternatives include other mood stabilizers (divalproex and carbamazepine), other SGAs (olanzapine, aripiprazole, risperidone, ziprasidone, asenapine, and clozapine), ECT, and adjunctive psychotherapy. Consistent with this assessment, guidelines commonly consider these treatments to be lower than first-line priority options (Goodwin and Consensus Group of the British Association for Psychopharmacology 2009; Grunze et al. 2010; National Institute for Health and Clinical Excellence 2006; Yatham et al. 2013).

Some Tier III options have mitigating advantages, such as bipolar disorder preventive treatment indications, enhanced safety/tolerability, or familiarity of use, that might make them attractive for selected patients, and in certain circumstances some of these interventions may be considered early on (e.g., psychotherapy or ECT for pregnant women with acute bipolar depression). For some of these treatments (e.g., adjunctive psychotherapy), advances in research, familiarity, and/or availability may ultimately be sufficient to merit their consideration for placement in higher tiers.

Adjunctive Antidepressants

The role of antidepressants in the management of bipolar disorder continues to be controversial (Geddes and Miklowitz 2013). European and Canadian experts have been more enthusiastic than their American counterparts regarding the utility of these agents in bipolar disorder, believing that antidepressants are effective in acute bipolar depression and that they do not entail a substantively increased risk of TEAS (Gijsman et al. 2004; Goodwin and Consensus Group of the British Association for Psychopharmacology 2009; Grunze et al. 2010; National Institute for Health and Clinical Excellence 2006; Yatham et al. 2013). American experts have been less sanguine about these agents, raising concerns regarding efficacy as well as the risks of TEAS and cycle acceleration (Calabrese et al. 2004; Ghaemi et al. 2003; Ostacher et al. 2010; Suppes et al. 2005). Nevertheless, on both sides of the Atlantic Ocean, there is general consensus that antidepressants in patients with bipolar I disorder need to be administered with concurrent mood stabilizers or antimanic agents (Goodwin and Consensus Group of the British Association for Psychopharmacology 2003; Suppes et al. 2005), although on occasion antidepressant monotherapy (without an antimanic agent) has been advocated for patients with bipolar II disorder (Amsterdam and Shults 2008).

Arguably, the most noteworthy recent development in this controversial area has been the 2013 publication of the ISBD Antidepressant Use in Bipolar Disorders Task Force Consensus Report (Pacchiarotti et al. 2013).

Integrating clinical research evidence and the experience of 65 bipolar expert task force members, consensus was reached for 12 statements regarding the use of antidepressants in bipolar disorder (summarized in Table 2–4). The majority (9) of these 12 statements focus on limiting the use of antidepressants, using terms such as *avoid, discontinue,* or *discourage,* whereas only a minority (three) of these statements focus on permissible uses of antidepressants.

The task force noted marked incongruity between the wide use of and the weak evidence base supporting a role for antidepressants in bipolar disorder, stating specifically that there was insufficient evidence for treatment benefits of antidepressants combined with mood stabilizers. The task force did, however, acknowledge that some individual bipolar patients could benefit from antidepressants, with risks of TEAS being greater with tricyclic and tetracyclic antidepressants and norepinephrine-serotonin reuptake inhibitors compared with serotonin reuptake inhibitors and bupropion, and in bipolar I compared with bipolar II disorder. Hence, the task force stated that in bipolar I patients, antidepressants should be prescribed only as an adjunct to mood stabilizers (rather than as monotherapy).

Another noteworthy recent development was the 2011 publication of the largest meta-analysis to date of controlled trials of antidepressants for acute bipolar depression (Sidor and Macqueen 2011). The authors compiled results of six double-blind, placebo-controlled studies of primarily adjunctive antidepressants (added to antimanic agents) in acute bipolar depression (approximately 90% of patients had bipolar I disorder) that included 416 patients taking antidepressants and 608 receiving placebo. However, one study (the olanzapine plus fluoxetine registration study) accounted for approximately 42% of these patients (Tohen et al. 2003), and another contributed approximately 32% of the patients (Sachs et al. 2007), so that the remaining four studies accounted for only approximately 26% of all patients (Amsterdam and Shults 2005; Cohn et al. 1989; Nemeroff et al. 2001; Shelton and Stahl 2004). In this meta-analysis, antidepressants compared with placebo had a favorable (triple-digit) NNH for TEAS of 209 (Figure 2–6, right; Table 2–1); however, this was in the context of an unfavorable double-digit NNT for response/remission of 29 (Figure 2–6, left; Table 2–1). Thus, although antidepressants were more than seven times as likely to yield benefit (response/remission) as harm (mood switch) compared with placebo (LHH=7.3; Table 2–1), this favorable benefit:harm ratio was offset by inadequate efficacy, consistent with adjunctive antidepressants lacking FDA approval for acute bipolar depression and continuing to be Tier III treatment options.

TABLE 2–4. Summary of 12 consensus statements of International Society for Bipolar Disorders Antidepressant Use in Bipolar Disorders Task Force Consensus Report

Adjunctive antidepressants for acute bipolar depression	*Permissible* if history of positive antidepressant response *Avoid* if ≥ 2 manic symptoms, psychomotor agitation, or rapid cycling
Adjunctive antidepressants for bipolar preventive treatment	*Permissible* if depressive relapse after stopping antidepressant
Antidepressant monotherapy for acute bipolar depression	*Avoid* in bipolar I disorder *Avoid* in bipolar I and II depression if ≥ 2 manic symptoms
Antidepressant switching to mania or hypomania, mixed features, or rapid cycling	*Discontinue* if antidepressant-emergent mania or hypomania or psychomotor agitation *Discourage* if prior antidepressant-emergent mania or hypomania or mixed features *Avoid* if high number of episodes or rapid cycling
Antidepressant use in mixed states	*Avoid* in manic and depressive episodes with mixed features *Avoid* in patients with predominantly mixed states *Discontinue* if mixed state emerges
Antidepressants with increased switch risk (SNRIs and TCAs)	*Permissible* only if other antidepressants already tried and patient closely monitored

Note. SNRI=serotonin-norepinephrine reuptake inhibitor; TCA=tricyclic antidepressant.
Source. Adapted from Pacchiarotti et al. 2013.

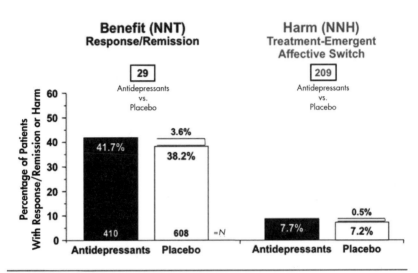

FIGURE 2–6. Benefits and harms of antidepressants (primarily adjunctive) in acute bipolar depression.

Note. In this six-study meta-analysis, antidepressants (primarily adjunctive) were more than sevenfold as likely to yield benefit as harm compared with placebo (i.e., had NNH >7×NNT), but at the cost of inadequate efficacy. NNH = number needed to harm; NNT=number needed to treat.

*P<0.01 vs. placebo.

Source. Data from Sidor and Macqueen 2011.

Not included in Sidor and Macqueen's (2011) antidepressant meta-analysis was an 8-week multicenter, randomized, double-blind, placebo-controlled trial in depressed patients (65% with bipolar I disorder and 35% with bipolar II disorder) described in the text (although not illustrated) in *Handbook of Diagnosis and Treatment of Bipolar Disorders* (Ketter 2010), and now illustrated in Figure 2–7 (McElroy et al. 2011). In this quetiapine manufacturer–sponsored study, paroxetine 20 mg/day (the conservative paroxetine dosing was a limitation) had a favorable (negative double-digit) NNH for somnolence of –44 (i.e., somnolence was numerically less common than with placebo) (Figure 2–7, right); however, this was in the context of an unfavorable (double-digit) NNT for response of 46 (Figure 2–7, left). Thus, paroxetine had a similarly low likelihood of yielding benefit (response) and harm (somnolence) compared with placebo, in the setting of inadequate efficacy (not significantly different from placebo), consistent with paroxetine being a Tier III (rather than Tier I or II)

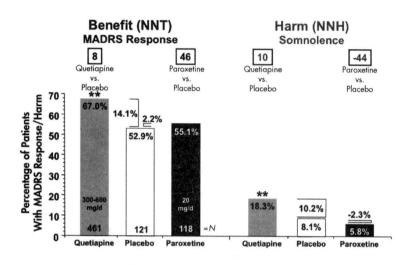

FIGURE 2–7. Benefits and harms of paroxetine (and quetiapine) in acute bipolar depression.

Note. Paroxetine (double-digit NNT and negative double-digit NNH) and quetiapine (single-digit NNT and near-single-digit NNH) were both similarly likely to yield benefit and harm (i.e., had NNTs that were similar to their NNHs). However, quetiapine (but not paroxetine) had adequate efficacy and thus was approved by the U.S. Food and Drug Administration for acute bipolar depression (also see Figure 2–2, *right*). MADRS=Montgomery-Åsberg Depression Rating Scale; NNH = number needed to harm (for somnolence vs. placebo); NNT=number needed to treat (for response vs. placebo).
**P<0.01 vs. placebo.
Source. Data from McElroy et al. 2011.

option for acute bipolar depression. In contrast, in this study quetiapine had an unfavorable (near single-digit) NNH for somnolence of 10 (Figure 2–7, right), although this was in the context of a favorable (single-digit) NNT for response of 8 (Figure 2–7, left). Thus, like paroxetine, quetiapine was similarly likely to yield benefit (response) and harm (somnolence) compared with placebo, although quetiapine had adequate efficacy (significantly superior to that of placebo), which is consistent with it being a Tier I option for acute bipolar depression. In this study, TEAS rates were 8.9% with placebo and 10.7% with paroxetine (NNH=54, not significantly different from the rate with placebo) but only 3.1% with quetiapine (NNH=–18, significantly lower than the rate with placebo).

Figure 2–7 includes assessment of the risk of somnolence with paroxetine versus quetiapine. Although somnolence was the harm with the lowest positive NNH for quetiapine, it was not so for paroxetine. Indeed, the harm with the lowest positive NNH for paroxetine was nausea, which occurred in 12.4% with paroxetine versus 5.6% with placebo (NNH = 14.8), and yielded an unfavorable LHH of 0.3 (Table 2–1), indicating that for paroxetine compared with placebo, nausea was three times as likely as response. This example demonstrates how findings of NNH and LHH analyses vary, depending of the harm selected, thus emphasizing the importance of individualizing such assessments.

Also not included in the Sidor and Macqueen (2011) antidepressant meta-analysis were four recent papers examining antidepressant monotherapy in acute bipolar II depression (Amsterdam and Shults 2010; Amsterdam et al. 2009, 2010, 2013). However, in a fashion similar to that noted in *Handbook of Diagnosis and Treatment of Bipolar Disorders* (Ketter 2010) for earlier such studies (Amsterdam and Shults 2005, 2008; Amsterdam et al. 1998, 2004), small sample sizes and other methodological limitations made interpretation of these more recent studies challenging.

Adjunctive Modafinil and Armodafinil

Racemic modafinil and its *R*-isomer armodafinil are stimulant-like low-affinity dopamine transporter inhibitors approved for improving wakefulness in adults with excessive sleepiness associated with narcolepsy, obstructive sleep apnea, and shift-work sleep disorder (Physicians' Desk Reference 2014). As described in *Handbook of Diagnosis and Treatment of Bipolar Disorders* (Ketter 2010), in a 6-week, multicenter, randomized, double-blind, placebo-controlled study in 85 patients with bipolar depression inadequately responsive to a mood stabilizer with or without concomitant antidepressant therapy, adjunctive modafinil (mean dosage 177 mg/day) versus placebo had a favorable (single-digit) NNT for response compared with placebo of 5, and a favorable (double-digit) NNH for headache compared with placebo of 14 (Frye et al. 2007). Thus, adjunctive modafinil compared with placebo not only was efficacious but was more than twice as likely to yield benefit (response) as harm (headache).

A recent positive multicenter, randomized, double-blind, placebo-controlled trial of adjunctive armodafinil for acute bipolar I depression (Ketter et al. 2013), combined with this older adjunctive modafinil data, has resulted in adjunctive modafinil and armodafinil being promoted from Tier IV in *Handbook of Diagnosis and Treatment of Bipolar Disorders* (Ketter 2010) to Tier III in the current volume.

Specifically, in a recent 8-week, multicenter, randomized, double-blind, placebo-controlled trial in adults with acute bipolar I depression, adjunctive armodafinil 150 mg/day (added to lithium, valproate, olanza-

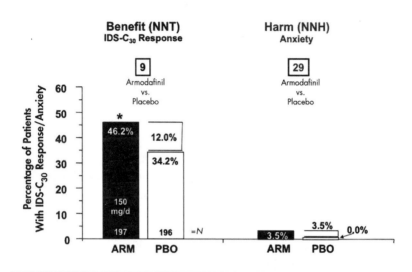

FIGURE 2–8. Benefits and harms of adjunctive armodafinil for acute bipolar I depression.

Note. Adjunctive armodafinil was more than three times as likely to yield benefit (IDS-C$_{30}$ response) as harm (anxiety) compared with placebo in acute bipolar I depression (i.e., had NNH>3×NNT), with adequate efficacy in this trial but not in two subsequent trials. IDS-C$_{30}$=Inventory of Depressive Symptomatology–Clinician-rated 30-item version; NNH=number needed to harm (for anxiety vs. placebo); NNT=number needed to treat (for IDS-C$_{30}$ response vs. placebo). *P<0.05 vs. placebo.

Source. Data from Ketter et al. 2013.

pine, risperidone, aripiprazole, or mood stabilizer plus ziprasidone) versus placebo had a favorable (single-digit) NNT for response compared with placebo of 9 (Figure 2–8, left; Table 2–1 legend footnote *g*) as well as a favorable (double-digit) NNH for anxiety compared with placebo of 29 (Figure 2–8, right; Table 2–1 legend footnote *g*) (Ketter et al. 2013). Hence, in this acute bipolar depression trial, adjunctive armodafinil compared with placebo not only was efficacious but was more than three times as likely to yield benefit (response) as harm (anxiety).

Unfortunately, in two subsequent acute bipolar I depression trials (Frye et al. 2013, 2014), adjunctive armodafinil, although well tolerated, was no more efficacious than placebo. Therefore, as of early 2015, adjunctive armodafinil was not FDA approved for acute bipolar I depression, and the manufacturer had discontinued development of armodafinil for this indication.

On the basis of pooled data from all three adjunctive armodafinil 150 mg/day studies, headache had the lowest positive NNH (30.4; see

Table 2–1) and NNT rose to an unfavorable 14.9, but LHH remained a favorable 2.0 (Table 2–1). Thus, although armodafinil was twice as likely to yield benefit (response) as harm (headache) compared with placebo, this favorable benefit:harm ratio was offset by inadequate efficacy, consistent with armodafinil being a Tier III option for acute bipolar depression.

Other Mood Stabilizers

As of early 2015, the other mood stabilizers (divalproex and carbamazepine), compared with lithium and lamotrigine, differed in that they continued to have less evidence supporting their use in acute bipolar depression and lacked FDA approval for bipolar disorder preventive treatment, but were similar in that they lacked FDA approval for acute bipolar depression treatment.

Although two recent meta-analyses found that divalproex in acute bipolar depression yielded a favorable (single-digit) NNT for response compared with placebo of 5, these were based on a pooled sample size of only 142 patients (Bond et al. 2010; Smith et al. 2010), less than one-seventh of that with lamotrigine ($N=1,071$; Figure 2–5, left). In spite of the limited controlled data supporting efficacy, some treatment guidelines (Goodwin and Consensus Group of the British Association for Psychopharmacology 2009; Grunze et al. 2010; Malhi et al. 2009), but not others (Kasper et al. 2008; National Institute for Health and Clinical Excellence 2006; Yatham et al. 2013), considered divalproex a first-line treatment for acute bipolar depression.

In contrast, treatment guidelines uniformly did not consider carbamazepine a first-line treatment for acute bipolar depression (Goodwin and Consensus Group of the British Association for Psychopharmacology 2009; Grunze et al. 2010; Kasper et al. 2008; Malhi et al. 2009; National Institute for Health and Clinical Excellence 2006; Yatham et al. 2013).

In summary, although divalproex (a proprietary formulation of valproate) and carbamazepine are commonly better tolerated than SGAs (Figure 2–1), the limited systematic efficacy data support consideration of these medications as merely alternative treatments for acute bipolar depression, consistent with these mood stabilizers remaining in Tier III.

Other Second-Generation Antipsychotics

As of early 2015, SGAs as a class continued to be important treatment options for acute mania (with six having FDA approval as monotherapy ± adjunctive therapy) and had become increasingly important for bipolar disorder preventive treatment (with five having FDA approval as monotherapy and/or adjunctive therapy). In contrast, SGAs appeared to lack a class effect for utility in acute bipolar depression, with only three having gained FDA approval. Specifically, as of early 2015, olanzapine monotherapy, aripiprazole monotherapy, ziprasidone monotherapy and adjunctive therapy, risperidone, asenapine, and clozapine continued to lack FDA approval for acute bipolar depression. On the basis of efficacy limitations and/or safety/tolerability challenges, these other SGAs remained in Tier III. Indeed, most guidelines consider these treatments to be lower than first-line priority options (Goodwin and Consensus Group of the British Association for Psychopharmacology 2009; Grunze et al. 2010; National Institute for Health and Clinical Excellence 2006; Yatham et al. 2013). For example, the 2013 CANMAT and ISBD collaborative update of CANMAT guidelines for the management of patients with bipolar disorder considered olanzapine monotherapy to be third-line because of tolerability limitations, and did not recommend aripiprazole monotherapy and ziprasidone monotherapy and adjunctive therapy as interventions because of their efficacy and tolerability limitations (Yatham et al. 2013).

Olanzapine monotherapy.   Olanzapine's utility in acute bipolar I depression has continued to be limited by its substantial side-effect risks (e.g., weight gain/metabolic problems), combined with its having only modest acute antidepressant effects, which were less robust than those of the olanzapine plus fluoxetine combination. In two multicenter RCTs (Tohen et al. 2003, 2012), olanzapine monotherapy compared with placebo yielded similarly unfavorable (single-digit) NNHs for at least 7% weight gain compared with placebo (6 in the first study and 5 in the second study; Figure 2–9, Harm). Moreover, olanzapine monotherapy (although it had statistically significant superiority to placebo) also had unfavorable (double-digit) NNTs for response compared with placebo (12 in the first study and 11 in the second study; Figure 2–9, Benefit). Thus, although olanzapine monotherapy was slightly superior to placebo, this modest efficacy was offset by substantial tolerability challenges, being approximately twice as likely to yield harm (weight gain) as benefit (response) compared with placebo (LHH for pooled data was 0.5; Table 2–1), consistent with it continuing to be a Tier III treatment option.

Aripiprazole monotherapy.   As noted in *Handbook of Diagnosis and Treatment of Bipolar Disorders* (Ketter 2010), aripiprazole monotherapy was not effective for the treatment of acute bipolar I depression (Thase et al. 2008) (NNT=44; Table 2–1), and in view of its SGA side-effect profile, this treatment has remained in Tier III.

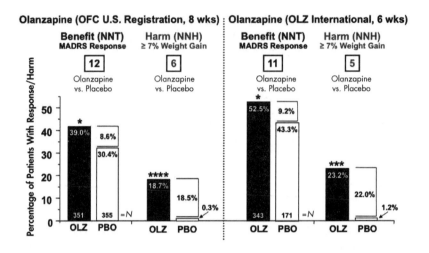

FIGURE 2–9.   Benefits and harms of the second-generation antipsychotic olanzapine as monotherapy for acute bipolar I depression.

Note.   Olanzapine was approximately twice as likely to yield harm (weight gain) as benefit (response) compared with placebo (i.e., had NNT approximately twice NNH), so that tolerability challenges offset olanzapine's modest (albeit statistically significant) efficacy, and olanzapine lacks U.S. Food and Drug Administration approval for acute bipolar depression. MADRS=Montgomery-Åsberg Depression Rating Scale; NNT=number needed to treat (for MADRS response vs. placebo); NNH=number needed to harm (for ≥7% weight gain vs. placebo); OFC=olanzapine+fluoxetine combination; OLZ=olanzapine; PBO = placebo.
*P<0.05, ***P<0.001, ****P<0.0001 vs. placebo.

Source.   Adapted from Ketter TA: *Handbook of Diagnosis and Treatment of Bipolar Disorders.* Washington, DC, American Psychiatric Publishing, 2010. Copyright 2010, American Psychiatric Publishing. Used with permission. OFC U.S. registration trial data (*left*) from Tohen et al. 2003. OLZ international trial data (*right*) from Tohen et al. 2012.

Risperidone.   As of early 2015, risperidone continued to lack an FDA indication for acute bipolar depression and, in view of its SGA side-effect profile, has remained in Tier III.

Ziprasidone.   Multicenter, randomized, double-blind, placebo-controlled trials found ziprasidone monotherapy (Lombardo et al. 2012) and adjunctive therapy (Sachs et al. 2011) to be no better than placebo for acute bipolar depression. Therefore, as of early 2015, ziprasidone lacked an acute bipolar depression indication and, in view of its SGA side-effect profile, has remained in Tier III.

However, in a five-center, 6-week study in 73 patients (approximately 60% with bipolar II disorder and 40% with unipolar major depressive disorder) with a current major depressive episode co-occurring with two or three mood elevation symptoms, approximately half of whom were taking antidepressants±mood stabilizers, adjunctive ziprasidone (approximately 130 mg/day) yielded a significantly higher MADRS response rate compared with placebo (52.9% vs. 28.9%, $P=0.04$) and thus a favorable single-digit NNT of 5 (Patkar et al. 2012). The most common side effects were headache and drowsiness, which occurred in approximately 15% of patients taking either adjunctive ziprasidone or adjunctive placebo.

Clozapine. As of early 2015, clozapine lacked any indication for bipolar disorder and, in view of its SGA side-effect profile, has remained in Tier III. However, potential antidepressant properties remain of interest, because clozapine is the only agent approved for decreasing suicidal behavior in patients with schizophrenia (Meltzer et al. 2003).

Electroconvulsive Therapy

As of early 2015, ECT remained an important option for treatment-resistant depression, supported by multiple RCTs, although these had commonly been in heterogeneous samples of patients with bipolar and unipolar depression. This evidence-base limitation, along with the expense and potential side effects, was consistent with ECT remaining a Tier III option for acute bipolar depression. Nevertheless, for patients with severe, psychotic, catatonic, or acutely suicidal depression, or with depression during pregnancy, ECT remains reasonable to consider and offer as an early option.

Adjunctive Psychotherapy

Data from controlled trials continue to indicate the importance of adjunctive (added to pharmacotherapy) psychosocial interventions in the management of bipolar disorder. The most-studied interventions have been family focused therapy (FFT) (Miklowitz 2010), cognitive-behavioral therapy (CBT) (Lam et al. 2010; Ramirez Basco and Rush 2005), interpersonal and social rhythm therapy (IPSRT) (Frank 2005), and group psychoeducation (Colom et al. 2006), with research continuing to provide evidence of efficacy for bipolar disorder preventive treatment more often than for acute bipolar depression (Geddes and Miklowitz 2013). More recent research has begun to examine the roles of dialectical behavior therapy (DBT)

(Van Dijk et al. 2013) and group mindfulness-based cognitive therapy (MBCT) (Weber et al. 2010; Williams et al. 2008).

As of early 2015, the largest psychosocial intervention study in acute bipolar depression remained the Systematic Treatment Enhancement Program for Bipolar Disorder (STEP-BD), a 9-month, multicenter, randomized, controlled effectiveness trial. In one study, 163 patients who received adjunctive intensive (thirty 50-minute sessions over 9 months) CBT, FFT, or IPSRT, compared with 130 patients who received a much more limited brief (three 50-minute sessions) psychoeducation control intervention (called collaborative care), had a higher recovery rate (64.4% and 51.5%, respectively; NNT=8) (Miklowitz et al. 2007). In contrast, in another STEP-BD multicenter, randomized, controlled study in acute bipolar depression, the effectiveness of adjunctive antidepressants (added to mood stabilizers) was no better or worse than that of adjunctive placebo, with both interventions yielding only modest recovery rates (23.5% and 27.3%, respectively) (Sachs et al. 2007).

A post hoc analysis of this STEP-BD adjunctive intensive psychotherapy in acute bipolar depression study found intensive psychotherapies superior to collaborative care in participants with (66% and 49% recovered, respectively; NNT=6) but not without (64% and 62% recovered, respectively; NNT=50) a lifetime anxiety disorder, and with one (84% and 53% recovered, respectively; NNT=4) but not with more than one (54% and 46% recovered, respectively; NNT=13) lifetime anxiety disorder (Deckersbach et al. 2014). Thus, comorbidities may affect patients' responses to intensive psychotherapy.

Unfortunately, some other studies assessing CBT and IPSRT separately were less encouraging than the above-mentioned pooled CBT/FFT/IPSRT STEP-BD intensive psychotherapy study. For example, an acute and preventive treatment study assessed CBT in 253 patients with highly recurrent or severe bipolar disorder, with approximately two-thirds of patients having either a current mood episode (primarily depressive) or psychiatric comorbidity/high recurrence (at least 30 prior episodes) (Scott et al. 2006). In this 18-month study, adjunctive CBT (22 sessions over 6 months, followed by 2 sessions in the next 6 months) compared with a no-adjunctive-psychotherapy control condition did not significantly improve mood outcomes in the overall sample, although CBT yielded improved mood outcomes among a subset of patients with fewer than 12 prior mood episodes.

Similarly, in the acute treatment phase of the pivotal IPSRT study (Frank et al. 2005), 175 patients with bipolar I disorder and current acute mood episodes (56% depressed, 44% elevated) who were randomly assigned to receive IPSRT compared with intensive clinical management (ICM; included support/education regarding bipolar disorder, sleep, medications, and side effects) did not have significant differences in time to remission and remission rate (70% vs. 72%), perhaps because ICM was an effective active control intervention that entailed substantive psychoeducation and supportive therapy elements.

Recent research has begun to examine the possibilities of roles for adjunctive DBT (Goldstein et al. 2007; Van Dijk et al. 2013) and adjunctive group MBCT (Weber et al. 2010; Williams et al. 2008) in patients with bipolar disorder.

Unfortunately, access to therapists with training in adjunctive psychotherapy modalities remains limited, hindering the dissemination of these valuable treatments, which therefore remain in Tier III.

Tier IV: Novel Adjunctive Treatments

Treatment resistance or intolerance is sufficiently common in patients with bipolar disorders that even the armamentarium in Tiers I–III is insufficient to meet clinical needs, so that adjunctive treatments with even more limited evidence of efficacy and/or safety/tolerability than the above-mentioned treatments may be considered. Treatment guidelines uniformly consider these modalities, if mentioned at all, to be low-priority interventions (Goodwin and Consensus Group of the British Association for Psychopharmacology 2009; Grunze et al. 2010; Hirschfeld 2007; Keck et al. 2004; National Institute for Health and Clinical Excellence 2006; Suppes et al. 2005; Yatham et al. 2013).

Nevertheless, some Tier IV options could prove attractive for carefully selected patients, after consideration of treatments on Tiers I–III (e.g., in patients experiencing inadequate efficacy and/or safety/tolerability with Tier I–III treatments). For some of these treatments, advances in research may ultimately provide sufficient evidence to merit their consideration for placement in higher tiers. Indeed, as noted earlier (see "Adjunctive Modafinil and Armodafinil"), a recent positive multicenter, randomized, double-blind, placebo-controlled trial of adjunctive armodafinil for acute bipolar I depression (Ketter et al. 2013), combined with older adjunctive modafinil data, resulted in adjunctive modafinil and armodafinil being promoted from Tier IV in *Handbook of Diagnosis and Treatment of Bipolar Disorders* (Ketter 2010) to Tier III in this volume. Although other recent advances in novel adjunctive treatments for acute bipolar depression have been limited, some merit updating.

Adjunctive Supraphysiologic Levothyroxine

A recent study suggested gender-specific (i.e., in women but not in men) antidepressant effects for supraphysiologic doses of levothyroxine in bipolar disorder. Thus, among 62 (32 female, 30 male) patients with acute bipolar depression, adjunctive supraphysiologic (300 μg/ day) levothyroxine yielded an NNT for Hamilton Depression Rating Scale (HDRS) response compared with placebo of 10 (36% vs. 26%, $P = 0.4$) (Stamm et al. 2014). However, in a secondary analysis, in women (but not in men) supraphysiologic levothyroxine was significantly better than placebo in decreasing HDRS score, and high baseline thyroid-stimulating hormone levels predicted better levothyroxine antidepressant effect. Because of the small sample size and methodological limitations of this study, adjunctive supraphysiologic levothyroxine has remained in Tier IV.

Adjunctive Sleep Deprivation and Light Therapy

A recent naturalistic open-label study found that multimodal therapy (starting or continuing lithium and combining with sleep deprivation and light therapy) might offer rapid benefit for acute bipolar depression and suicidality (i.e., after one total sleep deprivation cycle, comprising a period of 36 hours awake followed by recovery sleep and next morning bright light) (Benedetti et al. 2014). Among inpatients with acute bipolar depression, lithium initiation (in 65.2%) or continuation (in 34.8%), along with 1 week with three consecutive total sleep deprivation–morning bright light cycles, yielded a 70.1% HDRS response rate after the first week. Multimodal therapy was generally adequately tolerated, with 98.6% (141/ 143) of patients completing a 2-week regimen (the second week involved continued lithium and morning bright light but not sleep deprivation) and only 1.4% (2/143) experiencing TEAS. Because of methodological limitations (i.e., lack of a control group), adjunctive sleep deprivation and light therapy (even in combination) have remained in Tier IV.

Adjunctive Ramelteon

Ramelteon is a melatonin MT_1/MT_2 receptor agonist with an FDA indication for insomnia treatment (Physicians' Desk Reference 2014) that is commonly well tolerated. Very limited data suggesting that ramelteon has adjunctive therapeutic effects in acute bipolar I depression may merit exploration.

In an 8-week, single-center, randomized, double-blind, placebo-controlled assessment of 21 bipolar I disorder patients with mild to moderate mood elevation symptoms and sleep disturbance despite mood stabilizer and/or SGA therapy, adjunctive ramelteon 8 mg at bedtime compared with placebo was well tolerated and yielded significantly greater improvement in depressive symptoms according to the Clinical Global Impressions Scale Modified for Bipolar Illness (CGI-BP) but *not* according to the Inventory for Depressive Symptomatology (IDS) (McElroy et al. 2011). Also, in a 24-week, single-center, randomized, double-blind, placebo-controlled bipolar I disorder preventive treatment study, among 83 euthymic bipolar I disorder patients with sleep disturbance despite mood stabilizer, antipsychotic, and/or antidepressant therapy, adjunctive ramelteon 8 mg at bedtime compared with placebo was well tolerated and yielded a significantly less likelihood of mood episode recurrence; the NNTs for recurrence prevention compared with placebo were 5 for any episode, 7 for depressive episodes, and 20 for manic/mixed episodes (Norris et al. 2013).

Importantly, *neither* of these adjunctive ramelteon studies enrolled patients with acute bipolar I depression. Thus, results of two 6-week multicenter, randomized, double-blind, placebo-controlled adjunctive studies of ramelteon sublingual formulation (TAK-375SL) in acute bipolar I depression, which are registered on ClinicalTrials.gov (NCT01467700—added to lithium or valproate; and NCT01677182—added to lithium, valproate, olanzapine, risperidone, aripiprazole, or ziprasidone), will be needed to ascertain whether adjunctive ramelteon may ultimately have a role in the treatment of acute bipolar I depression. For the time being, however, adjunctive ramelteon is in Tier IV.

Nutriceuticals

A recent review of adjunctive nutriceuticals concluded that controlled studies did not support their routine use in the treatment of acute bipolar depression (Rakofsky and Dunlop 2014). This review concluded that omega-3 fatty acids had the strongest evidence of efficacy for acute bipolar depression, although some studies were negative. However, a meta-analysis of five RCTs (Frangou et al. 2006, 2007; Gracious et al. 2010; Keck et al. 2006; Stoll et al. 1999) suggested that adjunctive omega-3 fatty acids were superior to placebo for bipolar depression, with a small but statistically significant effect size of 0.34 (Sarris et al. 2012). This effect size was the same as that in the adjunctive lurasidone in acute bipolar I depression study, which had an NNT for response compared with

placebo of 7 (Loebel et al. 2014a). In their review of adjunctive nutriceuticals in acute bipolar depression,) stated that systematic data weakly
(not necessarily significantly) supported efficacy for vitamin C, cytidine, N-acetylcysteine, and inositol, but were negative for folic acid,
choline, and cytidine combined with omega-3 fatty acids. Finally, in a
study in 31 unipolar and 17 bipolar depression patients with methamphetamine dependence, adjunctive citicoline 2,000 mg/day compared
with placebo for 12 weeks was well tolerated and yielded significantly
greater improvement in depression (but not in methamphetamine use)
(Brown and Gabrielson 2012). Accordingly, as of early 2015, taken together, systematic data were consistent with adjunctive nutriceuticals remaining in Tier IV.

Other Novel Adjunctive Treatments

Because of ongoing limitations related to efficacy, tolerability, and/or
feasibility, adjunctive pramipexole, topiramate, stimulants, vagus nerve
stimulation, and transcranial magnetic stimulation remain on Tier IV.

Tier V: Research Treatments

As of early 2015, research suggested that two very innovative treatments—
adjunctive ketamine and adjunctive deep brain stimulation (DBS)—
could have promise but were thus far too novel and carried too substantive safety/tolerability risks to be considered clinical (as opposed to research) tools.

Adjunctive Ketamine

As of early 2015, ketamine had FDA approval as an intravenous (more
often than intramuscular) general anesthetic but lacked FDA approval
for mood disorders (Physicians' Desk Reference 2014). The U.S. prescribing information for ketamine includes a special note stating that
approximately 12% of patients may have emergence reactions that may
involve hallucinations, delirium, confusion, excitement, and irrational
behavior; the information also includes statements that ketamine has been
associated with abuse and dependence. Indeed, ketamine is a Schedule III
controlled substance.

Recent studies, however, suggest that ketamine, which has N-methyl-
D-aspartate (NMDA) antagonist effects, may have rapid antidepressant
effects in acute bipolar (and unipolar) depression. Specifically, in two National Institute of Mental Health–funded crossover studies—one in 18 pa-

tients (Diazgranados et al. 2010) and the other a replication in 15 patients (Zarate et al. 2012) with nonpsychotic bipolar I or II depression resistant to retrospective open antidepressant and to prospective open lithium or valproate—adjunctive (added to lithium or valproate) intravenous infusions of ketamine hydrochloride (0.5 mg/kg) compared with placebo (order randomized, 2 weeks apart) yielded greater MADRS improvement that was evident by 40 minutes and persisted through day 3, and rates of response at any point of 71% versus 6% (NNT=2) and 79% versus 0% (NNT=2), respectively. The replication study also found that ketamine could rapidly attenuate suicidal ideation. In these small studies, ketamine was well tolerated, with the most common adverse effect being dissociative symptoms, which occurred only at the 40-minute point.

Although research data have yielded substantial hope regarding the clinical treatment potential of adjunctive ketamine (or agents with similar antiglutamatergic mechanisms) in not only bipolar but also unipolar (Murrough et al. 2013) treatment-resistant depression, considerable caution has been advocated prior to clinically disseminating such approaches, because efficacy and safety/tolerability still need to be established in more representative groups of patients for whom adjunctive ketamine is likely to be used (Rush 2013; Schatzberg 2014). Thus, prior to clinical dissemination, additional research with larger groups of generalizable patients with acute bipolar depression is needed not only to confirm efficacy but also to assess risks of noteworthy potential harms such as abuse (De Luca et al. 2012) and the triggering and/or exacerbating of psychotic/manic symptoms (Moore et al. 2013).

Adjunctive Deep Brain Stimulation

Adjunctive (added to stable pharmacotherapy) DBS is a research tool for treatment-resistant depression that involves placement of cerebral electrodes in regions implicated in the neural circuitry underlying depression (Schlaepfer and Bewernick 2013). This modality entails substantive risks of adverse effects related to surgical cerebral electrode placement, device malfunctioning, and the stimulation itself, with the risk of mood elevation being an additional concern in patients with bipolar disorder (Schlaepfer and Bewernick 2013).

A meta-analysis of four observational (open) studies (Holtzheimer et al. 2012; Kennedy et al. 2011; Lozano et al. 2012; Puigdemont et al. 2012) found that DBS targeting the subgenual (subcallosal) cingulate cortex (SCC) in a total of 66 patients with severe, chronic, treatment-resistant (unipolar more than bipolar) depression yielded a significant decrease in depression scores between 3 and 6 months (but no significant change from 6 to 12 months), with a 12-month response rate of 39.9% and a 12-month dropout rate of 10.8% (Berlim et al. 2014). The authors concluded that adjunctive DBS applied to the SCC had adequate acceptability and was potentially efficacious, because the 12-month response rate for (primarily pharmacological) treatment as usual for treatment-resistant depression had been estimated to be only 11.6% (Dunner et al. 2006).

As of early 2015, studies had focused primarily on adjunctive DBS in the SCC in treatment-resistant unipolar depression, although some reports included small numbers of treatment-resistant bipolar depression patients (Holtzheimer et al. 2012; Torres et al. 2013) and targeted brain areas other than the SCC, such as the anterior limb of the internal capsule and the nucleus accumbens (Schlaepfer and Bewernick 2013). Additional research assessing the efficacy and safety/tolerability of adjunctive DBS in larger numbers of patients with treatment-resistant bipolar depression is needed to determine whether or not it merits clinical application.

■ Conclusion

Even though depression is the most pervasive abnormal mood state in patients with bipolar disorder, as of early 2015 there were still only three FDA-approved treatments (all with SGA components and thus substantive tolerability challenges) for acute bipolar depression, and controversy continued regarding the optimal approach to this challenge. The use of adjunctive antidepressants in acute bipolar depression continued to be one of the most controversial areas in the management of bipolar disorder. Development of agents with not only adequate efficacy but also acceptable safety/tolerability remained a crucial unmet need in the management of acute bipolar depression.

■ References

Adler C, Ketter T, Frye MA, et al: Randomized, double-blind, placebo-controlled trial of adjunctive armodafinil (150 mg/day) in adults with bipolar I depression: safety and primary efficacy findings. Paper presented at the 167th Annual Meeting of the American Psychiatric Association, New York, NY, May 3–7, 2014

Akobeng AK: Communicating the benefits and harms of treatments. Arch Dis Child 93(8):710–713, 2008 18456681

American Psychiatric Association: Diagnostic and Statistical Manual of Mental Disorders, 5th Edition. Washington, DC, American Psychiatric Association, 2013

Amsterdam JD, Shults J: Comparison of fluoxetine, olanzapine, and combined fluoxetine plus olanzapine initial therapy of bipolar type I and type II major depression—lack of manic induction. J Affect Disord 87(1):121–130, 2005 15923042

Amsterdam JD, Shults J: Comparison of short-term venlafaxine versus lithium monotherapy for bipolar II major depressive episode: a randomized open-label study. J Clin Psychopharmacol 28(2):171–181, 2008 18344727

Amsterdam JD, Shults J: Efficacy and mood conversion rate of short-term fluoxetine monotherapy of bipolar II major depressive episode. J Clin Psychopharmacol 30(3):306–311, 2010 20473068

Amsterdam JD, Garcia-España F, Fawcett J, et al: Efficacy and safety of fluoxetine in treating bipolar II major depressive episode. J Clin Psychopharmacol 18(6):435–440, 1998 9864074

Amsterdam JD, Shults J, Brunswick DJ, et al: Short-term fluoxetine monotherapy for bipolar type II or bipolar NOS major depression—low manic switch rate. Bipolar Disord 6(1):75–81, 2004 14996144

Amsterdam JD, Wang CH, Shwarz M, et al: Venlafaxine versus lithium monotherapy of rapid and non-rapid cycling patients with bipolar II major depressive episode: a randomized, parallel group, open-label trial. J Affect Disord 112(1–3):219–230, 2009 18486235

Amsterdam JD, Wang G, Shults J: Venlafaxine monotherapy in bipolar type II depressed patients unresponsive to prior lithium monotherapy. Acta Psychiatr Scand 121(3):201–208, 2010 19694630

Amsterdam JD, Luo L, Shults J: Effectiveness and mood conversion rate of short-term fluoxetine monotherapy in patients with rapid cycling bipolar II depression versus patients with nonrapid cycling bipolar II depression. J Clin Psychopharmacol 33(3):420–424, 2013 23609385

Benedetti F, Riccaboni R, Locatelli C, et al: Rapid treatment response of suicidal symptoms to lithium, sleep deprivation, and light therapy (chronotherapeutics) in drug-resistant bipolar depression. J Clin Psychiatry 75(2):133–440, 2014 24345382

Berlim MT, McGirr A, Van den Eynde F, et al: Effectiveness and acceptability of deep brain stimulation (DBS) of the subgenual cingulate cortex for treatment-resistant depression: a systematic review and exploratory meta-analysis. J Affect Disord 159:31–38, 2014 24679386

Bond DJ, Lam RW, Yatham LN: Divalproex sodium versus placebo in the treatment of acute bipolar depression: a systematic review and meta-analysis. J Affect Disord 124(3):228–234, 2010 20044142

Brown ES, Gabrielson B: A randomized, double-blind, placebo-controlled trial of citicoline for bipolar and unipolar depression and methamphetamine dependence. J Affect Disord 143(1–3):257–260, 2012 22974472

Calabrese JR, Bowden CL, Sachs GS, et al: A double-blind placebo-controlled study of lamotrigine monotherapy in outpatients with bipolar I depression. Lamictal 602 Study Group. J Clin Psychiatry 60(2):79–88, 1999 10084633

Calabrese JR, Sullivan JR, Bowden CL, et al: Rash in multicenter trials of lamotrigine in mood disorders: clinical relevance and management. J Clin Psychiatry 63(11):1012–1019, 2002 12444815

Calabrese JR, Kasper S, Johnson G, et al: International Consensus Group on Bipolar I Depression Treatment Guidelines. J Clin Psychiatry 65(4):571–579, 2004 15119923

Calabrese JR, Keck PE Jr, Macfadden W, et al: A randomized, double-blind, placebo-controlled trial of quetiapine in the treatment of bipolar I or II depression. Am J Psychiatry 162(7):1351–1360, 2005 15994719

Calabrese JR, Huffman RF, White RL, et al: Lamotrigine in the acute treatment of bipolar depression: results of five double-blind, placebo-controlled clinical trials. Bipolar Disord 10(2):323–333, 2008 18271912

Cohn JB, Collins G, Ashbrook E, et al: A comparison of fluoxetine imipramine and placebo in patients with bipolar depressive disorder. Int Clin Psychopharmacol 4(4):313–322, 1989 2607128

Colom F, Vieta E, Scott J: Psychoeducation Manual for Bipolar Disorder. New York, Cambridge University Press, 2006

Deckersbach T, Peters AT, Sylvia L, et al: Do comorbid anxiety disorders moderate the effects of psychotherapy for bipolar disorder? Results from STEP-BD. Am J Psychiatry 171(2):178–186, 2014 24077657

De Fruyt J, Deschepper E, Audenaert K, et al: Second generation antipsychotics in the treatment of bipolar depression: a systematic review and meta-analysis. J Psychopharmacol 26(5):603–617, 2012 21940761

De Luca MT, Meringolo M, Spagnolo PA, et al: The role of setting for ketamine abuse: clinical and preclinical evidence. Rev Neurosci 23(5–6):769–780, 2012 23159868

Diazgranados N, Ibrahim L, Brutsche NE, et al: A randomized add-on trial of an N-methyl-D-aspartate antagonist in treatment-resistant bipolar depression. Arch Gen Psychiatry 67(8):793–802, 2010 20679587

Dunner DL, Rush AJ, Russell JM, et al: Prospective, long-term, multicenter study of the naturalistic outcomes of patients with treatment-resistant depression. J Clin Psychiatry 67(5):688–695, 2006 16841617

Frangou S, Lewis M, McCrone P: Efficacy of ethyl-eicosapentaenoic acid in bipolar depression: randomised double-blind placebo-controlled study. Br J Psychiatry 188:46–50, 2006 16388069

Frangou S, Lewis M, Wollard J, et al: Preliminary in vivo evidence of increased N-acetyl-aspartate following eicosapentanoic acid treatment in patients with bipolar disorder. J Psychopharmacol 21(4):435–439, 2007 16891338

Frank E: Treating Bipolar Disorder: A Clinician's Guide to Interpersonal and Social Rhythm Therapy. New York, Guilford, 2005

Frank E, Kupfer DJ, Thase ME, et al: Two-year outcomes for interpersonal and social rhythm therapy in individuals with bipolar I disorder. Arch Gen Psychiatry 62(9):996–1004, 2005 16143731

Frye MA, Grunze H, Suppes T, et al: A placebo-controlled evaluation of adjunctive modafinil in the treatment of bipolar depression. Am J Psychiatry 164(8):1242–1249, 2007 17671288

Frye MA, Ketter TA, Yang R: Efficacy and safety of armodafinil as an adjunctive therapy for the treatment of major depression associated with bipolar I disorder. Paper presented at the 10th International Conference on Bipolar Disorder, Miami Beach, FL, June 13–16, 2013

Frye MA, Ketter T, Adler C, et al: Randomized, double-blind, placebo-controlled trial of adjunctive armodafinil (150 mg/day) in adults with bipolar I depression: safety and secondary efficacy findings. Paper presented at the 167th Annual Meeting of the American Psychiatric Association, New York, NY, May 3–7, 2014

Geddes JR, Miklowitz DJ: Treatment of bipolar disorder. Lancet 381(9878):1672–1682, 2013 23663953

Geddes JR, Calabrese JR, Goodwin GM: Lamotrigine for treatment of bipolar depression: independent meta-analysis and meta-regression of individual patient data from five randomised trials. Br J Psychiatry 194(1):4–9, 2009 19118318

Ghaemi SN, Hsu DJ, Soldani F, et al: Antidepressants in bipolar disorder: the case for caution. Bipolar Disord 5(6):421–433, 2003 14636365

Gijsman HJ, Geddes JR, Rendell JM, et al: Antidepressants for bipolar depression: a systematic review of randomized, controlled trials. Am J Psychiatry 161(9):1537–1547, 2004 15337640

Goldstein TR, Axelson DA, Birmaher B, et al: Dialectical behavior therapy for adolescents with bipolar disorder: a 1-year open trial. J Am Acad Child Adolesc Psychiatry 46(7):820–830, 2007 17581446

Goodwin GM; Consensus Group of the British Association for Psychopharmacology: Evidence-based guidelines for treating bipolar disorder: recommendations from the British Association for Psychopharmacology. J Psychopharmacol 17(2):149–173, discussion 147, 2003 12870562

Goodwin GM; Consensus Group of the British Association for Psychopharmacology: Evidence-based guidelines for treating bipolar disorder: revised second edition—recommendations from the British Association for Psychopharmacology. J Psychopharmacol 23(4):346–388, 2009 19329543

Goodwin GM, Bowden CL, Calabrese JR, et al: A pooled analysis of 2 placebo-controlled 18-month trials of lamotrigine and lithium maintenance in bipolar I disorder. J Clin Psychiatry 65(3):432–441, 2004 15096085

Gracious BL, Chirieac MC, Costescu S, et al: Randomized, placebo-controlled trial of flax oil in pediatric bipolar disorder. Bipolar Disord 12(2):142–154, 2010 20402707

Grunze H, Vieta E, Goodwin GM, et al; WFSBP Task Force On Treatment Guidelines For Bipolar Disorders: The World Federation of Societies of Biological Psychiatry (WFSBP) guidelines for the biological treatment of bipolar disorders: update 2010 on the treatment of acute bipolar depression. World J Biol Psychiatry 11(2):81–109, 2010 20148751

Haeberle A, Greil W, Russmann S, et al: Mono- and combination drug therapies in hospitalized patients with bipolar depression. Data from the European drug surveillance program AMSP. BMC Psychiatry 12:153, 2012 22998655

Hirschfeld RM: Guideline watch (November 2005): practice guideline for the treatment of patients with bipolar disorder, 2nd edition. Focus 5(1):34–39, 2007

Holtzheimer PE, Kelley ME, Gross RE, et al: Subcallosal cingulate deep brain stimulation for treatment-resistant unipolar and bipolar depression. Arch Gen Psychiatry 69(2):150–158, 2012 22213770

Hooshmand F, Miller S, Dore J, et al: Trends in pharmacotherapy in patients referred to a bipolar specialty clinic, 2000–2011. J Affect Disord 155:283–287, 2014 24314912

Kasper S, Calabrese JR, Johnson G, et al: International Consensus Group on the evidence-based pharmacologic treatment of bipolar I and II depression. J Clin Psychiatry 69(10):1632–1646, 2008 19192447

Keck PE, Perlis RH, Otto MW, et al: The expert consensus guideline series: medication treatment of bipolar disorder 2004. Postgrad Med Special Report 1–120, 2004

Keck PE Jr, Mintz J, McElroy SL, et al: Double-blind, randomized, placebo-controlled trials of ethyl-eicosapentanoate in the treatment of bipolar depression and rapid cycling bipolar disorder. Biol Psychiatry 60(9):1020–1022, 2006 16814257

Kennedy SH, Giacobbe P, Rizvi SJ, et al: Deep brain stimulation for treatment-resistant depression: follow-up after 3 to 6 years. Am J Psychiatry 168(5):502–510, 2011 21285143

Ketter TA: Handbook of Diagnosis and Treatment of Bipolar Disorders. Washington, DC, American Psychiatric Publishing, 2010

Ketter TA, Citrome L, Wang PW, et al: Treatments for bipolar disorder: can number needed to treat/harm help inform clinical decisions? Acta Psychiatr Scand 123(3):175–189, 2011 21133854

Ketter TA, Calabrese JR, Yang R, et al: A double-blind, placebo-controlled, multicenter trial of adjunctive armodafinil for the treatment of major depression associated with bipolar I disorder. Paper presented at the 10th International Conference on Bipolar Disorder, Miami Beach, FL, June 13–16, 2013

Lam DH, Jones SH, Hayward P: Cognitive Therapy for Bipolar Disorder: A Therapist's Guide to Concepts, Methods, and Practice, 2nd Edition. Chichester, UK, Wiley-Blackwell, 2010

Laupacis A, Sackett DL, Roberts RS: An assessment of clinically useful measures of the consequences of treatment. N Engl J Med 318(26):1728–1733, 1988 3374545

Loebel A, Cucchiaro J, Silva R, et al: Lurasidone as adjunctive therapy with lithium or valproate for the treatment of bipolar I depression: a randomized, double-blind, placebo-controlled study. Am J Psychiatry 171(2):169–177, 2014a 24170221

Loebel A, Cucchiaro J, Silva R, et al: Lurasidone monotherapy in the treatment of bipolar I depression: a randomized, double-blind, placebo-controlled study. Am J Psychiatry 171(2):160–168, 2014b 24170180

Lombardo I, Sachs G, Kolluri S, et al: Two 6-week, randomized, double-blind, placebo-controlled studies of ziprasidone in outpatients with bipolar I depression: did baseline characteristics impact trial outcome? J Clin Psychopharmacol 32(4):470–478, 2012 22722504

Lozano AM, Giacobbe P, Hamani C, et al: A multicenter pilot study of subcallosal cingulate area deep brain stimulation for treatment-resistant depression. J Neurosurg 116(2):315–322, 2012 22098195

Malhi GS, Adams D, Lampe L, et al; Northern Sydney Central Coast Mental Health Drug and Alcohol; NSW Health Clinical Redesign Program; CADE Clinic, University of Sydney: Clinical practice recommendations for bipolar disorder. Acta Psychiatr Scand Suppl (439):27–46, 2009 19356155

McElroy SL, Winstanley EL, Martens B, et al: A randomized, placebo-controlled study of adjunctive ramelteon in ambulatory bipolar I disorder with manic symptoms and sleep disturbance. Int Clin Psychopharmacol 26(1):48–53, 2011 20861739

Meltzer HY, Alphs L, Green AI, et al; International Suicide Prevention Trial Study Group: Clozapine treatment for suicidality in schizophrenia: International Suicide Prevention Trial (InterSePT). Arch Gen Psychiatry 60(1):82–91, 2003 12511175

Miklowitz DJ: Bipolar Disorder: A Family Focused Treatment Approach, 2nd Edition. New York, Guilford, 2010

Miklowitz DJ, Otto MW, Frank E, et al: Intensive psychosocial intervention enhances functioning in patients with bipolar depression: results from a 9-month randomized controlled trial. Am J Psychiatry 164(9):1340–1347, 2007 17728418

Moore JW, Cambridge VC, Morgan H, et al: Time, action and psychosis: using subjective time to investigate the effects of ketamine on sense of agency. Neuropsychologia 51(2):377–384, 2013 22813429

Murrough JW, Iosifescu DV, Chang LC, et al: Antidepressant efficacy of ketamine in treatment-resistant major depression: a two-site randomized controlled trial. Am J Psychiatry 170(10):1134–1142, 2013 23982301

National Institute for Health and Clinical Excellence: Bipolar Disorder: The Management of Bipolar Disorder in Adults, Children and Adolescents, in Primary and Secondary Care. National Clinical Practice Guideline Number 38. London, The British Psychological Society and Gaskell, 2006

Nemeroff CB, Evans DL, Gyulai L, et al: Double-blind, placebo-controlled comparison of imipramine and paroxetine in the treatment of bipolar depression. Am J Psychiatry 158(6):906–912, 2001 11384898

Norris ER, Karen Burke, Correll JR, et al: A double-blind, randomized, placebo-controlled trial of adjunctive ramelteon for the treatment of insomnia and mood stability in patients with euthymic bipolar disorder. J Affect Disord 144(1–2):141–147, 2013 22963894

Ostacher MJ, Perlis RH, Nierenberg AA, et al; STEP-BD Investigators: Impact of substance use disorders on recovery from episodes of depression in bipolar disorder patients: prospective data from the Systematic Treatment Enhancement Program for Bipolar Disorder (STEP-BD). Am J Psychiatry 167(3):289–297, 2010 20008948

Pacchiarotti I, Bond DJ, Baldessarini RJ, et al: The International Society for Bipolar Disorders (ISBD) task force report on antidepressant use in bipolar disorders. Am J Psychiatry 170(11):1249–1262, 2013 24030475

Patkar A, Gilmer W, Pae CU, et al: A 6 week randomized double-blind placebo-controlled trial of ziprasidone for the acute depressive mixed state. PloS One 7(4): e34757, 2012

Physicians' Desk Reference 2015, 69th Edition. Montvale, NJ, PDR Network, 2014

Puigdemont D, Pérez-Egea R, Portella MJ, et al: Deep brain stimulation of the subcallosal cingulate gyrus: further evidence in treatment-resistant major depression. Int J Neuropsychopharmacol 15(1):121–133, 2012 21777510

Rakofsky JJ, Dunlop BW: Review of nutritional supplements for the treatment of bipolar depression. Depress Anxiety 31(5):379–390, 2014 24353094

Ramirez Basco M, Rush A: Cognitive-Behavioral Therapy for Bipolar Disorders, 2nd Edition. New York, Guilford, 2005

Rush AJ: Ketamine for treatment-resistant depression: ready or not for clinical use? Am J Psychiatry 170(10):1079–1081, 2013 23982324

Sachs GS, Nierenberg AA, Calabrese JR, et al: Effectiveness of adjunctive antidepressant treatment for bipolar depression. N Engl J Med 356(17):1711–1722, 2007 17392295

Sachs GS, Ice KS, Chappell PB, et al: Efficacy and safety of adjunctive oral ziprasidone for acute treatment of depression in patients with bipolar I disorder: a randomized, double-blind, placebo-controlled trial. J Clin Psychiatry 72(10):1413–1422, 2011 21672493

Sarris J, Mischoulon D, Schweitzer I: Omega-3 for bipolar disorder: meta-analyses of use in mania and bipolar depression. J Clin Psychiatry 73(1):81–86, 2012 21903025

Schatzberg AF: A word to the wise about ketamine. Am J Psychiatry 171(3):262–264, 2014 24585328

Schlaepfer TE, Bewernick BH: Deep brain stimulation for major depression. Handb Clin Neurol 116:235–243, 2013 24112897

Scott J, Paykel E, Morriss R, et al: Cognitive-behavioural therapy for severe and recurrent bipolar disorders: randomised controlled trial. Br J Psychiatry 188:313–320, 2006 16582056

Shelton RC, Stahl SM: Risperidone and paroxetine given singly and in combination for bipolar depression. J Clin Psychiatry 65(12):1715–1719, 2004 15641878

Sidor MM, Macqueen GM: Antidepressants for the acute treatment of bipolar depression: a systematic review and meta-analysis. J Clin Psychiatry 72(2):156–167, 2011 21034686

Smith LA, Cornelius VR, Azorin JM, et al: Valproate for the treatment of acute bipolar depression: systematic review and meta-analysis. J Affect Disord 122(1–2):1–9, 2010 19926140

Stamm TJ, Lewitzka U, Sauer C, et al: Supraphysiologic doses of levothyroxine as adjunctive therapy in bipolar depression: a randomized, double-blind, placebo-controlled study. J Clin Psychiatry 75(2):162–168, 2014 24345793

Stang A, Poole C, Bender R: Common problems related to the use of number needed to treat. J Clin Epidemiol 63(8):820–825, 2010 19880287

Stoll AL, Severus WE, Freeman MP, et al: Omega 3 fatty acids in bipolar disorder: a preliminary double-blind, placebo-controlled trial. Arch Gen Psychiatry 56(5):407–412, 1999 10232294

Straus SE: Individualizing treatment decisions. The likelihood of being helped or harmed. Eval Health Prof 25(2):210–224, 2002 12026754

Suppes T, Dennehy EB, Hirschfeld RM, et al; Texas Consensus Conference Panel on Medication Treatment of Bipolar Disorder: The Texas implementation of medication algorithms: update to the algorithms for treatment of bipolar I disorder. J Clin Psychiatry 66(7):870–886, 2005 16013903

Thase ME, Macfadden W, Weisler RH, et al; BOLDER II Study Group: Efficacy of quetiapine monotherapy in bipolar I and II depression: a double-blind, placebo-controlled study (the BOLDER II study). J Clin Psychopharmacol 26(6):600–609, 2006 17110817

Thase ME, Jonas A, Khan A, et al: Aripiprazole monotherapy in nonpsychotic bipolar I depression: results of 2 randomized, placebo-controlled studies. J Clin Psychopharmacol 28(1):13–20, 2008 18204335

Tohen M, Vieta E, Calabrese J, et al: Efficacy of olanzapine and olanzapine-fluoxetine combination in the treatment of bipolar I depression. Arch Gen Psychiatry 60(11):1079–1088, 2003 14609883

Tohen M, McDonnell DP, Case M, et al: Randomised, double-blind, placebo-controlled study of olanzapine in patients with bipolar I depression. Br J Psychiatry 201(5):376–382, 2012 22918966

Torres CV, Ezquiaga E, Navas M, et al: Deep brain stimulation of the subcallosal cingulate for medication-resistant type I bipolar depression: case report. Bipolar Disord 15(6):719–721, 2013 23930934

Van Dijk S, Jeffrey J, Katz MR: A randomized, controlled, pilot study of dialectical behavior therapy skills in a psychoeducational group for individuals with bipolar disorder. J Affect Disord 145(3):386–393, 2013 22858264

Weber B, Jermann F, Gex-Fabry M, et al: Mindfulness-based cognitive therapy for bipolar disorder: a feasibility trial. Eur Psychiatry 25(6):334–337, 2010 20561769

Williams JM, Alatiq Y, Crane C, et al: Mindfulness-based cognitive therapy (MBCT) in bipolar disorder: preliminary evaluation of immediate effects on between-episode functioning. J Affect Disord 107(1–3):275–279, 2008 17884176

Yatham LN, Kennedy SH, Parikh SV, et al: Canadian Network for Mood and Anxiety Treatments (CANMAT) and International Society for Bipolar Disorders (ISBD) collaborative update of CANMAT guidelines for the management of patients with bipolar disorder: update 2013. Bipolar Disord 15(1):1–44, 2013 23237061

Young AH, McElroy SL, Bauer M, et al: A double-blind, placebo-controlled study of quetiapine and lithium monotherapy in adults in the acute phase of bipolar depression (EMBOLDEN I). J Clin Psychiatry 71(2):150–162, 2010 20122369

Zarate CA Jr, Brutsche NE, Ibrahim L, et al: Replication of ketamine's antidepressant efficacy in bipolar depression: a randomized controlled add-on trial. Biol Psychiatry 71(11):939–946, 2012 22297150

3 Treatment of Acute Manic and Mixed Episodes

Terence A. Ketter, M.D.
Shefali Miller, M.D.

Manic episodes continue to constitute substantial diagnostic and therapeutic challenges, particularly when there is a mixture of not only mood elevation symptoms but also depressive symptoms. As discussed in Chapter 1, "Diagnosis and Treatment of Bipolar Disorder," arguably one of the most important recent diagnostic advances in bipolar disorder was the publication of DSM-5 in 2013 (American Psychiatric Association 2013), which superseded DSM-IV-TR (American Psychiatric Association 2000), adding a "with mixed features" specifier for manic, hypomanic (or depressive) episodes. Moreover, DSM-5 stipulates that concurrent syndromal manic and major depressive symptoms be considered as a manic episode with mixed features. Thus, DSM-IV-TR mixed episodes have been eliminated in favor of manic episodes with mixed features in DSM-5.

This DSM-5 innovation entails a considerably more inclusive approach to mixed symptom phenomenology compared with the relatively exclusive or restricted approach of DSM-IV-TR, which only had full mixed episodes (syndromal manic episode concurrent with syndromal major depressive episode). Thus, DSM-5 includes the following patterns of mixed symptoms not included in DSM-IV-TR: 1) syndromal manic episode with subsyndromal depressive symptoms (as manic episode with mixed features); 2) syndromal hypomanic episode with syndromal or subsyndromal depressive symptoms (as hypomanic episode with mixed features); and 3) syndromal major depressive episode with subsyndromal mood elevation symptoms (as major depressive episode with mixed features).

The DSM-5 broadening of the options for classifying mood elevation episodes with varying degrees of depressive symptoms has facilitated diagnosis but has raised therapeutic challenges because the preexisting therapeutic evidence base most often addressed the DSM-IV-TR constructs of manic episodes and mixed episodes, rather than manic episodes with subsyndromal depressive symptoms or hypomanic episodes with syndromal or subsyndromal depressive symptoms. Accordingly, the old DSM-IV-TR terminology of manic and mixed episodes is used in this chapter.

Since the 2010 publication of *Handbook of Diagnosis and Treatment of Bipolar Disorders* (Ketter 2010), there have been important developments regarding the treatment of acute (DSM-IV-TR) manic and mixed episodes. These developments include approval by the U.S. Food and Drug Administration (FDA) of asenapine monotherapy (McIntyre et al. 2009, 2010) and adjunctive (added to lithium or valproate) therapy (Szegedi et al. 2012) for acute manic and mixed episodes, as well as the completion of multicenter, randomized, double-blind, placebo-controlled trials assessing the utility of cariprazine monotherapy (Calabrese et al. 2014; Starace et al. 2012), ziprasidone adjunctive (added to lithium or valproate) therapy (Sachs et al. 2012a, 2012b), paliperidone monotherapy (Berwaerts et al. 2012; Vieta et al. 2010a), and paliperidone adjunctive (added to lithium or valproate) therapy (Berwaerts et al. 2011) for acute manic and mixed episodes. In addition, in 2012, the FDA approved inhaled loxapine for acute agitation associated with bipolar I disorder (and schizophrenia) (Kwentus et al. 2012). Table 3–1 summarizes the current evidence base for the treatment of acute manic and mixed episodes and agitation associated with bipolar disorder.

The FDA-approved treatments are generally supported by at least two multicenter, randomized, double-blind, placebo-controlled clinical trials. In most instances, these are 3-week inpatient studies of patients with very limited psychiatric and medical comorbidities. In these trials, in aggregate, the agents with FDA indications for the monotherapy treatment of acute mania yielded rates of response (at least 50% improvement in mania ratings) of approximately 50%, as compared with approximately 30% with placebo, thus representing a 20% increase in response rate (Figure 3–1, left). Patients receiving either active treatment or placebo also received additional substantial psychosocial/behavioral interventions (acute psychiatric hospitalization) and more modest pharmacotherapy (as-needed benzodiazepine for approximately 1 week), accounting for a portion of both the active drug and placebo responses. Similarly, in aggregate, response rates for two-drug combination therapy (with olanzapine, risperidone, quetiapine, aripiprazole, or asenapine added to lithium or valproate) exceeded those of monotherapy (with lithium or valproate) by approximately 18% (Figure 3–1, right).

TABLE 3–1. Evidence-based treatments for acute (DSM-IV-TR) manic and mixed episodes and agitation associated with bipolar disorder

	Manic episodes	Mixed episodes	With or without psychotic features	Agitation associated with bipolar I disorder
Mood stabilizers				
Lithium	1970	–	+	
Divalproex	1994		+	
Divalproex ER	2005	2005	2005	
Carbamazepine ERC	2004	2004		
First-generation antipsychotics				
Chlorpromazine	1973			
Haloperidol	+	+	+	
Loxapine (inhaled)				2012
Second-generation antipsychotics				
Olanzapine	2000, 2003*	2000, 2003*	+	2004
Risperidone	2003, 2003*	2003, 2003*	+	
Quetiapine	2004*		+	
Quetiapine XR	2008*	2008*	+	
Ziprasidone	2004	2004	2004	(2000 schizophrenia, not bipolar)
Aripiprazole	2004*	2004*	2004*	2006
Asenapine	2009, 2010*	2009, 2010*	2009, 2010*	
Cariprazine	+	+	+	

Note. **Boldface** indicates U.S. Food and Drug Administration (FDA)-approved treatments. Dates signify year of initial approval in the United States. +=effective, –=not effective in multicenter, randomized, double-blind, placebo-controlled trials; ER=extended-release formulation; ERC=extended-release capsule formulation; XR=extended-release formulation. *Added to lithium or valproate increases antimanic efficacy.

Source. Adapted from Ketter 2010. Copyright 2010, American Psychiatric Publishing. Used with permission.

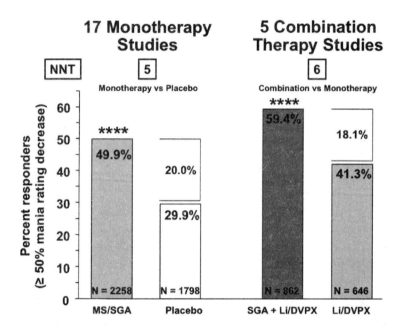

FIGURE 3–1.   Overview of 22 acute mania studies, with pooled response rates and numbers needed to treat for response.

Note.   On average, monotherapy yielded a 20% increase in pooled response rate compared with placebo (approximately 50% vs. 30%). Active drug and placebo rates are in part related to both groups also having acute hospitalization and a few days of rescue benzodiazepine. Monotherapy compared with placebo had an NNT for response of 5 (i.e., 100/20.0=5). Combination therapy yielded an approximately 18% increase in pooled response rate compared with monotherapy (approximately 59% vs. 41%) and an NNT for response of 6 (i.e., 100/ 18.1=5.5→6, rounded up). DVPX=divalproex; Li=lithium; MS=mood stabilizer (lithium, divalproex, or carbamazepine extended-release capsule formulation); NNT = number needed to treat; SGA=second-generation antipsychotic (olanzapine, risperidone, quetiapine, aripiprazole, ziprasidone [monotherapy only], or asenapine).

[****]$P<0.0001$ versus placebo or Li/DVPX monotherapy.

Source.   Data are pooled from 17 monotherapy studies (listed in legend to Figure 3–2) and five combination therapy (SGA plus lithium/divalproex) studies (Sachs et al. 2002; Szegedi et al. 2012; Tohen et al. 2002; Vieta et al. 2008; Yatham et al. 2004).

■ Treatment of Acute Mania: Balancing the Likelihood of Benefit and Harm

Clinicians and patients are faced with diverse options for the treatment of acute manic and mixed episodes (Table 3–1). It is crucial to determine, in making treatment decisions, which choice optimizes the benefit:harm risk ratio for the individual patient. This assessment can be quantitative and based on the results of controlled clinical trials, which can be interpreted in terms of metrics called the *number needed to treat* (NNT), the *number needed to harm* (NNH), and the *likelihood to help or harm* (LHH). Please refer to Chapter 2, "Treatment of Acute Bipolar Depression," for more detailed descriptions of NNT, NNH, and LHH definitions and calculations.

In brief, the NNT for response (which in this chapter is a ≥50% decrease in mania severity) for two treatments is defined as the reciprocal of the difference in the response rates (RRs) of two treatments—that is, $NNT = 1/(RR_{treatment\ 1} - RR_{treatment\ 2})$. The NNT for response represents the number of patients a provider expects to treat to obtain one additional response with one treatment compared with another. Thus, for monotherapy of acute mania with an FDA-approved agent, NNT = 100%/(49.9%−29.9%)=100%/20.0%=5. Similarly, for FDA-approved two-drug combination therapy (i.e., olanzapine, quetiapine, risperidone, aripiprazole, or asenapine combined with lithium or divalproex) compared with monotherapy with lithium or divalproex, NNT=100%/(59.4%−41.3%)=100%/18.1%=5.5→6(rounded up). Hence, clinicians can expect to obtain one additional response for every five patients treated with monotherapy with an approved agent compared with no approved agent (Figure 3–1, left), as well as one additional response for every six patients treated with an approved two-drug combination compared with lithium or valproate monotherapy (Figure 3–1, right). NNTs, NNHs, LHHs, and selected side-effect rates for selected acute mania monotherapy treatments (some with and some without FDA approval) are provided in Table 3–2.

Comparisons suggest that monotherapy response rates and NNTs are more similar than different across individual approved agents, and across mood stabilizers compared with second-generation antipsychotics (SGAs) (Figure 3–2, Table 3–2). However, there are substantive differences in tolerability profiles and NNHs of approved agents (Figure 3–2, Table 3–2). Noteworthy adverse-effect and NNH differences be-

TABLE 3–2.   Numbers needed to treat, numbers needed to harm, likelihood to help or harm, and selected harm (side-effect) rates for selected acute mania monotherapy treatments

Medication	NNT	NNH	LHH	Harm	BMH (%)
Mood stabilizers					
Lithium[1,2]	3.9	12.1	3.1	Vomiting[a]	11.2
Divalproex ER[1,3]	6.1	6.6	1.1	Somnolence[b]	29.5
Carbamazepine ERC[4–6]	3.9	3.2	0.8	Dizziness[c]	43.5
Second-generation antipsychotics					
Olanzapine[7,8]	4.4	4.5	1.0	Somnolence[d]	35.2
Risperidone[9–11]	4.1	6.2	1.5	EPS[e]	22.6
Quetiapine[12–14]	4.9	5.5	1.1	Som/Sed[f]	23.9
Ziprasidone[15,16]	6.3	5.0	0.8	Somnolence[g]	29.7
Aripiprazole[17,18]	4.7	8.1	1.7	Somnolence[h]	20.2
Asenapine[19,20]	7.7	5.1	0.7	Sedation[i]	28.1
Cariprazine[21,22,u]	5.2	6.1	1.2	Akathisia[j]	20.5
First-generation antipsychotics					
Haloperidol[23–25,u]	4.3	3.3	0.8	EPS[k]	40.8

Note. **Boldface** indicates drug names for U.S. Food and Drug Administration (FDA)–approved acute mania treatments. BMH=blind medication harm rate; ER=extended-release formulation; ERC=extended-release capsule formulation; LHH (NNH/NNT)=likelihood to help or harm compared with placebo; NNH = number needed to harm (for clinically relevant side effect with lowest NNH compared with placebo); NNT=number needed to treat (for antimanic response compared with placebo). NNTs, NNHs, and LHHs are rounded up to the next higher first decimal place (in contrast to being rounded up to the next higher integer in the text and figures).
[a]Somnolence with lithium: NNH=26.6, LHH=6.8, BMH=11.9%; ≥7% weight gain with lithium (in patients with baseline body mass index <25) (Bowden et al. 2005): NNT=3.9, NNH=13.0, LHH=3.3, BMH=16.9%.
[b]≥7% weight gain with divalproex ER (Bowden et al. 2006): NNT=7.1, NNH=16.7, LHH=2.3, BMH=9.0%.
[c]Somnolence with carbamazepine: NNH=5.4, LHH=1.4, BMH=31.4%; ≥7% weight gain with carbamazepine: NNH=23.0, LHH=7.4, BMH=5.3%.
[d]≥7% weight gain with olanzapine not reported in olanzapine registration studies, but reported by McIntyre et al. (2009, 2010): NNT=4.2, NNH=6.5, LHH=1.5, BMH = 16.1%.

TABLE 3–2. **Numbers needed to treat, numbers needed to harm, likelihood to help or harm, and selected harm (side-effect) rates for selected acute mania monotherapy treatments** *(continued)*

---

[e]EPS indicates extrapyramidal disorder (Smulevich et al. 2005; Khanna et al. 2005)/hyperkinesia (Hirschfeld et al. 2004); somnolence with risperidone (Hirschfeld et al. 2004; Smulevich et al. 2005): NNT=5.8, NNH=8.7, LHH=1.5, BMH=15.6%; ≥7% weight gain with risperidone: not reported.

[f]Som/Sed indicates somnolence (Bowden et al. 2005; McIntyre et al. 2005) or sedation (Cutler et al. 2011); ≥7% weight gain with quetiapine: NNH=8.3, LHH=1.7, BMH=15.7%.

[g]≥7% weight gain with ziprasidone (Potkin et al. 2005): NNT=5.9, NNH=70.9, LHH=12.1, BMH=4.8%; akathisia with ziprasidone: NNH=20.5, LHH=3.2, BMH=10.0%.

[h]≥7% weight gain with aripiprazole: NNH=−127.8, LHH=−26.9, BMH=1.1%; akathisia with aripiprazole: NNH=9.1, LHH=1.9, BMH=14.4%; nausea with aripiprazole: NNH=11.1, LHH=2.3, BMH=22.1%.

[i]Somnolence with asenapine: NNH=6.3, LHH=0.8, BMH=21.1%; ≥7% weight gain with asenapine: NNH=16.6, LHH=2.2, BMH=6.6%.

[j]Somnolence with cariprazine: NNH=49.4, LHH=9.5, BMH=4.2%; ≥7% weight gain with cariprazine: NNH=−943.6, LHH=−181.5, BMH=1.8%.

[k]EPS indicates extrapyramidal symptom–related (McIntyre et al. 2005)/extrapyramidal disorder (Smulevich et al. 2005)/extrapyramidal symptoms (Vieta et al. 2010a); tremor with haloperidol: NNH=11.1; LHH=2.6; BMH=13.3%; somnolence with haloperidol: NNH=15.1, LHH=3.5, BMH=9.7%; ≥7% weight gain with haloperidol (McIntyre et al. 2005; Vieta et al. 2010a): NNT=4.3, NNH=49.9, LHH=11.5, BMH=5.4% (McIntyre et al. 2005).

[u]Interventions lacking FDA approval for acute mania.

Source. Data from [1]Bowden et al. 1994 [2]Bowden et al. 2005; [3]Bowden et al. 2006; [4]Weisler et al. 2004a; [5]Weisler et al. 2005; [6]Weisler et al. 2006; [7]Tohen et al. 1999; [8]Tohen et al. 2000; [9]Hirschfeld et al. 2004; [10]Khanna et al. 2005; [11]Smulevich et al. 2005; [12]Bowden et al. 2005; [13]McIntyre et al. 2005; [14]Cutler et al. 2011; [15]Keck et al. 2003b; [16]Potkin et al. 2005; [17]Keck et al. 2003a; [18]Sachs et al. 2006; [19]McIntyre et al. 2009; [20]McIntyre et al. 2010; [21]Calabrese et al. 2014; [22]Ketter et al. 2014; [23]McIntyre et al. 2005; [24]Smulevich et al. 2005; [25]Vieta et al. 2010a.

---

tween individual agents are described in Figure 3–2 and Table 3–2, as well as in this chapter and in other chapters in this volume.

In addition to the above-mentioned data regarding mood stabilizers and SGAs, there have been multiple controlled trials of anticonvulsants in acute mania. However, as discussed in relevant sections later in this chapter, to date only divalproex, carbamazepine, and possibly oxcarbazepine appear effective.

NNTs for response for individual agents ranged from 4 to 8, related to differences in response rates for active drugs and placebo across studies. Pooled analysis of mood stabilizer monotherapies compared with placebo yielded response rates of approximately 50% and 28%, respectively,

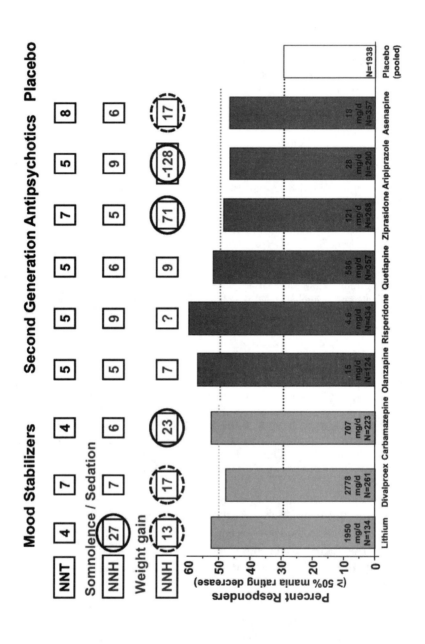

FIGURE 3–2. Overview of acute mania monotherapy registration and related studies, with numbers needed to treat for response, numbers needed to harm for somnolence/sedation and weight gain, and response rates.

Note. Solid and dashed circles indicate NNHs with low and moderate sedation/somnolence/weight gain risks, respectively. ? indicates data not reported. NNTs for response for individual agents ranged from 4 to 8, related to differences in response rates for active drugs and placebo across studies. Pooled analysis of mood stabilizer monotherapies compared with placebo yielded response rates of approximately 50% and 28%, respectively, and a pooled NNT for response of 5 (100/22.3=4.5→5, rounded up). Pooled analysis of second-generation antipsychotics (SGAs) compared with placebo yielded response rates of approximately 51% and 35%, respectively, and a pooled NNT for response of 7 (100/16.3 = 6.1→7, rounded up). Thus, a somewhat higher pooled placebo response rate in studies of SGAs (as opposed to mood stabilizers) yielded a somewhat higher pooled NNT for response for active drugs.

Aside from lithium (which more often yields vomiting than somnolence; see Table 3–2), NNHs for somnolence/sedation were comparable to NNTs for response, reflecting the sedative actions of approved treatments when dosed aggressively as in acute mania (Table 3–2). Carbamazepine, ziprasidone, and aripiprazole appeared to less often yield problems with weight gain compared with other agents, although these medications have different side effects that can substantively limit their utility, such as dizziness with carbamazepine (Table 3–2), akathisia with ziprasidone (Table 3–2 legend footnote *g*), and akathisia and nausea with aripiprazole (Table 3–2 legend footnote *h*). Context of effects is crucial—for example, somnolence/sedation for extremely agitated patients early in the inpatient treatment of acute mania may not yield prohibitive problems but may become increasingly unacceptable as mania resolves and discharge approaches. NNT=number needed to treat; NNH=number needed to harm.

Source. Data are pooled from controlled trials of the mood stabilizers lithium (Bowden et al. 1994, 2005), divalproex (Bowden et al. 1994, 2006), and carbamazepine (Weisler et al. 2004a, 2005); the second-generation antipsychotics olanzapine (Tohen et al. 1999, 2000), risperidone (Hirschfeld et al. 2004; Khanna et al. 2005; Smulevich et al. 2005), quetiapine (Bowden et al. 2005; Cutler et al. 2011; McIntyre et al. 2005), ziprasidone (Keck et al. 2003b; Potkin et al. 2005), aripiprazole (Keck et al. 2003a; Sachs et al. 2006), and asenapine (McIntyre et al. 2009, 2010); and placebo (Bowden et al. 1994, 2005, 2006; Cutler et al. 2011; Hirschfeld et al. 2004; Keck et al. 2003a, 2003b; Khanna et al. 2005; McIntyre et al. 2005, 2009, 2010; Potkin et al. 2005; Sachs et al. 2006; Tohen et al. 1999, 2000; Weisler et al. 2004a, 2005).

and a pooled NNT for response of 5 ($100/22.3=4.5\rightarrow5$, rounded up). A pooled analysis of SGAs compared with placebo yielded response rates of approximately 51% and 35%, respectively, and a pooled NNT for response of 7 ($100/16.3=6.1\rightarrow7$, rounded up). Thus, a somewhat higher pooled placebo response rate in studies of SGAs (as opposed to mood stabilizers) yielded a somewhat higher pooled NNT for response for SGAs, in spite of similar response rates for active drugs.

Aside from lithium (which more often yields vomiting than somnolence; Table 3–2), NNHs for somnolence/sedation were comparable to NNTs for response, reflecting the sedative actions of approved treatments when dosed aggressively as in acute mania (Table 3–2). Compared with other agents, carbamazepine, ziprasidone, and aripiprazole appeared to yield problems with weight gain less often, although these medications have different side effects that can substantively limit their utility, such as dizziness with carbamazepine (Table 3–2), akathisia with ziprasidone (Table 3–2, legend footnote g), and akathisia and nausea with aripiprazole (Table 3–2, legend footnote h). Context of effects is crucial—for example, somnolence/sedation for extremely agitated patients early in the inpatient treatment of acute mania may not yield prohibitive problems but may become increasingly unacceptable as mania resolves and discharge approaches.

Treatment selection in evidence-based medicine requires not only considering controlled and observational data regarding treatment efficacy/effectiveness and safety/tolerability, but also integrating individual patient characteristics. Efficacy may be particularly crucial in patients with severe, urgent, or treatment-resistant illness (commonly encountered during acute mania). High-priority acute mania treatments include those with the best matches to current episode characteristics (e.g., mixed or psychotic features), illness polarity predominance, episode sequence (e.g., mania then depression then well interval vs. depression then mania then well interval vs. continuous cycling), illness course (e.g., rapid cycling), and other illness characteristics predicting treatment responses (e.g., "classical" bipolar I disorder without mood-incongruent delusions and without comorbidity, which predicts potential lithium response), taking into account psychiatric and medical comorbidities. High-priority acute mania treatments include those with current acute or prior acute/preventive antimanic efficacy, taking into account psychiatric comorbidity and integrating first-degree relative efficacy information. High-priority preventive treatments also include those with adequate current and prior acute/preventive safety/tolerability and those best matching other characteristics predicting safety/tolerability (e.g., avoiding use of carbamazepine in Asians with the human leukocyte antigen [HLA] allele HLA-

B*1502, which is a biomarker for risk of serious rash), taking into account medical comorbidity and integrating first-degree relative safety/tolerability data. Finally, integrating preferences of patients and significant others is crucial, because these can impact positive and negative placebo responses as well as adherence.

In this chapter, we review the treatment of acute mania, emphasizing findings of controlled studies. Such work is helping to refine knowledge regarding lithium, divalproex, and carbamazepine; to appreciate the utility of SGAs; and to understand the limitations of newer anticonvulsants in acute mania. Thus, in addition to the mood stabilizers lithium, divalproex, and carbamazepine, we consider two main categories of potential treatment options for acute mania: SGAs and newer anticonvulsants. SGAs generally appear effective for acute mania (Table 3–3). In contrast, newer anticonvulsants appear to have diverse psychotropic profiles, and although they (with the possible exception of oxcarbazepine) are not effective for acute mania (Table 3–3; see also Table 3–4 in the later subsection "Other Anticonvulsants"), they may have utility for other aspects of bipolar disorders or comorbid conditions.

■ An Updated Five-Tier Approach to Acute Mania

Interventions for the treatment of acute mania are reviewed below, using the five-tier system presented in Table 3–3, which is an update of that published in *Handbook of Diagnosis and Treatment of Bipolar Disorders* (Ketter 2010). This system is a hybrid approach, combining evidence-based medical information regarding efficacy and safety/tolerability with more empirical constructs, such as familiarity and patient acceptability, to prioritize treatments in a fashion broadly consistent with American clinical practice and treatment guidelines.

Tier I treatment options, as of early 2015, had FDA approval for the treatment of acute mania and were supported by the most compelling evidence of efficacy. However, tolerability limitations (particularly in bipolar disorder preventive treatment) of at least some Tier I treatments may lead clinicians and patients, after comparing the risks and benefits, to consider other treatments.

The Tier II treatment option cariprazine, as of early 2015, lacked FDA approval for treatment of acute mania but had compelling evidence of efficacy and safety/tolerability that could make it, if ultimately approved, attractive for at least some patients with bipolar disorder.

TABLE 3–3. An updated five-tier approach to the management of acute mania

Tier	Priority	Name	Treatment Options

I	High	FDA approved	Mood stabilizers
			  Lithium, divalproex
			SGAs (monotherapy and adjunctive)
			  Olanzapine, risperidone, quetiapine, ziprasidone (monotherapy), aripiprazole, **asenapine**
			Other SGAs
			  Cariprazine (monotherapy)

II	High	Unapproved	

III	Intermediate	Other options	Other mood stabilizers
			  Carbamazepine
			First-generation antipsychotics
			  Chlorpromazine, thioridazine, thiothixene, pimozide, haloperidol, **loxapine (inhaled)**
			Other SGAs
			  Ziprasidone (adjunctive), paliperidone, clozapine
			Adjunctive benzodiazepines
			Electroconvulsive therapy

IV	Low	Novel adjuncts	Other mood stabilizers
			  Lamotrigine[a]
			Other anticonvulsants
			  Oxcarbazepine, gabapentin,[a] topiramate,[a] tiagabine,[b] levetiracetam,[b] zonisamide,[b] pregabalin,[b] rufinamide,[b] lacosamide,[b] vigabatrin,[b] ezogabine,[b] clobazam,[b] perampanel,[b,c] eslicarbazepine[b]
			Adjunctive psychotherapy

V	None[d]	Research treatment	**Tamoxifen**

Note. **Boldface** indicates treatments with important new developments. FDA=U.S. Food and Drug Administration; SGA=second-generation antipsychotic. [a]Ineffective in controlled acute mania trials, as of early 2015. [b]Not assessed in controlled acute mania trials, as of early 2015. [c]Boxed behavioral toxicity warning. [d]Not yet clinical options.

Source. Adapted from Ketter 2010. Copyright 2010, American Psychiatric Publishing. Used with permission.

Tier III treatment options, as of early 2015, lacked FDA approval for the treatment of acute mania and/or had substantive tolerability limitations and/or less compelling evidence of efficacy than Tier I or II options. In general, treatment guidelines have not considered these modalities to be first-line interventions but have cited them as intermediate-priority options. However, some Tier III options have mitigating advantages that might make them attractive for selected patients, and in certain circumstances, some of these interventions may be considered early on (e.g., electroconvulsive therapy [ECT] in pregnant women).

Tier IV treatment options, as of early 2015, lacked FDA approval for the treatment of acute mania and had even more limited evidence of efficacy than Tier I, II, or III options. Indeed, some of these interventions have been proved to be ineffective in acute mania but may have utility for comorbid conditions. In general, treatment guidelines consider these modalities to be low-priority interventions.

The new Tier V is reserved for innovative treatments that research suggests could have promise but that are thus far too novel and carry too substantive safety/tolerability risks to be considered clinical (as opposed to research) tools. Thus far, only tamoxifen has been included in this tier.

Tier I: FDA-Approved Acute Mania Treatments

As of early 2015, FDA-approved acute mania treatments included three mood stabilizers (lithium, divalproex, and carbamazepine), six SGAs (olanzapine, risperidone, quetiapine, ziprasidone, aripiprazole, and asenapine), and the first-generation antipsychotic (FGA) chlorpromazine. Recently, the FDA approved an inhaled formulation of the FGA loxapine for acute agitation associated with bipolar I disorder (and schizophrenia). A few of these FDA-approved acute mania treatments have been placed in Tier III rather than Tier I (i.e., carbamazepine due to drug interactions, and chlorpromazine and inhaled loxapine due to adverse effects). Since the publication of *Handbook of Diagnosis and Treatment of Bipolar Disorders* (Ketter 2010), asenapine (as monotherapy and added to lithium or valproate) has received FDA approval for the treatment of acute mania and has thus been promoted from Tier II to Tier I. Tier I options have favorable efficacy (single-digit NNTs; Figure 3–2), although some may also have safety/tolerability challenges. Thus, tolerability limitations of some Tier I treatments may lead clinicians and patients, after comparing the risks and benefits, to consider other treatments.

Mood Stabilizers

Mood stabilizers are considered foundational treatments for bipolar disorder, and three of these agents (lithium, divalproex, and carbamazepine) have FDA indications for the treatment of acute mania. The first-line acute mania treatment options, lithium and divalproex, are discussed in this section, and the alternative treatment carbamazepine is discussed in the later section on Tier III treatments. The other mood stabilizer, lamotrigine, is ineffective in acute mania, as discussed in the section on Tier IV treatments.

Lithium. Lithium, first reported to have efficacy in acute mania by John Cade in 1949, was widely used for the treatment of mania in Europe in the 1960s and received FDA approval for the monotherapy treatment of manic episodes of manic-depressive illness in 1970, based on placebo-controlled trials using randomized (Maggs 1963; Schou et al. 1954) and nonrandomized (Goodwin et al. 1969; Stokes et al. 1971) crossover designs. In addition, six early randomized acute mania trials compared lithium with the FGA chlorpromazine (Johnson et al. 1971; Platman 1970; Prien et al. 1972; Shopsin et al. 1975; Spring et al. 1970; Takahashi et al. 1975), the latter of which the FDA approved for acute mania monotherapy in 1973. Early studies generally reported comparable efficacy of lithium and FGAs in acute mania, with lithium having advantages later in treatment for achieving remission sufficient to permit discharge, but disadvantages earlier in treatment with respect to rapid control of agitation in highly active patients (Garfinkel et al. 1980; Johnson et al. 1968, 1971; Prien et al. 1972; Shopsin et al. 1975). However, a meta-analysis of five controlled acute mania trials (Johnson et al. 1968, 1971; Shopsin et al. 1975; Spring et al. 1970; Takahashi et al. 1975) found the pooled response rate with lithium (89%) to be superior to that with FGAs (38%) (Janicak et al. 1992). In the few studies that combined FGAs with lithium, the combination appeared to yield enhanced therapeutic effects over monotherapy (Garfinkel et al. 1980; Small et al. 1995).

Contemporary FDA-approved acute mania treatments are supported by at least two multicenter, randomized, double-blind, placebo-controlled clinical trials. Such methodologies are considered superior to that used in early lithium acute mania studies. These methodological differences may have eventually contributed to perceptions that lithium efficacy and tolerability in acute mania was less well established compared to newer agents. Indeed, meta-analyses have emphasized the efficacy of SGAs compared with lithium and other mood stabilizers for acute mania (Cipriani et al. 2011; Tarr et al. 2011).

However, lithium's efficacy and tolerability in acute mania have been confirmed in studies using contemporary methodology (Bowden et al. 1994, 2005) (Figure 3–3). The multicenter, randomized, double-blind, placebo-controlled divalproex acute mania registration study (Bowden et al. 1994) and a similar study of quetiapine (Bowden et al. 2005) both included lithium active comparator arms to assess assay sensitivity. In these studies, lithium (with mean concentrations of 0.8 and 1.2 mEq/L, consistent with treatment guidelines [American Psychiatric Association 2002]), demonstrated superior efficacy compared with placebo in a fashion similar to that seen with divalproex and quetiapine. In the divalproex study, antimanic response rates were 49% with lithium, 48% with divalproex (P=not significant [NS] vs. lithium), and 25% with placebo (P=0.025 vs. lithium, and P=0.004 vs. divalproex) (Bowden et al. 1994). Similarly, in the quetiapine study, response rates were 53.1% with lithium, 53.3% with quetiapine (P=NS vs. lithium), and 27.4% with placebo (P< 0.001 vs. lithium and quetiapine) (Bowden et al. 2005). Hence, NNTs for response compared with placebo for lithium were identical to those seen with divalproex (NNT=5; Figure 3–3, left) and quetiapine (NNT=4; Figure 3–3, right).

Moreover, the tolerability for somnolence and weight gain of lithium was superior to that of quetiapine and comparable to that of divalproex, although lithium was associated with other tolerability challenges, such as tremor, thyroid-stimulating hormone (TSH) elevation, vomiting, and adverse-effect discontinuation. In the quetiapine study (Bowden et al. 2005), rates of somnolence were 9.2% with lithium, 19.6% with quetiapine (P<0.05 vs. lithium), and 3.1% with placebo (P=NS vs. lithium, P<0.001 vs. quetiapine), yielding a more favorable NNH for somnolence compared with placebo for lithium versus quetiapine (17 vs. 7). Similarly, rates of weight gain were 6.1% with lithium, 15.0% with quetiapine (P<0.05 vs. lithium), and 1.0% with placebo (P=NS vs. lithium, P<0.001 vs. quetiapine), yielding a more favorable NNH for weight gain compared with placebo for lithium versus quetiapine (20 vs. 9). However, lithium had other noteworthy tolerability limitations, such as tremor (NNH=7 vs. 68 with quetiapine) and TSH elevation (NNH=7 vs. –844 with quetiapine). Also, in the divalproex study (Bowden et al. 1994), rates of somnolence were 19% with both lithium and divalproex (P=NS) and 15% with placebo (P=NS vs. lithium and divalproex), yielding identical NNHs for somnolence with lithium and divalproex (both 25). Rates of weight gain with lithium, divalproex, and placebo were not reported, indicating that they were all less than 15% and not significantly different from one another. Once again, lithium had other noteworthy tolerability limita-

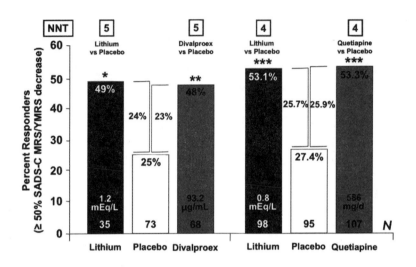

FIGURE 3–3.   Double-blind lithium versus placebo versus divalproex or quetiapine acute mania monotherapy studies, showing response rates and numbers needed to treat.

Note.   SADS-C MRS=Schedule for Affective Disorders and Schizophrenia— Change Version Mania Rating Scale; YMRS=Young Mania Rating Scale.
*$P<0.05$, **$P<0.01$, ***$P<<0.001$ vs. placebo.
Source.   Data on left from Bowden et al. 1994. Data on right from Bowden et al. 2005.

tions, including vomiting (NNH=5 vs. 10 with divalproex) and adverse-effect discontinuation (NNH=12 vs. 33 with divalproex).

Considering multicenter, randomized, double-blind, placebo-controlled acute mania monotherapy registration studies of the mood stabilizers divalproex and carbamazepine, and the SGAs olanzapine, risperidone, quetiapine, ziprasidone, aripiprazole, and asenapine, lithium had comparable efficacy (NNT for response of 4, compared with 4–8 with other agents) (Figure 3–2, Table 3–2), superior tolerability with respect to sedation (NNH for sedation of 27, compared with 5–9 with other agents) (Figure 3–2; Table 3–2, footnote *a*), and intermediate tolerability with respect to weight gain (NNH for weight gain of 13, compared with 7–71 with most other agents) (Figure 3–2; Table 3–2, footnote *a*), but lithium had other tolerability challenges, such as having an NNH for vomiting of 13 (Table 3–2).

In summary, in head-to-head trials using contemporary methodology in patients with acute mania, lithium yielded efficacy similar to that of divalproex and quetiapine, and tolerability for somnolence and weight gain that was superior to that of quetiapine and similar to that of divalproex. However, for other side effects such as vomiting, tremor, and TSH elevation, lithium had inferior tolerability. Moreover, across trials using contemporary methodology in patients with acute mania, lithium compared with other approved agents yielded similar efficacy and similar to superior somnolence and weight gain tolerability, but inferior gastrointestinal (i.e., vomiting) tolerability.

Randomized, double-blind, placebo-controlled acute mania studies have indicated efficacy when lithium (or divalproex) is augmented with olanzapine (Tohen et al. 2002), risperidone (Sachs et al. 2002; Yatham et al. 2003), quetiapine (Sachs et al. 2004; Yatham et al. 2004), aripiprazole (Vieta et al. 2008), or asenapine (Szegedi et al. 2012). In these studies, addition of an SGA tended to yield more adverse effects. In view of findings from these studies, the 2002 revision of the American Psychiatric Association's (2002) "Practice Guideline for the Treatment of Patients With Bipolar Disorder" recommended combinations of SGAs and mood stabilizers as first-line interventions for the treatment of severe cases of acute mania.

Over time, it has become evident that although lithium provides impressive benefits in classic (pure) mania, it has substantial efficacy limitations in mixed episodes (Freeman et al. 1992; Keller et al. 1986; Secunda et al. 1985), dysphoric mania (Swann et al. 2002), secondary mania (Krauthammer and Klerman 1978), and rapid-cycling bipolar disorder (Kukopulos et al. 1980). Thus, agents other than lithium may be preferable in patients with such presentations.

In summary, lithium is a traditional treatment for acute mania. Despite lithium's efficacy and tolerability limitations and the emergence of multiple new treatment options, lithium remains a foundational treatment for bipolar disorder.

Divalproex. The anticonvulsant divalproex (a proprietary formulation of valproate) received FDA approval for the monotherapy treatment of manic episodes associated with bipolar disorder in 1994. By the late 1990s, divalproex had overtaken lithium as the most common treatment for acute mania, in part due to enhanced tolerability and in part due to a broader spectrum of efficacy. In 2005, an extended-release (ER) formulation of divalproex received a monotherapy indication for the treatment of acute manic and mixed episodes, and between 2003 and 2009, five SGAs (olanzapine, risperidone, quetiapine, aripiprazole, and asenapine) were approved for use in combination with divalproex (or lithium) for acute mania.

In a pooled analysis of multicenter, randomized, double-blind, placebo-controlled acute mania registration studies for divalproex (Bowden et al. 1994) and divalproex ER formulation (Bowden et al. 2006), the NNT for response ($\geq 50\%$ decrease in Schedule for Affective Disorders and Schizophrenia—Change Version Mania Rating Scale [SADS-C MRS] score) with divalproex ($N=261$, mean dose 2,778 mg/day; mean serum concentration 95.4 µg/mL) compared with placebo was 7, and the NNH for somnolence compared with placebo was also 7 (Figure 3–2, Table 3–2). In the divalproex ER formulation study (Bowden et al. 2006), the NNH for at least 7% weight gain compared with placebo was 17 (Figure 3–2; Table 3–2, legend footnote *b*).

Divalproex appears to have a broader spectrum of efficacy than lithium, yielding benefit in patients with histories of lithium failure (Bowden et al. 1994; Pope et al. 1991) and in patients with lithium-resistant illness subtypes, such as dysphoric manic episodes (Freeman et al. 1992; Swann et al. 1997) and multiple prior episodes (Swann et al. 2000).

Randomized, double-blind, placebo-controlled acute mania studies have indicated efficacy when divalproex (or lithium) is augmented with olanzapine (Tohen et al. 2002), risperidone (Sachs et al. 2002; Yatham et al. 2003), quetiapine (Delbello et al. 2002; Sachs et al. 2004; Yatham et al. 2004), aripiprazole (Vieta et al. 2008), or asenapine (Szegedi et al. 2012). In these studies, however, addition of an SGA tended to yield somewhat more adverse effects.

In summary, divalproex is an important treatment option for acute mania that may have efficacy and/or tolerability advantages over lithium.

Second-Generation Antipsychotics

For much of the 1970s and 1980s, FGAs were commonly used (often in combination with lithium) for the treatment of acute mania, but such usage changed as the tolerability limitations of FGAs became more evident and as new treatment options emerged. In the late 1990s and early 2000s, the SGAs, also referred to as *atypical antipsychotics,* overtook FGAs in treatment of acute mania primarily due to tolerability concerns of FGAs, and the impressive efficacy evidence base accumulated for SGAs. Between 2000 and 2009 six SGAs (olanzapine, risperidone, quetiapine, ziprasidone, aripiprazole, and asenapine) received FDA indications for acute mania monotherapy, while between 2003 and 2009 five SGAs (olanzapine, risperidone, quetiapine, aripiprazole, and asenapine) also received FDA indications for acute mania adjunctive (combined with lithium or valproate) therapy.

Olanzapine. Olanzapine received FDA approval for the treatment of acute manic or mixed episodes associated with bipolar disorder as monotherapy in adults in 2000, as combination therapy (with lithium or valproate) in adults in 2003, and as longer-term monotherapy in adults in 2004 (Tohen et al. 2006). In 2009, in spite of safety/tolerability limitations, olanzapine monotherapy received FDA approval for acute manic or mixed episodes associated with bipolar disorder in adolescents ages 13–17 years (Tohen et al. 2007). Olanzapine orally disintegrating tablet formulation received FDA approval for acute mania in 2000, and olanzapine rapid-acting injectable intramuscular formulation was indicated for the treatment of agitation associated with bipolar I mania (and schizophrenia) in adults in 2004.

In a pooled analysis of the two multicenter, randomized, double-blind, placebo-controlled acute mania registration studies for olanzapine monotherapy (Tohen et al. 1999, 2000), the NNT for Young Mania Rating Scale (YMRS) response with olanzapine ($N=124$, mean dosage = 15 mg/day) compared with placebo was 5, and the NNH for somnolence compared with placebo was also 5 (Figure 3–2, Table 3–2). Unfortunately, rates for at least 7% weight gain were not reported for these olanzapine monotherapy acute mania registration studies; however, in a pooled analysis of two multicenter, randomized, double-blind, placebo-controlled acute mania registration studies for asenapine monotherapy in which olanzapine monotherapy was an active comparator (McIntyre et al. 2009, 2010), the NNT for response with olanzapine ($N=394$, mean dosage = 15.9 mg/day) compared with placebo was again 5, whereas the NNH for at least 7% weight gain with olanzapine compared with placebo was 7 (Figure 3–2; Table 3–2, legend footnote *d*).

Adjunctive olanzapine (added to lithium or divalproex) was effective in acute mania trials and was approved by the FDA for this indication in 2004. However, with combination therapy compared with monotherapy, the efficacy benefit was accompanied by tolerability limitations such as sedation and weight gain. In contrast, adjunctive olanzapine (added to carbamazepine) was no better than adjunctive placebo added to carbamazepine in patients with manic and mixed episodes, but yielded more weight gain and higher serum triglyceride concentrations (Tohen et al. 2008).

In summary, olanzapine is effective for acute mania, both as monotherapy and as adjunctive (added to lithium or divalproex, but not carbamazepine) therapy. However, sedation, weight gain, and metabolic problems may limit the utility of this agent, particularly in longer-term treatment.

Risperidone.   Risperidone received FDA approval for the treatment of acute manic or mixed episodes associated with bipolar I disorder in adults as monotherapy as well as in combination with lithium or valproate in 2003, and as monotherapy for acute manic or mixed episodes associated with bipolar I disorder in children and adolescents ages 10–17 years in 2007 (Haas et al. 2009). Risperidone long-acting injectable formulation was approved for bipolar disorder preventive treatment as monotherapy and as adjunctive therapy (added to lithium or valproate) in 2009.

In a pooled analysis of three multicenter, randomized, double-blind, placebo-controlled risperidone monotherapy acute mania studies (Hirschfeld et al. 2004; Khanna et al. 2005; Smulevich et al. 2005), the NNT for YMRS response with risperidone ($N=434$, mean dosage$=4.6$ mg/day) compared with placebo was 5, whereas the NNH for extrapyramidal symptoms (EPS) compared with placebo was 7 (Table 3–2). In a pooled analysis of two of these acute mania studies, the NNH for somnolence with risperidone ($N=288$, mean dosage$=4.2$ mg/day, NNT$=6$) was 9 (Hirschfeld et al. 2004; Smulevich et al. 2005; Table 3–2, legend footnote *e*). Unfortunately, rates of at least 7% weight gain with risperidone in these controlled acute mania studies were not reported.

In addition, two multicenter, randomized, double-blind, placebo-controlled studies confirmed the efficacy of adjunctive (added to lithium or divalproex) risperidone in acute mania (Sachs et al. 2002; Yatham et al. 2003).

In summary, risperidone is effective for acute mania, both as monotherapy and as adjunctive therapy. However, side effects such as EPS, somnolence, weight gain, and metabolic problems may limit the utility of this agent.

Quetiapine.   Quetiapine received FDA approval for the treatment of acute manic episodes associated with bipolar disorder, either as monotherapy or as adjunctive therapy to lithium or divalproex in 2004. Patients with rapid-cycling and mixed episodes were not included in the quetiapine immediate-release formulation pivotal acute mania studies, so the efficacy of quetiapine immediate-release formulation for these subtypes remains to be established. However, a quetiapine extended-release (XR) formulation was approved by the FDA for the monotherapy or adjunctive (added to lithium or valproate) treatment of acute manic and mixed episodes in 2008. The FDA also approved quetiapine monotherapy for acute manic episodes associated with bipolar disorder in children and adolescents ages 10–17 years in 2009 (DelBello et al. 2007).

In a pooled analysis of three multicenter, randomized, double-blind, placebo-controlled quetiapine immediate-release (Bowden et al. 2005;

McIntyre et al. 2005) and XR (Cutler et al. 2011) formulation monotherapy acute mania studies, the NNT for YMRS response with quetiapine (N=357, mean dosage=586 mg/day) compared with placebo was 5, the NNH for sedation (Cutler et al. 2011) or somnolence (Bowden et al. 2005, McIntyre et al. 2005) compared with placebo was 6 (Figure 3–2, Table 3–2), and the NNH for at least 7% weight gain compared with placebo was 9 (Figure 3–2; Table 3–2, footnote *f*).

In addition, multicenter, randomized, double-blind, placebo-controlled data support the efficacy of adjunctive (added to lithium or divalproex) quetiapine in acute mania (Yatham et al. 2004).

In summary, quetiapine is effective for acute mania, both in monotherapy and as adjunctive (added to lithium or valproate) treatment. However, somnolence/sedation, weight gain, and metabolic problems can substantively limit the utility of this agent.

Ziprasidone.   Ziprasidone received FDA approval for the treatment of acute manic or mixed episodes associated with bipolar disorder, with or without psychotic features, as monotherapy in 2004. Although some controlled data supported the use of ziprasidone monotherapy for acute manic episodes associated with bipolar disorder in children and adolescents ages 10–17 years (DelBello et al. 2008), as of early 2015 ziprasidone lacked such an indication. Unlike for some other SGAs, adjunctive ziprasidone (added to lithium or valproate) was not effective for acute mania (Sachs et al. 2012a, 2012b) and did not receive FDA approval for this indication. A rapid-acting injectable intramuscular formulation of ziprasidone was approved for the treatment of acute agitation in patients with schizophrenia in 2002 but, as of early 2015, not for patients with bipolar disorder.

In a pooled analysis of the two multicenter, randomized, double-blind, placebo-controlled ziprasidone monotherapy acute mania registration studies (Keck et al. 2003b; Potkin et al. 2005), the NNT for YMRS response with ziprasidone (N=268, mean dosage=121 mg/day) compared with placebo was 7, and the NNH for somnolence compared with placebo was 5 (Figure 3–2, Table 3–2). In the one of these two studies that reported rates of at least 7% weight gain, the NNH for at least 7% weight gain for ziprasidone (N=139, NNT=6) compared with placebo was 71 (Potkin et al. 2005) (Figure 3–2; Table 3–2, footnote *g*). Although akathisia can be problematic with ziprasidone, the pooled NNH for this harm compared with placebo in these two registration studies was 21 (Table 3–2, footnote *g*).

Limited controlled data suggest that rapid-acting intramuscular ziprasidone might yield benefit in psychotic agitated patients with bipolar disorder and manic or mixed episodes with psychotic features or schizoaffective disorder, bipolar type (Daniel et al. 2004).

In summary, ziprasidone monotherapy has an FDA indication for acute mania. Weight gain and metabolic concerns appear to be much less problematic with ziprasidone than with some other SGAs, although sedation and akathisia may limit ziprasidone's utility.

Aripiprazole.   Aripiprazole received FDA approval for the treatment of acute manic or mixed episodes associated with bipolar disorder as monotherapy in adults in 2004 and in children and adolescents ages 10–17 years in 2008, and as adjunctive therapy (added to lithium or valproate) in adults, children, and adolescents in 2008. Aripiprazole orally disintegrating tablet and rapid-acting intramuscular injectable formulations were approved by the FDA for acute mania and for agitation associated with bipolar disorder, manic or mixed (or schizophrenia), respectively, in 2006.

In a pooled analysis of the two multicenter, randomized, double-blind, placebo-controlled aripiprazole monotherapy acute mania registration studies (Keck et al. 2003a; Sachs et al. 2006), the NNT for YMRS response with aripiprazole (N=260, mean dosage=28 mg/day) compared with placebo was 5, the NNH for somnolence compared with placebo was 9 (Figure 3–2, Table 3–2), and the NNH for at least 7% weight gain compared with placebo was –128 (i.e., weight gain with aripiprazole was nonsignificantly less common than with placebo) (Figure 3–2; Table 3–2, footnote *h*). Akathisia and nausea can be problematic with aripiprazole, and the pooled NNHs for these harms compared with placebo in these two studies were 10 and 12, respectively (Table 3–2, footnote *h*).

In addition, multicenter, randomized, double-blind, placebo-controlled trials confirmed the efficacy of adjunctive aripiprazole (added to lithium or valproate) oral formulation in acute mania (Vieta et al. 2008), and of aripiprazole rapid-acting injectable intramuscular formulation for agitation associated with manic or mixed episodes (Zimbroff et al. 2007).

In summary, aripiprazole is effective for acute mania, and although sedation, weight gain, and metabolic concerns may be less problematic with aripiprazole compared with some other SGAs, akathisia and nausea may limit its utility.

Asenapine.   In 2009, asenapine received FDA approval as monotherapy and as adjunctive therapy for the treatment of acute mania. Hence, asenapine has been promoted from Tier II in *Handbook of Diagnosis and Treatment of Bipolar Disorders* (Ketter 2010) to Tier I in the current volume.

In a pooled analysis of the two multicenter, randomized, double-blind, placebo-controlled asenapine monotherapy acute mania registration studies (McIntyre et al. 2002, 2010), the NNT for YMRS response with asenapine (N=357, mean dosage=18 mg/day) compared to placebo was 8, the NNH for sedation compared with placebo was 6 (Figure 3–2, Table 3–2), and the NNH for at least 7% weight gain compared with placebo was 17 (Figure 3–2; Table 3–2, footnote *i*). Head-to-head comparisons indicated that olanzapine compared with asenapine was more efficacious (NNT=11, $P<0.01$) but yielded more weight gain (NNH=11, $P<0.0001$).

In summary, asenapine is effective for acute mania, and although sedation, weight gain, and metabolic concerns may be less problematic with asenapine than with some other SGAs, these side effects can limit its utility in some patients.

Tier II: High-Priority Unapproved Acute Mania Treatments

As noted above, safety/tolerability limitations of some Tier I approved treatments for acute mania may lead clinicians and patients to consider other options. When assessing alternative treatments, one approach is to consider medications that have controlled data indicating efficacy, which may (or may not) ultimately receive FDA approval for the treatment of acute mania. Indeed, since the publication of *Handbook of Diagnosis and Treatment of Bipolar Disorders* (Ketter 2010), asenapine (as monotherapy and added to lithium or valproate) received FDA approval for the treatment of acute mania and was thus promoted from Tier II in the *Handbook* to Tier I in the current volume. As of early 2015, cariprazine had not been approved by the FDA for the treatment of acute mania or marketed in the United States, because the pivotal trials described below were still under FDA review. It is anticipated that in the near future the FDA will make a definitive determination regarding the approval of cariprazine for acute mania.

Cariprazine

The novel SGA cariprazine is a partial agonist at dopamine ($D_3>D_2$) and serotonin 5-HT_{1A} receptors that, as of early 2015, was still under consideration by the FDA for the monotherapy treatment of acute mania (as well as acute schizophrenia). This consideration was based on two positive 3-week, multicenter, randomized, double-blind, placebo-controlled acute mania trials (RGH-M32 and RGH-M33) (Calabrese et al. 2014; Ketter et al. 2014; Starace et al. 2012).

In a pooled analysis of two multicenter, randomized, double-blind, placebo-controlled cariprazine monotherapy acute mania studies (Calabrese et al. 2014; Ketter et al. 2014), the NNT for YMRS response with cariprazine (*N*=492, mean dosage=7.2 mg/day) compared with placebo was 6 (Figure 3–4, left), while the NNH for akathisia compared with placebo was 7 (Figure 3–4, right; Table 3–2). Importantly, cariprazine had a low propensity toward yielding somnolence (NNH=50) and at least 7% weight gain (NNH=–944; i.e., weight gain was nonsignificantly less common than with placebo) (Table 3–2, footnote *j*). Thus, cariprazine monotherapy may ultimately prove to have adequate tolerability, with a side-effect profile more like that of aripiprazole than that of older SGAs such as olanzapine, risperidone, and quetiapine. In a pooled analysis of the acute mania studies, akathisia was usually not problematic enough to yield discontinuation, so that cariprazine monotherapy had a favorable (double-digit) NNH for discontinuation due to akathisia compared with placebo of 34 (Ketter et al. 2014). Indeed, in a 20-week study, among 402 patients with bipolar I disorder taking open-label cariprazine (3–12 mg/day, mean 6.2 mg/day), 32.6% had akathisia, but this side effect led to discontinuation in only 4.7%, and the rates of somnolence and at least 7% weight gain (i.e., adverse effects of concern with other SGAs) were 5.7% and 9%, respectively (Ketter et al. 2013).

Tier III: Intermediate-Priority Unapproved Acute Mania Treatment Options

The management of acute mania is sufficiently challenging that clinical need may outstrip the evidence-based treatment options. In this section we consider other (in most instances unapproved) treatment options with tolerability limitations and/or more limited evidence of efficacy compared with the previously discussed Tier I and Tier II treatments. These alternatives include the mood stabilizer carbamazepine; the FGAs chlorpromazine, thioridazine, thiothixene, pimozide, haloperidol, and inhaled loxapine; the SGAs adjunctive ziprasidone, paliperidone, and clozapine; adjunctive benzodiazepines; and ECT. In general, treatment guidelines do not consider these modalities to be first-line interventions but cite them as intermediate-priority options (American Psychiatric Association 2002; Goodwin and Consensus Group of the British Association for Psychopharmacology 2003; Grunze et al. 2002; Keck et al. 2004; Suppes et al. 2005; Yatham et al. 2006). Some Tier III options, however, have mitigating advantages that might make them attractive for selected patients, and in certain circumstances, some of these interventions may be considered early on (e.g., ECT in pregnant women).

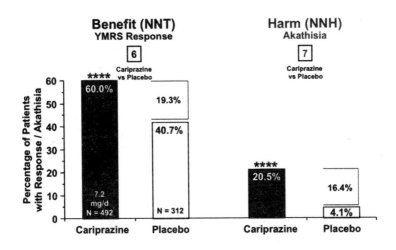

FIGURE 3–4. Benefits and harms of cariprazine in acute mania.

Note. Pooled 3-week double-blind cariprazine monotherapy versus placebo in acute mania trials, showing NNT, NNH, and response and akathisia rates. NNH=number needed to harm for somnolence versus placebo; NNT=number needed to treat for YMRS response versus placebo; YMRS=Young Mania Rating Scale.

****$P<0.0001$ versus placebo. Cariprazine monotherapy compared with placebo had superior efficacy but yielded more akathisia.

Source. Data from Calabrese et al. 2014; Ketter et al. 2014.

Other Mood Stabilizers

Although carbamazepine has FDA approval for the treatment of acute mania, complexity of its use related to drug interactions as well as tolerability limitations and having less compelling evidence of maintenance efficacy lead to its being considered an alternative rather than first-line antimanic agent. Nevertheless, inadequate efficacy and/or tolerability issues experienced with Tier I or II options may make carbamazepine an alternative worthy of consideration for selected patients.

Carbamazepine. In the 1980s, controlled carbamazepine studies using active comparator and on-off-on designs provided preliminary evidence of efficacy in acute mania. Because of economic concerns such as patent protection limitations and the high cost of obtaining FDA approval, a carbamazepine indication in acute mania was not initially sought in the United States but was obtained from agencies in several other countries. The absence of an FDA indication and complexity of use led carbamazepine to be considered an alternative rather than a first-line intervention in acute mania (American Psychiatric Association 2002). However, multicenter, randomized, double-blind, placebo-controlled trials confirmed the efficacy of a proprietary beaded, extended-release capsule formulation of carbamazepine in acute manic and mixed episodes (Weisler et al. 2004a, 2005), yielding an FDA indication for this formulation in 2004. However, as of early 2015, carbamazepine lacked an FDA indication for acute mania adjunctive treatment.

In a pooled analysis of the two multicenter, randomized, double-blind, placebo-controlled carbamazepine monotherapy acute mania registration studies (Weisler et al. 2004a, 2005, 2006), the NNT for YMRS response with carbamazepine ($N = 223$, mean dosage $= 707$ mg/day) compared with placebo was 4, the NNH for somnolence compared with placebo was 6 (Figure 3–2; Table 3–2, footnote c), and the NNH for at least 7% weight gain compared with placebo was 23 (Figure 3–2; Table 3–2, footnote c). Dizziness can be problematic with carbamazepine (particularly early in treatment), and the NNH for this harm compared with placebo in these studies was 4 (Table 3–2).

Older studies suggested utility for carbamazepine combined with lithium (Kramlinger and Post 1989) or antipsychotics (Okuma et al. 1989) in the treatment of acute mania. However, carbamazepine can increase the hepatic metabolism of multiple other agents, potentially compromising the efficacy of combination therapies (Ketter et al. 1991a, 1991b). In a subsequent study that reemphasized this point, carbamazepine yielded substantial decreases in blood risperidone concentrations, compromising efficacy of the combination in the treatment of acute mania (Yatham et al. 2003). In another combination therapy study, carbamazepine yielded lower-than-expected blood olanzapine concentrations, and even though this was addressed in part by a more aggressive olanzapine dosage, the efficacy of the olanzapine plus carbamazepine combination was still not significantly better than that of carbamazepine monotherapy in the treatment of acute mania (Tohen et al. 2008). Additionally, olanzapine plus carbamazepine compared with carbamazepine monotherapy yielded higher triglyceride levels and more frequent clinically significant ($\geq 7\%$) weight gain (24.6% for olanzapine plus carbamazepine vs. 3.4% for carbamazepine monotherapy).

In summary, carbamazepine is an option for acute mania that has drug interaction and tolerability limitations. Thus, carbamazepine is considered an intermediate-priority acute mania therapy by multiple treatment guidelines. Nevertheless, carbamazepine may be a useful treatment for acute mania in selected patients, particularly those who are not taking multiple other medications or who experience inadequate efficacy and/or tolerability with Tier I or II options.

First-Generation Antipsychotics

FGAs, also referred to as *typical antipsychotics*, have been superseded by SGAs, primarily because the latter have more favorable adverse-effect profiles. Multiple FGAs were approved by the FDA for the treatment of schizophrenia in the 1950s–1970s, but only one such agent, chlorpromazine, was eventually approved for acute mania.

Individual early studies found that FGAs compared with lithium tended to have comparable overall efficacy, with FGAs having advantages early in treatment for rapid control of agitation in highly active patients but disadvantages later in treatment for achieving remission of the full manic syndrome sufficient to permit discharge (Garfinkel et al. 1980; Johnson et al. 1968, 1971; Prien et al. 1972; Shopsin et al. 1975). In some studies, combining FGAs with lithium appeared to yield enhanced therapeutic effects (Garfinkel et al. 1980; Small et al. 1995).

FGAs were commonly used (often in combination with lithium) for the treatment of acute mania in the 1970s and 1980s, but this usage changed because of FGA tolerability limitations, such as acute EPS (Nasrallah et al. 1988), tardive dyskinesia (Kane and Smith 1982), and induction of dysphoria (Ahlfors et al. 1981), as well as the emergence of newer treatment options.

The rapid onset of action of FGAs was particularly evident with rapid-acting injectable intramuscular formulation administration. Indeed, use of rapid-acting injectable intramuscular formulation haloperidol (often combined with lorazepam injectable intramuscular formulation to enhance efficacy and with diphenhydramine injectable intramuscular formulation to decrease EPS) persisted even into the era of SGAs because it was a well-established, inexpensive, and generally well-tolerated treatment for acute agitation in bipolar I disorder. In 2012, an inhaled formulation of the FGA loxapine was approved by the FDA for the treatment of acute agitation in bipolar I disorder (and schizophrenia).

Chlorpromazine.   Chlorpromazine, the prototypical FGA, received FDA approval for schizophrenia in 1954 and for acute mania in 1973. Controlled trials demonstrated chlorpromazine's efficacy in acute mania as monotherapy (Post et al. 1980; Prien et al. 1972; Shopsin et al. 1975) and combined with lithium (Cookson et al. 1981; Janicak et al. 1988). However, the clinical utility of this low-potency FGA was limited by prominent sedation and hypotension, resulting in the increasing use of intermediate-potency and high-potency agents, particularly haloperidol.

Haloperidol.   The high-potency FGA haloperidol yields substantially less sedation and hypotension than chlorpromazine, albeit at the expense of more frequent EPS. Early trials suggested that haloperidol was effective in acute mania both as monotherapy (Garfinkel et al. 1980; Shopsin et al. 1975) and as an adjunct to lithium (Garfinkel et al. 1980).

In a pooled analysis of three multicenter, randomized, double-blind, placebo-controlled acute mania studies that included haloperidol monotherapy as an active comparator (McIntyre et al. 2005; Smulevich et al. 2005; Vieta et al. 2010b), the NNT for YMRS response with haloperidol (N=364 for efficacy, N=414 for safety/tolerability; maximum/ mean dosage=11.3 mg/day) compared with placebo was 5, and NNHs compared with placebo were 4 for EPS (Table 3–2), 16 for somnolence (Table 3–2, footnote k), and 50 for greater than 7% weight gain (Table 3–2, footnote k).

In acute agitation in schizophrenia or mania, rapid-acting injectable intramuscular haloperidol 5 mg compared with intramuscular lorazepam 2-mg injections every 30–60 minutes as needed appeared to have similar efficacy, although haloperidol yielded more EPS (Bieniek et al. 1998; Foster et al. 1997). Combining these agents appeared to yield more rapid benefit compared with either monotherapy, and perhaps even yielded fewer EPS compared with haloperidol monotherapy (Battaglia et al. 1997).

Inhaled loxapine.   In 2012, the FDA approved inhaled loxapine for acute agitation associated with bipolar I disorder, based on a multicenter, randomized, double-blind, placebo-controlled, parallel-group study of 314 inpatients with bipolar I disorder with acute agitation due to manic or mixed episodes, in whom inhaled loxapine (5 or 10 mg) was superior to inhaled placebo for decreasing Positive and Negative Syndrome Scale—Excited Component (PANSS-EC) score 2 hours after administration (Kwentus et al. 2012). Inhaled loxapine was generally well tolerated, so that in a pooled tolerability analysis of 259 inpatients with bipolar I disorder or schizophrenia, the inhaled loxapine 10-mg dose yielded NNHs compared with placebo of 11 for dysgeusia, 41 for sedation/somnolence, 44 for throat irritation, and 86 for EPS (Citrome 2013).

Among 1,095 study subjects without active airway disease who received inhaled loxapine during the clinical trial program, 1 (0.09%) required treatment with albuterol for bronchospasm, and 19 (1.7%) had cough (Citrome 2013). The FDA, in an effort to ensure that the benefits of inhaled loxapine outweighed the risk of bronchospasm, required a boxed warning describing the risk of bronchospasm with potential to lead to respiratory arrest and stipulated that inhaled loxapine only be available through a restricted Risk Evaluation and Mitigation Strategy program, in enrolled facilities with on-site access to equipment and personnel trained to manage acute bronchospasm, including advanced airway management.

In summary, some FGAs have evidence supporting their efficacy, but safety/tolerability concerns commonly result in FGAs being used only for patients who experience inadequate efficacy and/or tolerability with the mood stabilizers and SGAs listed in Tiers I and II.

Other Second-Generation Antipsychotics

As of early 2015, ziprasidone was the only SGA with an FDA acute mania indication as monotherapy but not as adjunctive (added to lithium or valproate) therapy, and clozapine, iloperidone, paliperidone, and lurasidone were the only SGAs with FDA schizophrenia but not acute mania indications. Limited data suggested that paliperidone had efficacy issues and clozapine had safety/tolerability limitations. In contrast, systematic data were lacking regarding the efficacy and safety/tolerability of lurasidone and iloperidone in acute mania.

Adjunctive ziprasidone. In a multicenter, randomized, double-blind, placebo-controlled study, ziprasidone (mean modal doses approximately 60 and 134 mg/day) added to lithium or valproate was not superior to adjunctive placebo (Sachs et al. 2012a), although methodological limitations could have contributed to the lack of separation from placebo (Sachs et al. 2012b).

Paliperidone. The first acute mania study of paliperidone (9-hydroxy-risperidone, the active metabolite of risperidone) was encouraging (Figure 3–5) in that flexibly dosed paliperidone monotherapy versus placebo yielded a favorable (single-digit) NNT for YMRS response compared with placebo of 5 (Figure 3–5, left) and a favorable (double-digit) NNH for somnolence compared with placebo of 17 (Figure 3–5, right) (Vieta et al. 2010a). Unfortunately, the second acute mania monotherapy study was discouraging, because paliperidone only modestly separated from placebo on the primary outcome measure and failed to separate from placebo on secondary outcomes (e.g., 12 mg/day yielded a YMRS response NNT of 12), and because there was a significant treatment-by-country interaction (Berwaerts et al. 2012). In view of efficacy findings driven largely by patients in Asia and Eastern Europe, paliperidone monotherapy was *not* approved for acute mania in the United States and the European Union. Moreover, paliperidone as adjunctive (added to lithium or valproate) therapy (median modal dose=6 mg/day) for acute manic or mixed episodes was not superior to placebo (NNT=17) (Berwaerts et

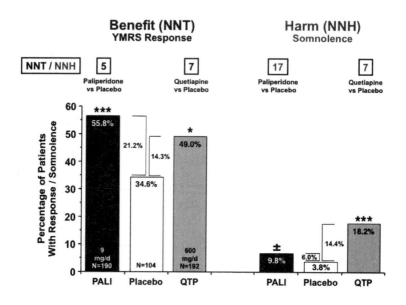

FIGURE 3–5. Benefits and harms of monotherapy with the second-generation antipsychotic paliperidone or quetiapine in acute mania.

Note. PALI monotherapy was more than three times as likely to yield benefit (YMRS response) than harm (somnolence) compared with placebo. In contrast, QTP monotherapy was similarly likely to yield benefit (YMRS response) and harm (somnolence) compared with placebo. NNH=number needed to harm for somnolence versus placebo; NNT=number needed to treat for YMRS response versus placebo. PALI=paliperidone; QTP=quetiapine; YMRS=Young Mania Rating Scale.

$\pm P<0.1$, $^*P<0.05$, $^{***}P<0.001$ vs. placebo.

Source. Data from Vieta et al. 2010a.

al. 2011). Therefore, as of early 2015, paliperidone had *not* received FDA approval for the treatment of acute mania, either as monotherapy or as adjunctive therapy, and accordingly has been placed on Tier III.

Clozapine. Although as of early 2015 clozapine lacked an FDA indication for acute mania, it remained of interest not only as the prototypical SGA but also as the only agent approved for treatment-resistant schizophrenia. However, clozapine's challenging adverse-effect profile continues to lead clinicians to commonly use it only for patients who experience inadequate efficacy with the mood stabilizers and SGAs in Tiers I and II or the FGAs in Tier III.

Adjunctive Benzodiazepines

Adjunctive benzodiazepines have antiagitation effects (Battaglia et al. 1997) and are commonly used in controlled acute mania trials to attenuate symptoms while not systematically interfering with separation of approved treatments from placebo. In aggregate, in contemporary acute mania trials, the control intervention of as-needed lorazepam, psychiatric hospitalization, and placebo yields an overall response rate of approximately 30%; adding an approved antimanic agent increases the overall response rate to approximately 50%.

The hypnotic (Andersen and Lingjaerde 1969) and anxiolytic (Ballenger et al. 1988) actions of benzodiazepines can be beneficial in patients with bipolar disorder. Thus, as with gabapentin and topiramate, although benzodiazepines do not appear to be effective as primary treatments for bipolar disorders, they may yield benefit in common comorbid problems, such as insomnia and anxiety disorders. Although benzodiazepines are generally well tolerated, care is indicated in patient selection because these agents have abuse potential and may yield disinhibition.

Electroconvulsive Therapy

Limited controlled data support ECT for acute mania (Mukherjee et al. 1994). Concerns based on case reports regarding the risks of delirium, seizures, and prolonged apnea resulted in recommendations that lithium not be combined with ECT (Small and Milstein 1990). Moreover, ECT is generally held in reserve for manic patients refractory to pharmacotherapy, because of the risk of cognitive adverse effects, stigma, consent challenges, and logistical concerns.

Tier IV: Novel Adjunctive Treatments

Tier IV includes novel adjunctive treatments that have even more limited evidence of efficacy than the treatments in Tiers I–III. The Tier IV treatments include other mood stabilizers, other anticonvulsants, and adjunctive psychotherapy. Very careful consideration is warranted when one is considering the specific role(s) of these treatments in patients with bipolar disorders. For example, for some of these interventions, controlled trials indicate inefficacy in acute mania but potential efficacy in other phases of bipolar disorder (e.g., lamotrigine for preventive treatment) or in the management of common comorbid conditions (e.g., gabapentin and topiramate for anxiety and alcohol use disorders, re-spectively). In general, treatment guidelines consider these modalities to be low-priority interventions or not recommended as interventions in the treatment of acute mania (American Psychiatric Association 2002; Goodwin and Consensus Group of the British Association for Psychopharmacology 2003; Grunze et al. 2002; Keck et al. 2004; Suppes et al. 2005; Yatham et al. 2006). Nevertheless, some Tier IV options could prove to be worthwhile adjuncts for very carefully selected patients, after consideration of Tier I–III treatments (e.g., in patients with prominent comorbid conditions).

Other Mood Stabilizers

The anticonvulsant lamotrigine has a distinctive psychotropic profile compared with other mood stabilizers, in that it has a bipolar disorder preventive treatment indication but lacks an acute indication, and it appears more effective in countering depressive as opposed to mood elevation symptoms. In the absence of an acute indication, clinicians may ponder the optimal timing of initiating lamotrigine therapy. In most instances, this will be during euthymia or syndromal or subsyndromal depression (on occasion immediately after an acute manic episode) rather than during acute mania.

Lamotrigine.   As of early 2015, lamotrigine, unlike the anticonvulsants divalproex and carbamazepine, did *not* appear effective in and lacked an FDA indication for acute mania (Bowden et al. 2000; Goldsmith et al. 2003). However, despite lamotrigine's inefficacy for acute mania, some providers opine that it may occasionally be worth considering as an adjunct as soon as standard therapy for acute mania has commenced, with the goal of preventing or delaying a postmania depression, although the strengths and limitations of such an approach need to be carefully considered on an individualized basis.

Other Anticonvulsants

The efficacy and tolerability limitations of lithium and antipsychotics, and the utility of valproate, carbamazepine, and lamotrigine in bipolar disorders, resulted in the assessment of several other anticonvulsants in acute mania. These other anticonvulsants appeared to have diverse psychotropic profiles. Although these anticonvulsants, aside from the possible exception of oxcarbazepine, have not been found effective for acute mania (Table 3–4), at least some of these medications (e.g., gabapentin,

TABLE 3–4.   Other anticonvulsants not proved effective in mania (as of early 2015)

Drug	Evidence
Oxcarbazepine	Negative underpowered placebo-controlled trial in pediatric acute mania that had an encouraging (but nonsignificant) number needed to treat for response (Wagner et al. 2006)
Gabapentin	Negative placebo-controlled trial of adjunctive therapy in acute mania or hypomania (Pande et al. 2000a)
Topiramate	Five negative placebo- and lithium-controlled adult monotherapy acute mania studies (Kushner et al. 2006)
Tiagabine	Negative open adjunctive treatment-resistant bipolar disorder study, with safety/tolerability concerns (Grunze et al. 1999)
Zonisamide	No published controlled bipolar disorder study
Levetiracetam	No published controlled bipolar disorder study
Pregabalin	No published controlled bipolar disorder study
Rufinamide	No published controlled bipolar disorder study
Lacosamide	No published controlled bipolar disorder study
Vigabatrin	No published controlled bipolar disorder study
Ezogabine (retigabine)	Negative open monotherapy acute mania study (Amann et al. 2006)
Clobazam	No published controlled bipolar disorder study
Perampanel	No published controlled bipolar disorder study, and has behavioral toxicity boxed warning
Eslicarbazepine	No published controlled bipolar disorder study

topiramate, and zonisamide) may be worth considering in selected patients with bipolar disorder for treatment of comorbid conditions (e.g., anxiety disorders, alcohol use disorders, obesity, or pain syndromes). However, administration of other anticonvulsants that lack evidence of efficacy for such comorbid conditions and/or have substantive safety limitations and/or have behavioral toxicity warnings in the U.S. prescribing information (e.g., tiagabine, levetiracetam, ezogabine, and perampanel) ought to be approached with considerable caution.

Oxcarbazepine.   Oxcarbazepine, a congener of carbamazepine with more favorable adverse-effect and drug interaction profiles, may differ from other newer anticonvulsants in that it may have efficacy in acute mania. Unfortunately, as of early 2015, there had been no positive large double-blind, placebo-controlled trial of oxcarbazepine in bipolar disorder. However, in a multicenter randomized, double-blind, placebo-controlled, 7-week, pediatric acute mania trial with limited sample size, although 59 patients taking oxcarbazepine and 56 taking placebo had statistically similar mean YMRS decreases from baseline to endpoint and YMRS response rates, oxcarbazepine yielded a nonsignificant but encouraging single-digit NNT for YMRS response compared with placebo of 7 (Wagner et al. 2006). Accordingly, oxcarbazepine is most often held in reserve for patients who experience tolerability issues with the more established therapies in Tiers I–III (Table 3–3, Table 3–4).

Gabapentin. Randomized, double-blind, placebo-controlled studies of gabapentin in acute bipolar disorder were discouraging (Frye et al. 2000; Pande et al. 2000a), so as of early 2015 gabapentin lacked an FDA indication for acute mania. However, gabapentin appeared effective in several comorbid conditions seen in patients with bipolar disorders, with double-blind, placebo-controlled trials indicating efficacy in alcohol dependence (Mason et al. 2014), anxiety disorders such as social phobia (Pande et al. 1999), and (in a post hoc analysis) moderate to severe panic disorder (Pande et al. 2000b), as well as in pain syndromes such as neuropathic pain (Serpell and Neuropathic Pain Study Group 2002), chronic daily headache (Spira and Beran 2003), and postherpetic neuralgia (Rowbotham et al. 1998), and received an FDA indication for the latter pain syndrome. Although gabapentin does not appear to be effective in acute mania, it may be worth considering as an adjunct for comorbid conditions in selected patients with bipolar disorder.

Topiramate. Although early open reports on topiramate in bipolar disorders were encouraging, results from later multicenter, randomized, double-blind, placebo-controlled studies were discouraging (Kushner et al. 2006). Therefore, as of early 2015, topiramate lacked an FDA indication for acute mania. However, topiramate appeared effective in several comorbid conditions seen in patients with bipolar disorders, with randomized, double-blind, placebo-controlled trials indicating efficacy in eating disorders such as obesity with or without diabetes mellitus (Bray et al. 2003; Rosenstock et al. 2007; Stenlöf et al. 2007; Toplak et al. 2007; Tremblay et al. 2007), obesity with binge eating disorder (Claudino et al. 2007; McElroy et al. 2003), obesity with bipolar disorder (McElroy et al. 2007), olanzapine-associated weight gain (Egger et al. 2007), and bulimia (Hoopes et al. 2003), as well as in alcohol dependence (Johnson et al. 2003, 2007), essential tremor (Ondo et al. 2006), chronic low back pain (Muehlbacher et al. 2006), borderline personality disorder (Loew et al. 2006), and the prevention of migraine headaches (Brandes et al. 2004; Silberstein et al. 2007). Weight loss has been consistently observed in controlled trials with topiramate, not only in patients with eating disorders but also in manic (Kushner et al. 2006) and depressed (McIntyre et al. 2002) patients with bipolar disorders. Thus, although not effective in acute mania, topiramate may be worth considering as an adjunct for comorbid conditions in selected patients with bipolar disorder.

Tiagabine. Tiagabine lacks controlled studies in bipolar disorder and any FDA indication for bipolar disorder treatment. Although some experience with open low-dose tiagabine in bipolar disorders was encouraging (Schaffer et al. 2002), other open reports suggested problems with efficacy and/or tolerability (Grunze et al. 1999; Suppes et al. 2002). In contrast, a small controlled trial reported that low-dose (≤16 mg/day) tiagabine was generally well tolerated and yielded benefit in generalized anxiety disorder (Rosenthal 2003). Thus, like gabapentin and topiramate, tiagabine does not appear to be effective as a primary treatment for bipolar disorder but may yield benefit in comorbid problems, such as generalized anxiety disorder. However, reports of tolerability problems suggest that considerable caution ought to be exercised with tiagabine in patients with bipolar disorder (Grunze et al. 1999; Suppes et al. 2002).

Zonisamide. As of early 2015, there are no controlled studies and only a few open reports of zonisamide in bipolar disorder (Kanba et al. 1994; McElroy et al. 2005). However, some controlled data suggest that zonisamide, like topiramate, may have utility in obesity and eating disorders (Gadde et al. 2003, 2007; McElroy et al. 2006).

Adjunctive Psychotherapy

Data from controlled trials indicate the importance of adjunctive psychosocial interventions in bipolar disorder, with the optimal time of administration being during euthymia or depression as opposed to during mania (Swartz and Frank 2001), a mood state that entails such marked cognitive and behavioral disruptions that psychological interventions may not be feasible.

Tier V: Research Treatments

As of early 2015, there were some very innovative treatments that research suggested could have promise for acute mania, but that were thus far too novel and/or carried too substantive safety/tolerability risks to be considered clinical (as opposed to research) tools. In this section we discuss one such treatment, tamoxifen.

Tamoxifen

Tamoxifen, a nonsteroidal antiestrogen used in breast cancer treatment (commonly at dosages of 20–40 mg/day), is also a protein kinase C inhibitor, a mechanism that may yield antimanic effects (DiazGranados and Zarate 2008). In two small double-blind, placebo-controlled acute mania studies, in which 32 patients took tamoxifen up to 80 mg/day (Yildiz et al. 2008) and 8 patients took up to 140 mg/day (Zarate et al. 2007), tamoxifen monotherapy appeared efficacious, with a pooled NNT for response compared with placebo of 3, and was either well tolerated (Yildiz et al. 2008) or yielded an NNH for decreased appetite compared with placebo of 2 (Zarate et al. 2007). Also, in a small double-blind, placebo-controlled acute mania study, in which 20 patients took adjunctive tamoxifen up to 80 mg/day added to lithium 1.0–1.2 mEq/L, tamoxifen appeared efficacious, with an NNT for response compared with placebo of 4, but an NNH for fatigue compared with placebo of 3 (Amrollahi et al. 2011). However, two even smaller double-blind, placebo-controlled adjunctive acute mania studies, in which 5 subjects took tamoxifen 40 mg/day added to lithium (Kulkarni et al. 2006) or 15 subjects took tamoxifen 40 mg/day added to lithium, valproate, or carbamazepine ± antipsychotics (Kulkarni et al. 2014), suggested efficacy and inefficacy, respectively.

Important limitations of these studies include tamoxifen's potent antiestrogen effects, which confound its putative protein kinase C inhibition psychotropic mechanism; its uncertain optimal acute mania dosing; and the lack of safety/tolerability data in larger numbers of patients with bipolar disorder. The use of tamoxifen in women with breast cancer, although commonly well tolerated (aside from yielding menopausal symptoms), entails small (triple- to quadruple-digit NNHs per patient-year compared with placebo) risks of endometrial cancer and cerebrovascular/pulmonary embolism. Thus, safety/tolerability concerns suggest the possibility that using tamoxifen as a third-line clinical intervention in acute mania (Yatham et al. 2009) may be premature (Shen et al. 2009). These considerations, combined with the broad array of other treatments for acute mania listed in Tiers I–IV, appear to indicate that for the time being tamoxifen ought to remain a research (rather than a clinical) tool for the treatment of acute mania, and so this agent has been placed in Tier V.

■ Conclusion

Clinical research has provided not only important additional options for acute mania treatment but also enhanced understanding of the efficacy and safety/tolerability of older agents. SGAs and anticonvulsants are the two main groups of non-lithium agents that have been investigated in acute mania. SGAs may commonly be effective for acute mania but vary importantly with respect to safety/tolerability. In contrast, anticonvulsants have more heterogeneous efficacy profiles, and although (aside from valproate, carbamazepine, and possibly oxcarbazepine) they are not efficacious for acute mania, a few (but not most) have efficacy for conditions that commonly co-occur in patients with bipolar disorder, combined with adequate safety/tolerability.

■ References

Ahlfors UG, Baastrup PC, Dencker SJ, et al: Flupenthixol decanoate in recurrent manic-depressive illness. A comparison with lithium. Acta Psychiatr Scand 64(3):226–237, 1981 7324992

Amann B, Sterr A, Vieta E, et al: An exploratory open trial on safety and efficacy of the anticonvulsant retigabine in acute manic patients. J Clin Psychopharmacol 26(5):534–536, 2006 16974202

American Psychiatric Association: Diagnostic and Statistical Manual of Mental Disorders, 4th Edition, Text Revision. Washington, DC, American Psychiatric Association, 2000

American Psychiatric Association: Practice guideline for the treatment of patients with bipolar disorder (revision). Am J Psychiatry 159(4)(Suppl):1–50, 2002 11958165

American Psychiatric Association: Diagnostic and Statistical Manual of Mental Disorders, 5th Edition. Washington, DC, American Psychiatric Association, 2013

Amrollahi Z, Rezaei F, Salehi B, et al: Double-blind, randomized, placebo-controlled 6-week study on the efficacy and safety of the tamoxifen adjunctive to lithium in acute bipolar mania. J Affect Disord 129(1–3):327–331, 2011 20843556

Andersen T, Lingjaerde O: Nitrazepam (Mogadon) as a sleep-inducing agent. An analysis based on a double-blind comparison with phenobarbitone. Br J Psychiatry 115(529):1393–1397, 1969 4902186

Ballenger JC, Burrows GD, DuPont RL Jr, et al: Alprazolam in panic disorder and agoraphobia: results from a multicenter trial. I. Efficacy in short-term treatment. Arch Gen Psychiatry 45(5):413–422, 1988 3282478

Battaglia J, Moss S, Rush J, et al: Haloperidol, lorazepam, or both for psychotic agitation? A multicenter, prospective, double-blind, emergency department study. Am J Emerg Med 15(4):335–340, 1997 9217519

Berwaerts J, Lane R, Nuamah IF, et al: Paliperidone extended-release as adjunctive therapy to lithium or valproate in the treatment of acute mania: a randomized, placebo-controlled study. J Affect Disord 129(1–3):252–260, 2011 20947174

Berwaerts J, Xu H, Nuamah I, et al: Evaluation of the efficacy and safety of paliperidone extended-release in the treatment of acute mania: a randomized, double-blind, dose-response study. J Affect Disord 136(1–2):e51–e60, 2012 20624657

Bieniek SA, Ownby RL, Penalver A, et al: A double-blind study of lorazepam versus the combination of haloperidol and lorazepam in managing agitation. Pharmacotherapy 18(1):57–62, 1998 9469682

Bowden CL, Brugger AM, Swann AC, et al; The Depakote Mania Study Group: Efficacy of divalproex vs lithium and placebo in the treatment of mania. JAMA 271(12):918–924, 1994 8120960

Bowden C, Calabrese J, Ascher J, et al: Spectrum of efficacy of lamotrigine in bipolar disorder: overview of double-blind placebo-controlled studies. Paper presented at the 39th Annual Meeting of the American College of Neuropsychopharmacology, San Juan, Puerto Rico, December 10–14, 2000

Bowden CL, Grunze H, Mullen J, et al: A randomized, double-blind, placebo-controlled efficacy and safety study of quetiapine or lithium as monotherapy for mania in bipolar disorder. J Clin Psychiatry 66(1):111–121, 2005 15669897

Bowden CL, Swann AC, Calabrese JR, et al; Depakote ER Mania Study Group: A randomized, placebo-controlled, multicenter study of divalproex sodium extended release in the treatment of acute mania. J Clin Psychiatry 67(10):1501–1510, 2006 17107240

Brandes JL, Saper JR, Diamond M, et al; MIGR-002 Study Group: Topiramate for migraine prevention: a randomized controlled trial. JAMA 291(8):965–973, 2004 14982912

Bray GA, Hollander P, Klein S, et al: A 6-month randomized, placebo-controlled, dose-ranging trial of topiramate for weight loss in obesity. Obes Res 11(6):722–733, 2003 12805393

Cade JFJ: Lithium salts in the treatment of psychotic excitement. Med J Aust 2(10):349–352, 1949 18142718

Calabrese J, Lu K, Laszlovszky I, et al: Efficacy of cariprazine in patients with acute manic or mixed episodes associated with bipolar I disorder: results from 2 phase III, placebo-controlled trials. Paper presented at the 16th Annual Conference of the International Society for Bipolar Disorders, Seoul, South Korea, March 18–21, 2014

Cipriani A, Barbui C, Salanti G, et al: Comparative efficacy and acceptability of antimanic drugs in acute mania: a multiple-treatments meta-analysis. Lancet 378(9799):1306–1315, 2011 21851976

Citrome L: Addressing the need for rapid treatment of agitation in schizophrenia and bipolar disorder: focus on inhaled loxapine as an alternative to injectable agents. Ther Clin Risk Manag 9:235–245, 2013 23723707

Claudino AM, de Oliveira IR, Appolinario JC, et al: Double-blind, randomized, placebo-controlled trial of topiramate plus cognitive-behavior therapy in binge-eating disorder. J Clin Psychiatry 68(9):1324–1332, 2007 17915969

Cookson J, Silverstone T, Wells B: Double-blind comparative clinical trial of pimozide and chlorpromazine in mania. A test of the dopamine hypothesis. Acta Psychiatr Scand 64(5):381–397, 1981 7051755

Cutler AJ, Datto C, Nordenhem A, et al: Extended-release quetiapine as monotherapy for the treatment of adults with acute mania: a randomized, double-blind, 3-week trial. Clin Ther 33(11):1643–1658, 2011 22054797

Daniel DG, Brook S, Warrington L, et al: Intramuscular ziprasidone in agitated psychotic patients. Paper presented at the 157th Annual Meeting of the American Psychiatric Association, New York, NY, May 1–6, 2004

Delbello MP, Schwiers ML, Rosenberg HL, et al: A double-blind, randomized, placebo-controlled study of quetiapine as adjunctive treatment for adolescent mania. J Am Acad Child Adolesc Psychiatry 41(10):1216–1223, 2002 12364843

DelBello MP, Findling RL, Earley WR, et al: Efficacy of quetiapine in children and adolescents with bipolar mania: a 3-week, double-blind, randomized, placebo-controlled trial. Paper presented at the 46th Annual Meeting of the American College of Neuropsychopharmacology, Boca Raton, Florida, December 9–13, 2007

DelBello MP, Findling RL, Wang PP, et al: Safety and efficacy of ziprasidone in pediatric bipolar disorder. Paper presented at the 55th Annual Convention and Scientific Program of the Society of Biological Psychiatry, Washington, DC, May 1–3, 2008

DiazGranados N, Zarate CA Jr: A review of the preclinical and clinical evidence for protein kinase C as a target for drug development for bipolar disorder. Curr Psychiatry Rep 10(6):510–519, 2008 18980735

Egger C, Muehlbacher M, Schatz M, et al: Influence of topiramate on olanzapine-related weight gain in women: an 18-month follow-up observation. J Clin Psychopharmacol 27(5):475–478, 2007 17873679

Foster S, Kessel J, Berman ME, et al: Efficacy of lorazepam and haloperidol for rapid tranquilization in a psychiatric emergency room setting. Int Clin Psychopharmacol 12(3):175–179, 1997 9248875

Freeman TW, Clothier JL, Pazzaglia P, et al: A double-blind comparison of valproate and lithium in the treatment of acute mania. Am J Psychiatry 149(1):108–111, 1992 1728157

Frye MA, Ketter TA, Kimbrell TA, et al: A placebo-controlled study of lamotrigine and gabapentin monotherapy in refractory mood disorders. J Clin Psychopharmacol 20(6):607–614, 2000 11106131

Gadde KM, Franciscy DM, Wagner HR 2nd, et al: Zonisamide for weight loss in obese adults: a randomized controlled trial. JAMA 289(14):1820–1825, 2003 12684361

Gadde KM, Yonish GM, Foust MS, et al: Combination therapy of zonisamide and bupropion for weight reduction in obese women: a preliminary, randomized, open-label study. J Clin Psychiatry 68(8):1226–1229, 2007 17854247

Garfinkel PE, Stancer HC, Persad E: A comparison of haloperidol, lithium carbonate and their combination in the treatment of mania. J Affect Disord 2(4):279–288, 1980 6450787

Goldsmith DR, Wagstaff AJ, Ibbotson T, et al: Lamotrigine: a review of its use in bipolar disorder. Drugs 63(19):2029–2050, 2003 12962521

Goodwin FK, Murphy DL, Bunney WE Jr: Lithium-carbonate treatment in depression and mania. A longitudinal double-blind study. Arch Gen Psychiatry 21(4):486–496, 1969 4896983

Goodwin GM; Consensus Group of the British Association for Psychopharmacology: Evidence-based guidelines for treating bipolar disorder: recommendations from the British Association for Psychopharmacology. J Psychopharmacol 17(2):149–173, discussion 147, 2003 12870562

Grunze H, Erfurth A, Marcuse A, et al: Tiagabine appears not to be efficacious in the treatment of acute mania. J Clin Psychiatry 60(11):759–762, 1999 10584764

Grunze H, Kasper S, Goodwin G, et al; World Federation of Societies of Biological Psychiatry Task Force on Treatment Guidelines for Bipolar Disorders: World Federation of Societies of Biological Psychiatry (WFSBP) guidelines for biological treatment of bipolar disorders. Part I: Treatment of bipolar depression. World J Biol Psychiatry 3(3):115–124, 2002 12478876

Haas M, Delbello MP, Pandina G, et al: Risperidone for the treatment of acute mania in children and adolescents with bipolar disorder: a randomized, double-blind, placebo-controlled study. Bipolar Disord 11(7):687–700, 2009 19839994

Hirschfeld RM, Keck PE Jr, Kramer M, et al: Rapid antimanic effect of risperidone monotherapy: a 3-week multicenter, double-blind, placebo-controlled trial. Am J Psychiatry 161(6):1057–1065, 2004 15169694

Hoopes SP, Reimherr FW, Hedges DW, et al: Treatment of bulimia nervosa with topiramate in a randomized, double-blind, placebo-controlled trial, part 1: improvement in binge and purge measures. J Clin Psychiatry 64(11):1335–1341, 2003 14658948

Janicak PG, Bresnahan DB, Sharma R, et al: A comparison of thiothixene with chlorpromazine in the treatment of mania. J Clin Psychopharmacol 8(1):33–37, 1988 3280617

Janicak PG, Newman RH, Davis JM: Advances in the treatment of mania and related disorders: a reappraisal. Psychiatr Ann 22:92–103, 1992

Johnson BA, Ait-Daoud N, Bowden CL, et al: Oral topiramate for treatment of alcohol dependence: a randomised controlled trial. Lancet 361(9370):1677–1685, 2003 12767733

Johnson BA, Rosenthal N, Capece JA, et al; Topiramate for Alcoholism Advisory Board; Topiramate for Alcoholism Study Group: Topiramate for treating alcohol dependence: a randomized controlled trial. JAMA 298(14):1641–1651, 2007 17925516

Johnson G, Gershon S, Hekimian LJ: Controlled evaluation of lithium and chlorpromazine in the treatment of manic states: an interim report. Compr Psychiatry 9(6):563–573, 1968 4883428

Johnson G, Gershon S, Burdock EI, et al: Comparative effects of lithium and chlorpromazine in the treatment of acute manic states. Br J Psychiatry 119(550):267–276, 1971 4936131

Kanba S, Yagi G, Kamijima K, et al: The first open study of zonisamide, a novel anticonvulsant, shows efficacy in mania. Prog Neuropsychopharmacol Biol Psychiatry 18(4):707–715, 1994 7938561

Kane JM, Smith JM: Tardive dyskinesia: prevalence and risk factors, 1959 to 1979. Arch Gen Psychiatry 39(4):473–481, 1982 6121548

Keck PE Jr, Marcus R, Tourkodimitris S, et al; Aripiprazole Study Group: A placebo-controlled, double-blind study of the efficacy and safety of aripiprazole in patients with acute bipolar mania. Am J Psychiatry 160(9):1651–1658, 2003a 12944341

Keck PE Jr, Versiani M, Potkin S, et al; Ziprasidone in Mania Study Group: Ziprasidone in the treatment of acute bipolar mania: a three-week, placebo-controlled, double-blind, randomized trial. Am J Psychiatry 160(4):741–748, 2003b 12668364

Keck PE, Perlis RH, Otto MW, et al: The expert consensus guideline series: medication treatment of bipolar disorder 2004. Postgrad Med Special Report 1–120, 2004

Keller MB, Lavori PW, Coryell W, et al: Differential outcome of pure manic, mixed/cycling, and pure depressive episodes in patients with bipolar illness. JAMA 255(22):3138–3142, 1986 3702024

Ketter TA: Handbook of Diagnosis and Treatment of Bipolar Disorders. Washington, DC, American Psychiatric Publishing, 2010

Ketter TA, Post RM, Worthington K: Principles of clinically important drug interactions with carbamazepine. Part I. J Clin Psychopharmacol 11(3):198–203, 1991a 2066459

Ketter TA, Post RM, Worthington K: Principles of clinically important drug interactions with carbamazepine. Part II. J Clin Psychopharmacol 11(5):306–313, 1991b 1765573

Ketter TA, Sachs GS, Lu K, et al: Long-term safety and tolerability of open-label cariprazine in patients with bipolar I disorder. Paper presented at the 10th International Conference on Bipolar Disorder, Miami Beach, FL, June 13–16, 2013

Ketter TA, Lu K, Debelle M, et al: Safety and tolerability of cariprazine in patients with acute manic or mixed episodes associated with bipolar I disorder: results from 2 phase III placebo-controlled trials. Paper presented at the 16th Annual Conference of the International Society for Bipolar Disorders, Seoul, South Korea, March 18–21, 2014

Khanna S, Vieta E, Lyons B, et al: Risperidone in the treatment of acute mania: double-blind, placebo-controlled study. Br J Psychiatry 187:229–234, 2005 16135859

Kramlinger KG, Post RM: Adding lithium carbonate to carbamazepine: antimanic efficacy in treatment-resistant mania. Acta Psychiatr Scand 79(4):378–385, 1989 2500006

Krauthammer C, Klerman GL: Secondary mania: manic syndromes associated with antecedent physical illness or drugs. Arch Gen Psychiatry 35(11):1333–1339, 1978 757997

Kukopulos A, Reginaldi D, Laddomada P, et al: Course of the manic-depressive cycle and changes caused by treatment. Pharmakopsychiatr Neuropsychopharmakol 13(4):156–167, 1980 6108577

Kulkarni J, Garland KA, Scaffidi A, et al: A pilot study of hormone modulation as a new treatment for mania in women with bipolar affective disorder. Psychoneuroendocrinology 31(4):543–547, 2006 16356651

Kulkarni J, Berk M, Wang W, et al: A four week randomised control trial of adjunctive medroxyprogesterone and tamoxifen in women with mania. Psychoneuroendocrinology 43:52–61, 2014 24703170

Kushner SF, Khan A, Lane R, Olson WH: Topiramate monotherapy in the management of acute mania: results of four double-blind placebo-controlled trials. Bipolar Disord 8(1):15–27, 2006 16411977

Kwentus J, Riesenberg RA, Marandi M, et al: Rapid acute treatment of agitation in patients with bipolar I disorder: a multicenter, randomized, placebo-controlled clinical trial with inhaled loxapine. Bipolar Disord 14(1):31–40, 2012 22329470

Loew TH, Nickel MK, Muehlbacher M, et al: Topiramate treatment for women with borderline personality disorder: a double-blind, placebo-controlled study. J Clin Psychopharmacol 26(1):61–66, 2006 16415708

Maggs R: Treatment of manic illness with lithium carbonate. Br J Psychiatry 109:56–65, 1963

Mason BJ, Quello S, Goodell V, et al: Gabapentin treatment for alcohol dependence: a randomized clinical trial. JAMA Intern Med 174(1):70–77, 2014 24190578

McElroy SL, Arnold LM, Shapira NA, et al: Topiramate in the treatment of binge eating disorder associated with obesity: a randomized, placebo-controlled trial. Am J Psychiatry 160(2):255–261, 2003 12562571

McElroy SL, Suppes T, Keck PE Jr, et al: Open-label adjunctive zonisamide in the treatment of bipolar disorders: a prospective trial. J Clin Psychiatry 66(5):617–624, 2005 15889949

McElroy SL, Kotwal R, Guerdjikova AI, et al: Zonisamide in the treatment of binge eating disorder with obesity: a randomized controlled trial. J Clin Psychiatry 67(12):1897–1906, 2006 17194267

McElroy SL, Frye MA, Altshuler LL, et al: A 24-week, randomized, controlled trial of adjunctive sibutramine versus topiramate in the treatment of weight gain in overweight or obese patients with bipolar disorders. Bipolar Disord 9(4):426–434, 2007 17547588

McIntyre RS, Mancini DA, McCann S, et al: Topiramate versus bupropion SR when added to mood stabilizer therapy for the depressive phase of bipolar disorder: a preliminary single-blind study. Bipolar Disord 4(3):207–213, 2002 12180276

McIntyre RS, Brecher M, Paulsson B, et al: Quetiapine or haloperidol as monotherapy for bipolar mania—a 12-week, double-blind, randomised, parallel-group, placebo-controlled trial. Eur Neuropsychopharmacol 15(5):573–585, 2005 16139175

McIntyre RS, Cohen M, Zhao J, et al: A 3-week, randomized, placebo-controlled trial of asenapine in the treatment of acute mania in bipolar mania and mixed states. Bipolar Disord 11(7):673–686, 2009 19839993

McIntyre RS, Cohen M, Zhao J, et al: Asenapine in the treatment of acute mania in bipolar I disorder: a randomized, double-blind, placebo-controlled trial. J Affect Disord 122(1–2):27–38, 2010 20096936

Muehlbacher M, Nickel MK, Kettler C, et al: Topiramate in treatment of patients with chronic low back pain: a randomized, double-blind, placebo-controlled study. Clin J Pain 22(6):526–531, 2006 16788338

Mukherjee S, Sackeim HA, Schnur DB: Electroconvulsive therapy of acute manic episodes: a review of 50 years' experience. Am J Psychiatry 151(2):169–176, 1994 8296883

Nasrallah HA, Churchill CM, Hamdan-Allan GA: Higher frequency of neuroleptic-induced dystonia in mania than in schizophrenia. Am J Psychiatry 145(11):1455–1456, 1988 2903686

Okuma T, Yamashita I, Takahashi R, et al: Clinical efficacy of carbamazepine in affective, schizoaffective, and schizophrenic disorders. Pharmacopsychiatry 22(2):47–53, 1989 2717658

Ondo WG, Jankovic J, Connor GS, et al; Topiramate Essential Tremor Study Investigators: Topiramate in essential tremor: a double-blind, placebo-controlled trial. Neurology 66(5):672–677, 2006 16436648

Pande AC, Davidson JR, Jefferson JW, et al: Treatment of social phobia with gabapentin: a placebo-controlled study. J Clin Psychopharmacol 19(4):341–348, 1999 10440462

Pande AC, Crockatt JG, Janney CA, et al; Gabapentin Bipolar Disorder Study Group: Gabapentin in bipolar disorder: a placebo-controlled trial of adjunctive therapy. Bipolar Disord 2(3 Pt 2):249–255, 2000a 11249802

Pande AC, Pollack MH, Crockatt J, et al: Placebo-controlled study of gabapentin treatment of panic disorder. J Clin Psychopharmacol 20(4):467–471, 2000b 10917408

Platman SR: A comparison of lithium carbonate and chlorpromazine in mania. Am J Psychiatry 127(3):351–353, 1970 4917856

Pope HG Jr, McElroy SL, Keck PE Jr, et al: Valproate in the treatment of acute mania. A placebo-controlled study. Arch Gen Psychiatry 48(1):62–68, 1991 1984763

Post RM, Jimerson DC, Bunney WE Jr, et al: Dopamine and mania: behavioral and biochemical effects of the dopamine receptor blocker pimozide. Psychopharmacology (Berl) 67(3):297–305, 1980 6155678

Potkin SG, Keck PE Jr, Segal S, et al: Ziprasidone in acute bipolar mania: a 21-day randomized, double-blind, placebo-controlled replication trial. J Clin Psychopharmacol 25(4):301–310, 2005 16012271

Prien RF, Caffey EM Jr, Klett CJ; Report of the Veterans Administration and National Institute of Mental Health Collaborative Study Group: Comparison of lithium carbonate and chlorpromazine in the treatment of mania. Arch Gen Psychiatry 26(2):146–153, 1972 4551257

Rosenstock J, Hollander P, Gadde KM, et al; OBD-202 Study Group: A randomized, double-blind, placebo-controlled, multicenter study to assess the efficacy and safety of topiramate controlled release in the treatment of obese type 2 diabetic patients. Diabetes Care 30(6):1480–1486, 2007 17363756

Rosenthal M: Tiagabine for the treatment of generalized anxiety disorder: a randomized, open-label, clinical trial with paroxetine as a positive control. J Clin Psychiatry 64(10):1245–1249, 2003 14658975

Rowbotham M, Harden N, Stacey B, et al: Gabapentin for the treatment of postherpetic neuralgia: a randomized controlled trial. JAMA 280(21):1837–1842, 1998 9846778

Sachs GS, Grossman F, Ghaemi SN, et al: Combination of a mood stabilizer with risperidone or haloperidol for treatment of acute mania: a double-blind, placebo-controlled comparison of efficacy and safety. Am J Psychiatry 159(7):1146–1154, 2002 12091192

Sachs G, Chengappa KN, Suppes T, et al: Quetiapine with lithium or divalproex for the treatment of bipolar mania: a randomized, double-blind, placebo-controlled study. Bipolar Disord 6(3):213–223, 2004 15117400

Sachs G, Sanchez R, Marcus R, et al; Aripiprazole Study Group: Aripiprazole in the treatment of acute manic or mixed episodes in patients with bipolar I disorder: a 3-week placebo-controlled study. J Psychopharmacol 20(4):536–546, 2006 16401666

Sachs GS, Vanderburg DG, Edman S, et al: Adjunctive oral ziprasidone in patients with acute mania treated with lithium or divalproex, part 2: influence of protocol-specific eligibility criteria on signal detection. J Clin Psychiatry 73(11):1420–1425, 2012a 23218158

Sachs GS, Vanderburg DG, Karayal ON, et al: Adjunctive oral ziprasidone in patients with acute mania treated with lithium or divalproex, part 1: results of a randomized, double-blind, placebo-controlled trial. J Clin Psychiatry 73(11):1412–1419, 2012b 23218157

Schaffer LC, Schaffer CB, Howe J: An open case series on the utility of tiagabine as an augmentation in refractory bipolar outpatients. J Affect Disord 71(1–3):259–263, 2002 12167526

Schou M, Juel-Nielsen N, Strömgren E, et al: The treatment of manic psychoses by the administration of lithium salts. J Neurol Neurosurg Psychiatry 17(4):250–260, 1954 13212414

Secunda SK, Katz MM, Swann A, et al: Mania. Diagnosis, state measurement and prediction of treatment response. J Affect Disord 8(2):113–121, 1985 3157719

Serpell MG; Neuropathic Pain Study Group: Gabapentin in neuropathic pain syndromes: a randomised, double-blind, placebo-controlled trial. Pain 99(3):557–566, 2002 12406532

Shen CC, Bai YM, Su TP: Comment to Dr. Yatham regarding tamoxifen listed as a third-line recommendation for the pharmacological treatment of acute mania. Bipolar Disord 11(7):773–775, author reply 775, 2009 19840002

Shopsin B, Gershon S, Thompson H, et al: Psychoactive drugs in mania. A controlled comparison of lithium carbonate, chlorpromazine, and haloperidol. Arch Gen Psychiatry 32(1):34–42, 1975 1089401

Silberstein SD, Lipton RB, Dodick DW, et al; Topiramate Chronic Migraine Study Group: Efficacy and safety of topiramate for the treatment of chronic migraine: a randomized, double-blind, placebo-controlled trial. Headache 47(2):170–180, 2007 17300356

Small JG, Milstein V: Lithium interactions: lithium and electroconvulsive therapy. J Clin Psychopharmacol 10(5):346–350, 1990 2258451

Small JG, Klapper MH, Marhenke JD, et al: Lithium combined with carbamazepine or haloperidol in the treatment of mania. Psychopharmacol Bull 31(2):265–272, 1995 7491378

Smulevich AB, Khanna S, Eerdekens M, et al: Acute and continuation risperidone monotherapy in bipolar mania: a 3-week placebo-controlled trial followed by a 9-week double-blind trial of risperidone and haloperidol. Eur Neuropsychopharmacol 15(1):75–84, 2005 15572276

Spira PJ, Beran RG; Australian Gabapentin Chronic Daily Headache Group: Gabapentin in the prophylaxis of chronic daily headache: a randomized, placebo-controlled study. Neurology 61(12):1753–1759, 2003 14694042

Spring G, Schweid D, Gray C, et al: A double-blind comparison of lithium and chlorpromazine in the treatment of manic states. Am J Psychiatry 126(9):1306–1310, 1970 4905019

Starace A, Bose A, Wang Q, et al: Cariprazine in the treatment of acute mania in bipolar disorder: a double-blind, placebo-controlled, phase III trial. Paper presented at the 165th Annual Meeting of the American Psychiatric Association, Philadelphia, PA, May 5–9, 2012

Stenlöf K, Rössner S, Vercruysse F, et al; OBDM-003 Study Group: Topiramate in the treatment of obese subjects with drug-naive type 2 diabetes. Diabetes Obes Metab 9(3):360–368, 2007 17391164

Stokes PE, Shamoian CA, Stoll PM, et al: Efficacy of lithium as acute treatment of manic-depressive illness. Lancet 1(7713):1319–1325, 1971 4103395

Suppes T, Chisholm KA, Dhavale D, et al: Tiagabine in treatment refractory bipolar disorder: a clinical case series. Bipolar Disord 4(5):283–289, 2002 12479659

Suppes T, Dennehy EB, Hirschfeld RM, et al; Texas Consensus Conference Panel on Medication Treatment of Bipolar Disorder: The Texas implementation of medication algorithms: update to the algorithms for treatment of bipolar I disorder. J Clin Psychiatry 66(7):870–886, 2005 16013903

Swann AC, Bowden CL, Morris D, et al: Depression during mania. Treatment response to lithium or divalproex. Arch Gen Psychiatry 54(1):37–42, 1997 9006398

Swann AC, Bowden CL, Calabrese JR, et al: Mania: differential effects of previous depressive and manic episodes on response to treatment. Acta Psychiatr Scand 101(6):444–451, 2000 10868467

Swann AC, Bowden CL, Calabrese JR, et al: Pattern of response to divalproex, lithium, or placebo in four naturalistic subtypes of mania. Neuropsychopharmacology 26(4):530–536, 2002 11927177

Swartz HA, Frank E: Psychotherapy for bipolar depression: a phase-specific treatment strategy? Bipolar Disord 3(1):11–22, 2001 11256459

Szegedi A, Calabrese JR, Stet L, et al; Apollo Study Group: Asenapine as adjunctive treatment for acute mania associated with bipolar disorder: results of a 12-week core study and 40-week extension. J Clin Psychopharmacol 32(1):46–55, 2012 22198448

Takahashi R, Sakuma A, Itoh K, et al: Comparison of efficacy of lithium carbonate and chlorpromazine in mania. Report of collaborative study group on treatment of mania in Japan. Arch Gen Psychiatry 32(10):1310–1318, 1975 1101844

Tarr GP, Glue P, Herbison P: Comparative efficacy and acceptability of mood stabilizer and second generation antipsychotic monotherapy for acute mania—a systematic review and meta-analysis. J Affect Disord 134(1–3):14–19, 2011 21145595

Tohen M, Sanger TM, McElroy SL, et al: Olanzapine versus placebo in the treatment of acute mania. The Olanzapine HGEH Study Group. Am J Psychiatry 156(5):702–709, 1999 10327902

Tohen M, Jacobs TG, Grundy SL, et al: Efficacy of olanzapine in acute bipolar mania: a double-blind, placebo-controlled study. The Olanzapine HGEH Study Group. Arch Gen Psychiatry 57(9):841–849, 2000 10986547

Tohen M, Chengappa KN, Suppes T, et al: Efficacy of olanzapine in combination with valproate or lithium in the treatment of mania in patients partially nonresponsive to valproate or lithium monotherapy. Arch Gen Psychiatry 59(1):62–69, 2002 11779284

Tohen M, Calabrese JR, Sachs GS, et al: Randomized, placebo-controlled trial of olanzapine as maintenance therapy in patients with bipolar I disorder responding to acute treatment with olanzapine. Am J Psychiatry 163(2):247–256, 2006 16449478

Tohen M, Kryzhanovskaya L, Carlson G, et al: Olanzapine versus placebo in the treatment of adolescents with bipolar mania. Am J Psychiatry 164(10):1547–1556, 2007 17898346

Tohen M, Bowden CL, Smulevich AB, et al: Olanzapine plus carbamazepine v. carbamazepine alone in treating manic episodes. Br J Psychiatry 192(2):135–143, 2008 18245032

Toplak H, Hamann A, Moore R, et al: Efficacy and safety of topiramate in combination with metformin in the treatment of obese subjects with type 2 diabetes: a randomized, double-blind, placebo-controlled study. Int J Obes (Lond) 31(1):138–146, 2007 16703004

Tremblay A, Chaput JP, Bérubé-Parent S, et al: The effect of topiramate on energy balance in obese men: a 6-month double-blind randomized placebo-controlled study with a 6-month open-label extension. Eur J Clin Pharmacol 63(2):123–134, 2007 17200837

Vieta E, T'joen C, McQuade RD, et al: Efficacy of adjunctive aripiprazole to either valproate or lithium in bipolar mania patients partially nonresponsive to valproate/lithium monotherapy: a placebo-controlled study. Am J Psychiatry 165(10):1316–1325, 2008 18381903

Vieta E, Nuamah IF, Lim P, et al: A randomized, placebo- and active-controlled study of paliperidone extended release for the treatment of acute manic and mixed episodes of bipolar I disorder. Bipolar Disord 12(3):230–243, 2010a 20565430

Vieta E, Ramey T, Keller D, et al: Ziprasidone in the treatment of acute mania: a 12-week, placebo-controlled, haloperidol-referenced study. J Psychopharmacol 24(4):547–558 2010b 19074536

Wagner KD, Kowatch RA, Emslie GJ, et al: A double-blind, randomized, placebo-controlled trial of oxcarbazepine in the treatment of bipolar disorder in children and adolescents. Am J Psychiatry 163(7):1179–1186, 2006 16816222

Warrington L, Lombardo I, Loebel A, et al: Ziprasidone for the treatment of acute manic or mixed episodes associated with bipolar disorder. CNS Drugs 21(10):835–849, 2007 17850172

Weisler RH, Kalali AH, Ketter TA; SPD417 Study Group: A multicenter, randomized, double-blind, placebo-controlled trial of extended-release carbamazepine capsules as monotherapy for bipolar disorder patients with manic or mixed episodes. J Clin Psychiatry 65(4):478–484, 2004a 15119909

Weisler RH, Warrington L, Dunn J, et al: Adjunctive ziprasidone in bipolar mania: short-term and long-term data. Paper presented at the 157th Annual Meeting of the American Psychiatric Association, New York, NY, May 1–6, 2004b

Weisler RH, Keck PE Jr, Swann AC, et al; SPD417 Study Group: Extended-release carbamazepine capsules as monotherapy for acute mania in bipolar disorder: a multicenter, randomized, double-blind, placebo-controlled trial. J Clin Psychiatry 66(3):323–330, 2005 15766298

Weisler RH, Hirschfeld R, Cutler AJ, et al; SPD417 Study Group: Extended-release carbamazepine capsules as monotherapy in bipolar disorder: pooled results from two randomised, double-blind, placebo-controlled trials. CNS Drugs 20(3):219–231, 2006 16529527

Yatham LN, Grossman F, Augustyns I, et al: Mood stabilisers plus risperidone or placebo in the treatment of acute mania. International, double-blind, randomised controlled trial. Br J Psychiatry 182:141–147, 2003 12562742

Yatham LN, Paulsson B, Mullen J, et al: Quetiapine versus placebo in combination with lithium or divalproex for the treatment of bipolar mania. J Clin Psychopharmacol 24(6):599–606, 2004 15538120

Yatham LN, Kennedy SH, O'Donovan C, et al; Guidelines Group, CANMAT: Canadian Network for Mood and Anxiety Treatments (CANMAT) guidelines for the management of patients with bipolar disorder: update 2007. Bipolar Disord 8(6):721–739, 2006 17156158

Yatham LN, Kennedy SH, Schaffer A, et al: Canadian Network for Mood and Anxiety Treatments (CANMAT) and International Society for Bipolar Disorders (ISBD) collaborative update of CANMAT guidelines for the management of patients with bipolar disorder: update 2009. Bipolar Disord 11(3):225–255, 2009 19419382

Yildiz A, Guleryuz S, Ankerst DP, et al: Protein kinase C inhibition in the treatment of mania: a double-blind, placebo-controlled trial of tamoxifen. Arch Gen Psychiatry 65(3):255–263, 2008 18316672

Zarate CA Jr, Singh JB, Carlson PJ, et al: Efficacy of a protein kinase C inhibitor (tamoxifen) in the treatment of acute mania: a pilot study. Bipolar Disord 9(6):561–570, 2007 17845270

Zimbroff DL, Marcus RN, Manos G, et al: Management of acute agitation in patients with bipolar disorder: efficacy and safety of intramuscular aripiprazole. J Clin Psychopharmacol 27(2):171–176, 2007 17414241

4 Bipolar Disorder Preventive Treatment

Terence A. Ketter, M.D.
Shefali Miller, M.D.
Jenifer Culver, Ph.D.

The recurrent episodic nature of bipolar disorder, and the dysfunction, morbidity, illness progression, and mortality associated with acute episodes, make prevention of new episodes a crucial goal. Recurrent mood disorders worsen with increasing number of episodes, in that episodes progress from reactive to stress to spontaneous, and become more frequent, more severe, and ultimately resistant to treatment—this has been termed the *kindling theory of mood disorders* (Post 1992). Thus, preventing episodes may prevent bipolar illness progression, including increasing severity of affective symptoms and cognitive and functional impairment. Naturalistic (Judd et al. 2002, 2003) and controlled (Vieta et al. 2009) data suggest that depressive compared with mood elevation symptoms are more pervasive over time.

Although most treated patients achieve symptomatic recovery (absence of affective symptoms), less than half may achieve functional recovery (absence of cognitive/functional impairment) within 2 years of a first manic/mixed episode (Tohen et al. 2003b). Hence, the goals of longer-term treatment need to include attaining and preserving not only full symptomatic recovery but also full functional recovery.

Lithium was approved by the U.S. Food and Drug Administration (FDA) for bipolar disorder preventive treatment in 1974 and for almost three decades was the only agent with such an approval (see Table 1–1 in Chapter 1, "Diagnosis and Treatment of Bipolar Disorder"). Lithium was perceived as being unique because it was effective in acute mania and bipolar disorder preventive treatment, as well as (perhaps to a lesser extent) in acute bipolar depression. In contrast, first-generation antipsychotics could relieve mania but might exacerbate depression, and older antidepressants could relieve depression but might exacerbate mania, and therefore these were considered unimodal agents. Considered the only bimodal agent, lithium could address not only acute episodes of either polarity but also the disorder as a whole over time (i.e., it could help prevent episodes). The term *mood stabilizer* was applied to lithium, distinguishing it from other classes of agents and emphasizing its role as "the" (as opposed to "a") comprehensive treatment for bipolar disorder.

After two decades, the notion that lithium was the only mood stabilizer was challenged, and divalproex received FDA approval for the treatment of acute mania (Bowden et al. 1994). Divalproex was not an antipsychotic, had efficacy in acute mania, did not appear to exacerbate depression, and, in spite of lacking an FDA indication for bipolar disorder preventive treatment (Bowden et al. 2000), was commonly used in longer-term bipolar disorder treatment and became referred to as a mood stabilizer. In a similar fashion, carbamazepine became referred to as an mood stabilizer.

In 2003, lamotrigine was approved by the FDA as the first alternative to lithium for bipolar disorder preventive treatment (Goodwin et al. 2004). Lamotrigine was distinctive in two important ways: 1) unlike lithium, divalproex, or carbamazepine, it could "stabilize mood from below," being more effective against depressive than mood elevation aspects of the illness (Ketter and Calabrese 2002); and 2) it received an FDA bipolar disorder preventive treatment indication despite lacking an FDA acute bipolar disorder indication (specifically, lamotrigine was not approved by the FDA for acute bipolar depression). Thus, lamotrigine became the third anticonvulsant to address a component (in this case preventive treatment) of bipolar disorder without exacerbating other aspects of the illness and also became referred to as a mood stabilizer. As of early 2015, there was still no consensus definition of the term *mood stabilizer*, and the FDA did not use the term, although agents with bipolar indications that were not antipsychotics—that is, lithium, divalproex, carbamazepine, and lamotrigine—were commonly referred to as such.

In 2004 and 2005, the second-generation antipsychotics (SGAs) olanzapine (Tohen et al. 2006) and aripiprazole (Keck et al. 2006), respectively, received FDA approval for bipolar disorder preventive treatment. Moreover, in 2008, quetiapine received the first adjunctive (added to lithium or valproate) bipolar disorder preventive treatment indication (Suppes et al. 2009). The FDA subsequently granted bipolar disorder preventive treatment approvals for risperidone long-acting injectable (LAI) formulation monotherapy (Quiroz et al. 2010) and adjunctive (added to lithium or valproate) therapy (Macfadden et al. 2009), ziprasidone adjunctive (added to lithium or valproate) therapy (Bowden et al. 2010) in 2009, and aripiprazole adjunctive (added to lithium or valproate) therapy (Marcus et al. 2011) in 2011. Finally, although lacking FDA approval for bipolar disorder preventive treatment, one multicenter, double-blind, placebo-controlled trial supported the efficacy of quetiapine monotherapy (Weisler et al. 2011), whereas another such trial failed to detect efficacy for aripiprazole when added to lamotrigine (Carlson et al. 2012).

These developments further challenged assumptions that antipsychotics were mere short-term adjuncts for acute mania that needed to be discontinued as quickly as possible to minimize the risks of tardive dyskinesia and exacerbation of depressive symptoms. Although as of early 2015, all SGAs assessed appeared effective in acute mania and prevention of mania and did not tend to exacerbate bipolar depression, only selected agents in this class (e.g., quetiapine, but not aripiprazole or ziprasidone) appeared to be effective in acute bipolar depression and able to prevent bipolar depression. The FDA approval of lurasidone for acute bipolar depression as monotherapy and adjunctive therapy in 2013 raised important questions regarding its efficacy in other phases of bipolar disorder, such as acute mania and bipolar disorder preventive treatment.

As of early 2015, the role of antidepressants (which were most often added to antimanic agents) in the preventive treatment of bipolar disorder continued to be a controversial issue (Pacchiarotti et al. 2013). In the past, these agents were considered mere short-term adjuncts for acute bipolar depression that needed to be discontinued as quickly as possible to minimize the risk of exacerbation of mood elevation symptoms. However, it appeared that a minority of patients with bipolar disorder (perhaps one in seven) had very good acute responses to adjunctive antidepressants and might also benefit from continuing such agents (along with antimanic medications) for prevention of depression (Altshuler et al. 2003). Although some clinicians emphasized the favorable somatic safety/tolerability profiles of antidepressants compared with mood stabilizers and SGAs, and invoked the multiphase treatment strategy (i.e., continuing effective and adequately tolerated acute treatments in efforts to prevent relapse) to advocate using adjunctive antidepressants as preventive agents in selected patients with bipolar disorder, other clinicians emphasized the risk of mood destabilization with longer-term antidepressants and advocated limiting exposure to these agents in patients with bipolar disorder (Pacchiarotti et al. 2013).

Thus, as of early 2015, five monotherapies (lithium, lamotrigine, olanzapine, aripiprazole, and risperidone LAI) and four adjunctive (added to lithium or divalproex) therapies (quetiapine, risperidone LAI, ziprasidone, and aripiprazole) had FDA approval for bipolar disorder preventive treatment. Two of these agents that were not antipsychotics (lithium and lamotrigine) along with divalproex and carbamazepine were referred to as mood stabilizers. In contrast, the five SGAs with evidence of preventive efficacy in bipolar disorder (olanzapine, aripiprazole, quetiapine, risperidone, and ziprasidone) were still called SGAs rather than mood stabilizers, despite all having not only acute mania indications but also evidence of efficacy for preventing mania. In addition to these advances in pharmacological preventive treatment, data continued to suggest that adjunctive (added to pharmacotherapy) psychosocial interventions could contribute importantly to recurrence prevention in patients with bipolar disorder.

■ Bipolar Disorder Preventive Treatment Phase

The bipolar disorder preventive treatment phase starts with symptomatic recovery (sustained remission of mood symptoms), so that, at least initially, even subsyndromal mood symptoms are absent and it is assumed that there is no current underlying mood episode. Ideally, this phase represents the vast majority of time spent in treatment; unfortunately, however, syndromal episode recurrences are common in bipolar disorder, marking an end to the preventive treatment phase and a return to the acute treatment phase. Accordingly, the duration of the bipolar disorder preventive treatment phase is commonly considered indefinite. In view of the highly recurrent nature of bipolar disorder, American guidelines tend to recommend preventive treatment after the first manic episode (American Psychiatric Association 2002; Keck et al. 2004; Suppes et al. 2005), whereas international/European guidelines are more conservative, with some tending to recommend bipolar disorder preventive treatment after the second or even third manic episode, depending on clinical circumstances (Goodwin and Consensus Group of the British Association for Psychopharmacology 2009; Grunze et al. 2013).

Clinical trial designs for bipolar disorder preventive treatment are more heterogeneous than those for acute mania or acute bipolar depression (Grunze et al. 2013; Ketter 2010). Currently, enriched discontinuation designs predominate because they enhance ability to detect preventive efficacy by using samples of patients enriched for current adequate acute efficacy and safety/tolerability with open stabilization treatment. However, such studies risk confounding true recurrences of new mood episodes with relapses into prior episodes (Tohen et al. 2006) and treatment discontinuation effects (Baldessarini et al. 1997), and (aside from use of lithium as an unenriched active comparator in some trials) fail to inform clinical decision making in instances where acute efficacy and safety/tolerability of the proposed bipolar disorder preventive treatment are not yet known. Most contemporary bipolar preventive treatment trials enroll patients with recent manic/mixed (rather than depressive) episodes, consistent with most interventions having greater acute antimanic compared with acute antidepressant efficacy. However, the degree of enrichment for acute efficacy can vary substantially in the duration of affective symptom remission. For example, in bipolar disorder preventive treatment studies of SGAs, durations of remission prior to randomization to continued SGA versus placebo have ranged from 2 weeks (with olanzapine monotherapy) (Tohen et al. 2006) to 12 weeks (with adjunctive quetiapine) (Suppes et al. 2009; Vieta et al. 2008).

The use of an open stabilization phase prior to a double-blind, placebo-controlled, randomized phase limits interpretation of safety/tolerability (i.e., number needed to harm [NNH]), because rates of adverse events of particular interest in the open stabilization phase may or may not be reported and, even if published, lack placebo control. The duration of most bipolar preventive trials, although far more substantial than for acute mania or acute bipolar depression trials, may still be insufficient to adequately detect very gradually emerging adverse effects (Grunze et al. 2013). Indeed, it has been suggested that adequate pharmacovigilance for safety/tolerability may need to last 5 years or longer (Grunze et al. 2013) and may be best obtained from national registries (Kessing et al. 2012), cohort/observational studies (Gitlin et al. 1995), comparative effectiveness trials (Licht et al. 2010), or postmarketing surveillance of community treatment populations (Safer and Zito 2013). In spite of these limitations, some investigators opine that safety/tolerability data from bipolar disorder preventive treatment registration trials may provide rapid economically and/or logistically feasible and useful preliminary longer-term safety/tolerability information regarding recently approved treatments (Citrome and Ketter 2013).

The therapeutic goals of the bipolar disorder preventive treatment phase include maintaining affective recovery and achieving and maintaining functional (including cognitive) recovery. Medication strategies prioritize safety/tolerability and include efforts to decrease medication burden by tapering down and discontinuing adjuncts that may no longer be necessary. Antidepressants are commonly discontinued but in some patients may be necessary to prevent depression (Altshuler et al. 2003). It is important that medication decreases be gradual to limit the risk of recurrence. For example, rapid (taking less than 2 weeks) as compared with gradual (taking more than 2 weeks) discontinuation of lithium has been associated with more rapid and more frequent recurrence (Baldessarini et al. 1997).

■ Bipolar Disorder Preventive Treatment: Balancing the Likelihood of Benefit and Harm

As of early 2015, five monotherapies (lithium, lamotrigine, olanzapine, aripiprazole, and risperidone LAI) had received FDA approval for bipolar disorder preventive treatment (Figure 4–1, left). Moreover, although not FDA approved for bipolar disorder preventive treatment, divalproex continued to be commonly used, and quetiapine monotherapy had controlled data supporting its use (Weisler et al. 2011) (Figure 4–1, right). In addition, controlled data suggested that paliperidone (which lacked any FDA bipolar indication) may have some efficacy in preventing manic/mixed episodes (Berwaerts et al. 2012). The FDA-approved bipolar disorder preventive treatment monotherapies, like approved treatments for other aspects of bipolar disorder, generally had single-digit numbers needed to treat (NNTs; Figure 4–1, left) for recurrence prevention compared with placebo, indicating that treating fewer than 10 patients with an FDA-approved agent compared with placebo could be expected to yield one less recurrence. In addition, divalproex monotherapy and quetiapine monotherapy had single-digit NNTs for recurrence prevention compared with placebo (Figure 4–1, right).

Also, four adjunctive (added to lithium/divalproex) therapies (quetiapine, risperidone LAI formulation, ziprasidone, and aripiprazole) had received FDA approval for bipolar disorder preventive treatment (Figure 4–2). These FDA-approved preventive adjunctive therapies most often had single-digit NNTs (Figure 4–2).

More detailed assessment of the preventive efficacy of selected bipolar disorder preventive treatment options is presented in Table 4–1. Although most approved interventions have single-digit NNTs for episode prevention, these agents have differential patterns of efficacy with respect to prevention of manic versus depressive episodes. Most agents have substantially lower (i.e., at least 50% lower) NNTs for mania versus depression prevention, suggesting that they may "stabilize mood from above" because of their more robust prevention of mania than depression. The most extreme examples of mania more than depression prevention are arguably risperidone LAI and paliperidone extended-release oral formulation, both of which had single-digit NNTs for mania prevention but negative NNTs for depression prevention, so that depressive recurrence was numerically more common with these agents than with placebo. In contrast, lamotrigine had a numerically lower NNT

TABLE 4–1. Numbers needed to treat for selected bipolar disorder preventive treatments

	Episode prevention	Mania prevention	Depression prevention
Mood stabilizers			
Lithium[1,2,3]	5	7	17
Divalproex[1,u]	8	22	11
Lamotrigine[2]	9	23	15
Atypical antipsychotics			
Olanzapine[4]	3	5	12
Aripiprazole[5]	6	6	64
Risperidone LAI[6]	4	4	–26
Quetiapine[3,u]	4	6	9
Paliperidone[7,u]	13	8	–17
Aripiprazole+lithium/ divalproex[8] *	10	13	42
Quetiapine+lithium/ divalproex[9]*	4	6	9
Ziprasidone+lithium/ divalproex[10]*	8	10	56
Risperidone LAI+treatment as usual[11]*	5	7	16

Note. **Boldface** drug names indicate FDA-approved bipolar disorder preventive treatments. **Boldface** NNTs are those of particular interest. LAI=long-acting injectable formulation.
[u]Unapproved treatments.
*Compared with lithium/divalproex monotherapy.
Source. Data from [1]Bowden et al. 2000; [2]Goodwin et al. 2004; [3]Weisler et al. 2011; [4]Tohen et al. 2006; [5]Keck et al. 2006; [6]Quiroz et al. 2010; [7]Berwaerts et al. 2012; [8]Marcus et al. 2011; [9]Suppes et al. 2013; [10]Bowden et al. 2010; [11]Macfadden et al. 2009.

for depression as compared to mania prevention, suggesting that lamotrigine may "stabilize mood from below." Curiously, in a multicenter preventive study, divalproex and lithium as an active comparator had numerically lower NNTs for depression compared to mania prevention (Bowden et al. 2000). However, this study had methodological limitations and failed in the sense that both lithium and divalproex failed to separate from placebo on the primary outcome measure (time to any

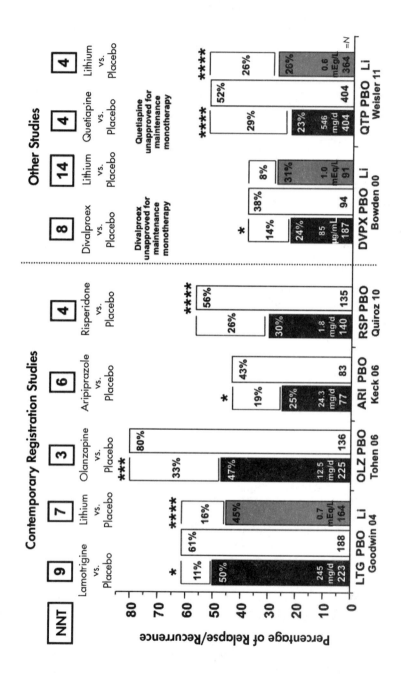

FIGURE 4–1.   Overview of selected bipolar disorder preventive treatment monotherapy studies, with numbers needed to treat (NNTs) for relapse/recurrence prevention, and rates.

Note.   Data from contemporary registration studies (*left*) and other studies (*right*). U.S. Food and Drug Administration (FDA)–approved bipolar disorder preventive treatments generally have single-digit NNTs (*left*). Divalproex and quetiapine are unapproved monotherapy treatments with single-digit NNTs. ARI=aripiprazole; DVPX=divalproex; Li=lithium; LTG=lamotrigine; OLZ=olanzapine; PBO = placebo; QTP=quetiapine; RSP=risperidone long-acting injectable formulation.

*P<0.05, ***P<0.001, ****P<0.0001 vs. placebo.

Source.   Data from Bowden et al. 2000; Goodwin et al. 2004; Keck et al. 2006; Quiroz et al. 2010; Tohen et al. 2006; Weisler et al. 2011.

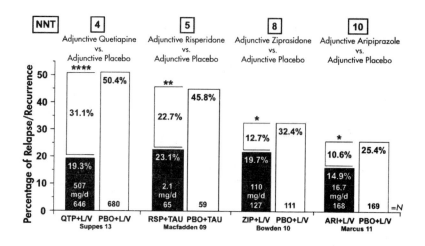

FIGURE 4–2. Overview of contemporary adjunctive (added to lithium or valproate) bipolar disorder preventive treatment registration studies, with numbers needed to treat (NNTs) for relapse/recurrence prevention, and rates.

Note. Approved treatments generally have single-digit NNTs. ARI = aripiprazole; L/V = lithium or valproate; PBO = placebo; QTP = quetiapine; RSP = risperidone long-acting injectable formulation; TAU = treatment as usual (mood stabilizers, antidepressants, anxiolytics); ZIP = ziprasidone.
$^*P<0.05$, $^{**}P<0.01$, $^{****}P<0.0001$ vs. adjunctive placebo.
Source. Data from Bowden et al. 2010; Macfadden et al. 2009; Marcus et al. 2011; Suppes et al. 2013.

mood episode recurrence), limiting interpretation of polarity of benefits. Of particular interest, quetiapine both as monotherapy and as adjunctive therapy had single-digit NNTs for both mania and depression prevention, suggesting that it may have a relatively balanced bimodal stabilizing action, consistent with quetiapine monotherapy having indications for both acute mania and acute bipolar depression.

For other bipolar disorder treatments that have demonstrated at least some efficacy in acute mania/depression, it may be hoped that continued use of such agents might prevent mania/depression (perhaps more than depression/mania).

The practice of evidence-based medicine entails considering not only efficacy data (i.e., giving higher priorities to treatments with lower NNTs) but also taking into account safety/tolerability data (i.e., giving higher priorities to treatments with higher NNHs). For example, as discussed in the following section on the four-tier approach, although SGAs generally have favorable NNTs, their safety/tolerability limitations suggest that in many instances these agents should be reserved for patients with inadequate efficacy with mood stabilizers.

Unfortunately, contemporary preventive trial methodology (which relies on uncontrolled prerandomization open mood stabilization with the intervention of interest) makes assessment of harms with longer-term treatment challenging. Indeed, it may be necessary to consider not only NNHs from the controlled randomized phase of bipolar disorder preventive treatment trials, but also rates of harms during the controlled randomized phase and the uncontrolled prerandomization open stabilization phase of such trials, and possibly even NNHs from acute treatment trials, when assessing longer-term safety/tolerability, keeping in mind that NNHs from randomized controlled trials may be insufficiently sensitive to adequately assess risks of some chronic and/or rare harms. Moreover, selection of the particular harm of greatest interest (for individual benefit vs. harm assessments) is highly personalized, depending on the severity of the harm and the vulnerability of the individual patient.

With these limitations kept in mind, Table 4–2 provides a listing of benefits (NNTs rounded to one decimal place for recurrence prevention from controlled randomized phases of bipolar preventive trials) and harms (NNHs rounded to one decimal place for the most common clinically relevant harms from the controlled randomized phase of such trials) compared with placebo, as well as the likelihood to help or harm (LHH=NNH/NNT, rounded to one decimal place).

Unfortunately, the LHH data in Table 4–2 appear to be inadequately sensitive, merely suggesting that most agents are more likely to yield help than harm (i.e., most LHHs range between 1.5 and 5.7). Rates of specific harms during the controlled randomized phase and during the uncontrolled prerandomization open stabilization phase of bipolar preventive trials and the totals thereof are also provided to facilitate more sensitive assessments of harm risk. Although the totals in the far right column of Table 4–2 appear to be in some instances informative (e.g., indicating that olanzapine may yield at least 7% weight gain in 51.1% of patients), in other instances they may be overly sensitive (e.g., indicating that lamotrigine may yield somnolence in 18% of patients) or still have inadequate sensitivity (e.g., for somnolence/sedation with quetiapine; see Table 4–2, legend footnotes *a* and *c*).

Taken together, these data indicate that there is a substantial unmet need for more accurate quantified personalized harm risk assessments in bipolar disorder preventive treatment.

TABLE 4–2. Numbers needed to treat, numbers needed to harm, likelihood to help or harm, and selected harm (side-effect) rates for selected bipolar disorder preventive treatments

Medication	NNT	NNH	LHH	Harm	BMH (%)	OMH (%)	BMH+OMH (%)
Mood stabilizers							
Lithium[1,2,3]	4.9	10.2	2.1	Tremor	27.7	Not applicable	>27.7
Divalproex[1,u]	7.1	3.5	0.5	Tremor	41.2	Not applicable	>41.2
Lamotrigine[2]	8.8	50.0	5.7	Somnolence	9.0	9	18.0
Second-generation antipsychotics							
Olanzapine[4]	3.0	7.2	2.4	Weight gain	16.1	35	51.1
Aripiprazole[5]	5.3	8.0	1.5	Weight gain	12.5	Not reported	>12.5
Risperidone LAI[6]	3.8	11.1	2.9	Weight gain	12.0	2 (oral), 15 (LAI)	29.0
Quetiapine[3,u]	3.5	12.5[a]	3.6	Weight gain[a]	10.6	16.8	27.4
Paliperidone[7,u]	12.1	29.8[b]	2.5	Somnolence[b]	3.4	12.4	15.8
Aripiprazole+lithium/divalproex[8*]	9.5	27.9	2.9	Tremor	6.0	13.8	19.8
Quetiapine+lithium/divalproex[9*]	3.2	15.3[c]	4.7	Weight gain[c]	9.3	23.9	33.2
Ziprasidone+lithium/divalproex[10*]	7.8	36.7[d]	4.7	Tremor[d]	6.3	12.5	18.8
Risperidone LAI+treatment as usual[11*]	4.4	6.9	1.6	Tremor	24.6	Not reported	>24.6

TABLE 4–2. Numbers needed to treat, numbers needed to harm, likelihood to help or harm, and selected harm (side-effect) rates for selected bipolar disorder preventive treatments (*continued*)

Note. **Boldface** indicates drug names of U.S. Food and Drug Administration (FDA)–approved bipolar disorder preventive treatments. BMH=blind medication harm rate; LAI=long-acting injectable formulation; LHH (NNH/NNT)=likelihood to help or harm compared with placebo; lithium/divalproex=lithium or divalproex; NNH=number needed to harm (for clinically relevant side effect with lowest NNH compared with placebo); NNT=number needed to treat (for recurrence prevention compared with placebo). OMH=open medication harm rate. NNTs, NNHs, and LHHs are rounded up to the next higher first decimal place (in contrast to being rounded up to the next higher integer in the text and figures).

Weight gain indicates ≥7% weight gain for all medications except lithium and divalproex.

*Compared with placebo+lithium/divalproex or with placebo+treatment as usual.

[a]Somnolence with quetiapine: NNT=3.5, NNH=40.4, LHH=11.5, BMH=6.7%, OMH=25.6%, BMH+OMH=32.3%.

[b]Extrapyramidal symptoms with paliperidone: OMH=34.0%. From open treatment baseline to randomized treatment endpoint: 29% paliperidone/paliperidone and 21% paliperidone/placebo had ≥7% weight gain (paliperidone/paliperidone NNH=12.5).

[c]Somnolence (Vieta et al. 2008)/sedation (Suppes et al. 2009) with adjunctive quetiapine: NNT=3.2, NNH=21.1, LHH=6.6, BMH=6.3%, OMH (sedation) (Suppes et al. 2013)=24.1%, BMH+OMH somnolence/sedation rate=30.4%.

[d]Sedation with adjunctive ziprasidone: OMH=22.9%.

[u]Interventions lacking FDA approval for bipolar disorder preventive treatment.

Source. Data from [1]Bowden et al. 2000; [2]Goodwin et al. 2004; [3]Weisler et al. 2011; [4]Tohen et al. 2006; [5]Keck et al. 2006; [6]Quiroz et al. 2010; [7]Berwaerts et al. 2012; [8]Marcus et al. 2011; [9]Suppes et al. 2013; [10]Bowden et al. 2010; [11]Macfadden et al. 2009.

As noted in Chapter 2, "Treatment of Acute Bipolar Depression," treatment selection in evidence-based medicine requires not only considering controlled and observational data regarding treatment efficacy/effectiveness and safety/tolerability but also integrating individual patient characteristics. Safety/tolerability may be particularly crucial in patients who have mild to moderate, nonurgent/non-treatment-resistant illness (which may be more commonly encountered during the bipolar disorder preventive treatment phase) and who have specific safety/tolerability concerns. High-priority preventive treatments include those with the best matches to individual patient illness efficacy characteristics, including those with current acute efficacy (consistent with the multiphase treatment strategy), prior acute efficacy, and current and prior preventive efficacy, and require taking into account psychiatric comorbidity, integrating efficacy data from first-degree relatives, and, if current efficacy data are lacking, treatments with efficacy in unenriched designs (e.g., lithium). High-priority preventive treatments also include those with current and prior acute and preventive safety/tolerability and those best matching other safety/tolerability characteristics (e.g., avoiding use of agents implicated in causing somnolence or weight gain/metabolic problems in patients already struggling with such challenges), and require taking into account patient medical comorbidity and safety/tolerability data from first-degree relatives. Finally, integrating preferences of patients and significant others is crucial, because these can impact positive and negative placebo responses as well as adherence.

■ An Updated Four-Tier Approach to Bipolar Preventive Treatment

Balancing benefit and risk is arguably even more crucial during the bipolar disorder preventive treatment phase than during the acute treatment phases, due to the longer duration of the phase and the absence of an acute episode to provide motivation for adherence. Clinicians need to integrate the efficacy data in Figures 4–1 and 4–2 and Tables 4–1 and 4–2 with safety/tolerability data, as described in Table 4–2 and throughout this section for bipolar disorder preventive treatment, as well as in Chapters 2 and 3 on the treatment of acute bipolar depression and acute mania, respectively.

Interventions for bipolar disorder preventive treatment are reviewed in the following subsections, using the four-tier system presented in Table 4–3, which is an update of that published in *Handbook of Diagnosis and Treatment of Bipolar Disorders* (Ketter 2010), integrating the polarity-specific preventive information in Table 4–1. This system is a hybrid approach, combining evidence-based medical information regarding efficacy and tolerability with more empirical constructs, such as familiarity and patient acceptability, to prioritize treatments in a fashion broadly consistent with American clinical practice and treatment guidelines.

Although most bipolar disorder preventive treatment interventions appear to be more robust in countering mood elevation compared with depression (Table 4–1), FDA bipolar disorder preventive treatment indications commonly state only limited information regarding predominant polarity preventive efficacy (i.e., ability to prevent mood elevation as opposed to depression). However, bipolar disorder preventive treatment selection needs to match polarity-specific information for interventions with that of individual patient illnesses. It is worth reiterating that quetiapine (adjunctive therapy as well as monotherapy) is the only agent with clearly established abilities to relieve and prevent both acute mood elevation and depression. In contrast, risperidone, paliperidone, and first-generation antipsychotics may, to varying degrees, prevent mania at the expense of increasing the risk of depression, whereas adjunctive antidepressants may prevent depression at the expense of increasing the risk of mood elevation.

As of early 2015, the seven Tier I treatment options had FDA approval for bipolar disorder preventive treatment and were supported by the most compelling evidence of efficacy. However, tolerability limitations of some Tier I treatments may lead clinicians and patients, after comparing the risks and benefits, to consider treatments in other tiers, particularly Tier II (e.g., divalproex). Indeed, in clinical practice and in some treatment guidelines (Suppes et al. 2005; Yatham et al. 2013), some Tier I treatments have been considered to have equal or even lower priority than some Tier II options.

Tier II treatment options, as of early 2015, lacked FDA approval for preventive treatment of bipolar disorder and had less compelling evidence of efficacy than Tier I options, but arguably had mitigating advantages such as tolerability, familiarity, or acute indications that might make them attractive for a substantial number of patients. In clinical practice and in some treatment guidelines (American Psychiatric Association 2002; Goodwin and Consensus Group of the British Association for Psychopharmacology 2009; Grunze et al. 2013; Keck et al. 2004; Suppes et al. 2005; Yatham et al. 2013), some of these medications (e.g., divalproex) have been considered first-line interventions, in spite of the absence of an FDA indication for bipolar disorder preventive treatment.

Tier III treatment options, as of early 2015, lacked FDA approval for bipolar disorder preventive treatment and had even less compelling evi-

TABLE 4–3. Integrated four-tier and predominant polarity approach to bipolar disorder preventive treatment

Tier	Priority	Description	Predominantly mood elevation prevention	Predominantly depression prevention

I	High	FDA approved	Mood stabilizers
			  Lithium
			SGAs
			  Olanzapine (monotherapy), aripiprazole (monotherapy/adjunctive), risperidone long-acting injectable formulation (monotherapy/adjunctive), quetiapine (adjunctive), ziprasidone (adjunctive)
				Mood stabilizers
				  Lamotrigine
				SGAs
				  Quetiapine (adjunctive)

II	High	Unapproved	SGAs
			  Quetiapine (monotherapy)
				Other mood stabilizers
				  Divalproex
				SGAs
				  Quetiapine (monotherapy)

TABLE 4–3. Integrated four-tier and predominant polarity approach to bipolar disorder preventive treatment

Tier	Priority	Description	Predominantly mood elevation prevention	Predominantly depression prevention
III	Intermediate	Unapproved	Other mood stabilizers Carbamazepine Other SGAs Olanzapine (adjunctive), ziprasidone (monotherapy), asenapine (monotherapy), paliperidone (monotherapy), clozapine (adjunctive)	Other SGAs Olanzapine plus fluoxetine, lurasidone (monotherapy or adjunctive) Adjunctive antidepressants Adjunctive psychotherapy Psychoeducation, cognitive-behavioral therapy, family focused therapy, interpersonal and social rhythm therapy
IV	Low	Novel adjunctive options		Electroconvulsive therapy Vagus nerve stimulation Transcranial magnetic stimulation

Note. FDA=U.S. Food and Drug Administration; SGA=second-generation antipsychotic.
Source. Adapted from Ketter TA: *Handbook of Diagnosis and Treatment of Bipolar Disorders.* Washington, DC, American Psychiatric Publishing, 2010. Copyright 2010, American Psychiatric Publishing. Used with permission.

dence of efficacy than Tier II options. Treatment guidelines generally continued to not consider Tier III agents, aside from adjunctive antidepressants (which were ranked highly by some but not all experts), to be first-line interventions but cited at least some of them as intermediate-priority options (American Psychiatric Association 2002; Goodwin and Consensus Group of the British Association for Psychopharmacology 2009; Grunze et al. 2013; Keck et al. 2004; Suppes et al. 2005; Yatham et al. 2013). Nevertheless, some Tier III options had mitigating advantages, such as tolerability, familiarity, or acute indications, that might make them attractive for selected patients, and in certain circumstances some of these interventions may be considered early on (e.g., psychotherapy in pregnant women). For some of these treatments (e.g., adjunctive psychotherapy), advances in research, familiarity, and/or availability may ultimately be sufficient to merit their consideration for placement in higher tiers.

Tier IV treatment options, as of early 2015, lacked FDA approval for preventive treatment of bipolar disorder and had even more limited evidence of efficacy than Tier I–III options. Treatment guidelines have uniformly considered these modalities to be low-priority interventions, if mentioned at all (American Psychiatric Association 2002; Goodwin and Consensus Group of the British Association for Psychopharmacology 2009; Grunze et al. 2013; Keck et al. 2004; Suppes et al. 2005; Yatham et al. 2013). Nevertheless, some Tier IV options could prove attractive for carefully selected patients, after consideration of treatments from Tiers I–III (e.g., for patients who are treatment resistant or intolerant to Tier I–III treatments). For some of these treatments, advances in research may ultimately provide sufficient evidence to merit their consideration for placement in higher tiers.

Tier I: FDA-Approved Bipolar Disorder Preventive Treatments

As of early 2015, the FDA-approved bipolar disorder preventive treatments were the mood stabilizers lithium and lamotrigine as monotherapy, and the SGAs olanzapine, aripiprazole, and risperidone LAI as monotherapy, and quetiapine, risperidone LAI, ziprasidone, and aripiprazole as adjunctive (added to lithium or divalproex) therapy. As described in greater detail in the following subsections, these options have favorable efficacy (generally single-digit NNTs; Figures 4–1 and 4–2, Tables 4–1 and 4–2), with most having more robust abilities to prevent or delay manic/mixed compared with depressive episodes (Tables 4–1 and 4–3). Two important exceptions to this profile are lamotrigine, which appears to have more robust antidepressant than antimanic actions, and quetiapine, which appears to have comparably robust antidepressant and antimanic actions. Safety/tolerability limitations of some Tier I treatments (e.g., SGAs) may lead clinicians and patients, after comparing the risks and benefits, to consider treatments in other tiers, particularly Tiers II and III. Indeed, in clinical practice and in some treatment guidelines, some Tier I treatments (e.g., olanzapine) have been considered to have equal or even lower priority than some Tier II options (e.g., divalproex) (Suppes et al. 2005; Yatham et al. 2013).

Mood Stabilizers

Mood stabilizers are considered foundational agents in the treatment of bipolar disorder. As of early 2015, two of these agents, lithium and lamotrigine, had been approved by the FDA for bipolar disorder preventive treatment. These agents appear to have distinctive and in some ways complementary efficacy and safety/tolerability profiles. Lithium provides more robust prevention of mood elevation than depression and has an acute mania indication, but it has tolerability limitations. In contrast, lamotrigine provides more robust prevention of depression than mood elevation and has generally good tolerability, but it lacks an acute bipolar disorder (specifically, an acute bipolar *depression*) indication.

Lithium.   Lithium monotherapy was approved by the FDA as bipolar disorder preventive treatment in 1974 and for almost three decades was the only approved preventive treatment. As of early 2015, neither carbamazepine nor valproate had obtained such approval. In the 1980s, 1990s, and 2000s, randomized controlled monotherapy bipolar disorder preventive trials found carbamazepine compared with lithium was most often similar (Bellaire et al. 1988; Coxhead et al. 1992; Placidi et al. 1986; Watkins et al. 1987), but on occasion inferior (Greil et al. 1997; Hartong et al. 2003) or superior (Lusznat et al. 1988); however, multicenter, randomized, double-blind, placebo-controlled carbamazepine bipolar disorder preventive studies were lacking. In the 1990s and 2000s, randomized controlled monotherapy bipolar disorder preventive trials found that valpromide compared with lithium was somewhat superior (Lambert and Venaud 1992) and valproate compared with lithium was similar (Bowden et al. 2000). However, in the latter study, perhaps because of methodological reasons, neither lithium nor valproate separated from placebo.

Subsequently, FDA bipolar disorder preventive treatment monotherapy indications were obtained for lamotrigine in 2003 (Goodwin et al. 2004) and for the SGAs olanzapine in 2004 (Tohen et al. 2006), aripiprazole in 2005 (Keck et al. 2006), and risperidone LAI in 2009 (Quiroz et al. 2010). Adjunctive (added to lithium or valproate) bipolar disorder preventive indications were also obtained for the SGAs quetiapine in 2008 (Suppes et al. 2009; Vieta et al. 2008), risperidone LAI in 2009 (Macfadden et al. 2009), ziprasidone in 2009 (Bowden et al. 2010), and aripiprazole in 2011 (Marcus et al. 2011). These developments challenged assumptions regarding longer-term bipolar disorder management, because FGAs previously were considered mere short-term adjuncts for acute mania that needed to be discontinued after the acute treatment phase to minimize the risks of tardive dyskinesia (Kane and Smith 1982) and exacerbation of depression (Ahlfors et al. 1981).

Contemporary FDA-approved bipolar disorder preventive treatments are supported by multicenter, randomized, double-blind, placebo-controlled clinical trials. Although one early placebo-controlled lithium bipolar preventive study had a large sample size and a multicenter, randomized, single-blind (participants and raters but not providers were blind) design (Prien et al. 1973), most early lithium maintenance studies involved small samples and/or older, less rigorous methodology (Baastrup et al. 1970; Coppen et al. 1971; Cundall et al. 1972; Dunner et al. 1976; Fieve et al. 1976; Hullin et al. 1972; Kane et al. 1982; Stallone et al. 1973). These methodological differences and limitations appeared to have contributed to emergence of the perception by some that lithium efficacy and tolerability in bipolar disorder preventive treatment was inadequately established (Moncrieff 1995).

Lithium's efficacy and tolerability in bipolar I disorder preventive treatment has been confirmed in two additional studies using contemporary methodology (Goodwin et al. 2004; Weisler et al. 2011) (Figure 4–3); however, perhaps for methodological reasons, one earlier study failed to demonstrate preventive benefit with either lithium or divalproex compared with placebo (Bowden et al. 2000). These multicenter, randomized, double-blind, placebo-controlled bipolar I disorder preventive treatment studies of lamotrigine (Goodwin et al. 2004), quetiapine (Weisler et al. 2011), and divalproex (Bowden et al. 2003) included lithium active comparator arms to assess assay sensitivity and did *not* require open stabilization with lithium. Indeed, two of these studies required open stabilization with agents other than lithium: lamotrigine in one instance (Goodwin et al. 2004) and quetiapine in the other (Weisler et al. 2011).

In the studies of lamotrigine (Goodwin et al. 2004) and quetiapine (Weisler et al. 2011), lithium, at mean concentrations of 0.7 and 0.6 mEq/ L, respectively—values consistent with the lower (better-tolerated) end of the therapeutic range in prior studies (Prien et al. 1973; Kane et al. 1982)

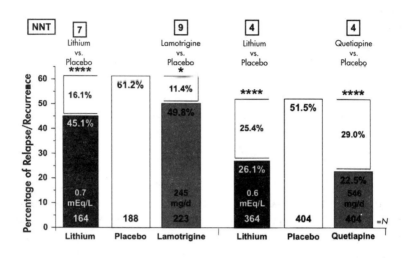

FIGURE 4–3. Double-blind lithium versus placebo versus lamotrigine/quetiapine bipolar I disorder preventive treatment monotherapy studies: numbers needed to treat for relapse/recurrence prevention, and rates.

Note. NNT=number needed to treat.
*P<0.05, ****P<0.0001 vs. placebo.
Source. Data on left from Goodwin et al. 2004 (pooled from Bowden et al. 2003; Calabrese et al. 2003). Data on right from Weisler et al. 2011.

and treatment guidelines (American Psychiatric Association 2002)—demonstrated superior overall efficacy (any mood episode recurrence prevention) compared with placebo in a fashion broadly similar to that seen with lamotrigine and quetiapine, despite patients having had open stabilization with these other agents rather than with lithium. Thus, in the lamotrigine registration studies (Goodwin et al. 2004), rates of any recurrence were 45.1% with lithium, 49.8% with lamotrigine (*P*=not significant [NS] for lithium vs. lamotrigine), and 61.2% with placebo (*P*<0.05 vs. lithium and lamotrigine), and in the quetiapine-lithium-placebo study (Weisler et al. 2011), 26.1% with lithium, 22.5% with quetiapine (*P*=NS for lithium vs. quetiapine), and 51.5% with placebo (*P*<0.0001 vs. lithium and quetiapine). Hence, the NNT to obtain one less patient with any recurrence compared with placebo for lithium was similar to that seen with lamotrigine (NNT=7 vs. 9) and identical to that seen with quetiapine (NNT=4). In these bipolar I disorder preventive treatment studies, lithium demonstrated substantially greater mania compared with depression prevention (NNT=8 and 49, respectively, in the pooled lamotrigine-lithium-placebo studies; and NNT=6 and 14, respectively, in the quetiapine-lithium-placebo study). In contrast, lamotrigine demonstrated somewhat less mania compared with depression prevention (NNT=23 and 15, respectively; Table 4–1), while quetiapine demonstrated comparable mania versus depression prevention (NNT=6 and 9, respectively; Table 4–1).

Compared with quetiapine, lithium yielded less somnolence and weight gain, but more thyroid-stimulating hormone (TSH) elevation, vomiting, and tremor (Weisler et al. 2011). Specifically, during the randomized preventive phase, rates of somnolence were 2.6% with lithium, 6.7% with quetiapine ($P=0.007$ vs. lithium), and 4.2% with placebo ($P = NS$ vs. lithium, $P<0.0001$ vs. quetiapine), yielding a superior NNH for somnolence compared with placebo with lithium versus quetiapine (–64 vs. 41). Importantly, 25.6% of patients taking quetiapine during the open stabilization phase had somnolence. Similarly, during the randomized preventive phase, rates of at least 7% weight gain were 5.4% with lithium, 10.6% with quetiapine ($P=0.007$ vs. lithium), and 2.6% with placebo ($P = NS$ vs. lithium, $P<0.0001$ vs. quetiapine), yielding a superior NNH for at least 7% weight gain compared with placebo for lithium versus quetiapine (36 vs. 13). Importantly, 16.8% of patients taking quetiapine during the open stabilization phase had at least 7% weight gain. However, during the randomized preventive phase, rates of potentially clinically significant TSH elevation (>5 µU/mL) were 20.1% with lithium, 3.1% with quetiapine ($P<0.0001$ vs. lithium), and 3.0% with placebo ($P<0.0001$ vs. lithium, $P=NS$ vs. quetiapine), yielding an inferior NNH for TSH elevation compared with placebo with lithium versus quetiapine (6 vs. 543). Similarly, during the randomized preventive phase, rates of vomiting were 11.2% with lithium, 2.0% with quetiapine ($P<0.0001$ vs. lithium), and 3.0% with placebo ($P<0.0001$ vs. lithium, $P=NS$ vs. quetiapine), yielding an inferior NNH for vomiting compared with placebo with lithium versus quetiapine (13 vs. –101). Moreover, during the randomized preventive phase, rates of tremor were 7.4% with lithium, 3.0% with quetiapine ($P = 0.0045$ vs. lithium), and 2.0% with placebo ($P=0.0002$ vs. lithium, $P=NS$ vs. quetiapine), yielding an inferior NNH for tremor compared with placebo for lithium versus quetiapine (19 vs. 101). Importantly, rates of TSH elevation, vomiting, and tremor were all less than 5.0% with quetiapine during the open stabilization phase.

Lithium as opposed to lamotrigine yielded similar somnolence and weight gain, but more diarrhea and tremor. Thus, in the lamotrigine registration studies (Goodwin et al. 2004), during the randomized preventive phase, lithium compared with lamotrigine yielded significantly more diarrhea (19% vs. 7%, NNH=9) and tremor (15% vs. 4%, NNH=10), and compared with placebo yielded significantly more diarrhea (19% vs.

8%, NNH=10), tremor (15% vs. 5%, NNH=10), nausea (20% vs. 11%, NNH=12), and somnolence (13% vs. 7%, NNH=17). However, rates of somnolence were 13% with lithium, 9% with lamotrigine (P=NS vs. lithium), and 7% with placebo (P=NS vs. lithium and lamotrigine) during the randomized preventive phase (and 9% with lamotrigine during the open stabilization phase), yielding comparable NNHs for somnolence compared with placebo for lithium and lamotrigine (17 vs. 50). Also, during the randomized preventive phase, rates of at least 7% weight gain were 11.8% with lithium, 10.9% with lamotrigine (P=NS vs. lithium), and 7.6% with placebo (P=NS vs. lithium and lamotrigine), yielding similar NNHs for at least 7% weight gain compared with placebo for lithium and lamotrigine (25 vs. 31) (Sachs et al. 2006).

Hence, during the randomized preventive phase, compared with placebo, the likelihood of recurrence prevention was similar to that of diarrhea/tremor with lithium (NNT=7 vs. NNH=10) but greater than that of somnolence with lamotrigine (NNT=9 vs. NNH=17) (Goodwin et al. 2004). Also, during the randomized preventive phase, compared with placebo, the likelihood of recurrence prevention was similar to that of TSH elevation with lithium (NNT=7 vs. NNH=6) but greater than that of weight gain with quetiapine (NNT=4 vs. NNH=13) (Weisler et al. 2011). During the randomized preventive phase, the rather high NNHs for quetiapine compared with placebo for somnolence and weight gain (41 and 13, respectively) are at variance with the rather high rates of these problems during the quetiapine open stabilization phase (25.6% and 16.8%, respectively).

In other multicenter, randomized, double-blind, placebo-controlled bipolar prevention monotherapy registration studies, SGAs demonstrated similar efficacy to prevent recurrence—with single-digit NNTs of 3 with olanzapine (Tohen et al. 2006), 6 with aripiprazole (Keck et al. 2006), and 4 with risperidone LAI (Quiroz et al. 2010)—to that seen with lithium in the above-mentioned studies (with NNTs to prevent recurrence of 4 [Weisler et al. 2011] and 7 [Goodwin et al. 2004]). In these SGA monotherapy bipolar preventive studies, the NNHs during the randomized preventive phase for at least 7% weight gain were 8 with olanzapine (35% during open stabilization) (Tohen et al. 2006), 8 with aripiprazole (percentage during open stabilization not reported) (Keck et al. 2006), and 12 with risperidone LAI (17% during open stabilization) (Quiroz et al. 2010), and were thus less favorable than the NNHs for weight gain compared with placebo seen with lithium: 36 in the study by Weisler et al. (2011) and 25 in the study by Sachs et al. (2006).

Thus, in head-to-head bipolar preventive trials using contemporary methodology, lithium yielded similar efficacy compared with quetiapine and lamotrigine, but variable tolerability: 1) compared with quetiapine, less somnolence and weight gain but more TSH elevation, vomiting, and tremor, and 2) compared with lamotrigine, comparable somnolence and weight gain, but more diarrhea and tremor (Table 4–2). Moreover, across bipolar preventive trials using contemporary methodology, lithium, when compared with approved SGAs, yielded similar efficacy and superior tolerability.

Finally, in a head-to-head multicenter, randomized, double-blind, placebo-controlled, bipolar I disorder preventive treatment monotherapy trial, lithium yielded comparable (in)efficacy versus divalproex (perhaps for methodological reasons, both failed to separate from placebo on time to any recurrence, although NNTs for prevention of any episode vs. placebo were 14 and 8 for lithium and divalproex, respectively), but variable safety/tolerability that entailed, compared with divalproex, more polyuria, diarrhea, and thirst (NNHs for lithium vs. divalproex=10, 11, and 12, respectively), but less sedation, infection, alopecia, and weight gain (NNHs for lithium vs. divalproex=−7, −7, −12, and −13, respectively) (Bowden et al. 2000).

In the last decade, randomized, open/single-blind (rater), comparative effectiveness trials have assessed longer-term treatment with lithium in a variety of paradigms, including lithium plus limited antidepressants/ antipsychotics versus lamotrigine plus limited antidepressants/antipsychotics in the Danish University Antidepressant Group 6th (DUAG-6) trial (Licht et al. 2010); lithium plus antidepressants/antipsychotics/ mood stabilizers (AAMS) versus valproate plus AAMS, and versus the lithium plus valproate combination plus AAMS in the Bipolar Affective Disorder Lithium/Anticonvulsant Evaluation (BALANCE) study (Geddes et al. 2010); moderate-dose lithium combined with Optimized Personal Treatment (OPT) versus OPT without lithium in the Lithium Treatment Moderate-Dose Use Study (LiTMUS) (Nierenberg et al. 2013); and lithium plus adjunctive personalized treatments (APT) versus quetiapine plus APT in the Clinical and Health Outcomes Initiative in Comparative Effectiveness for Bipolar Disorder (Bipolar CHOICE) study (Nierenberg et al. 2014).

In the DUAG-6 trial, adults with bipolar I disorder (not necessarily remitted), randomly assigned to receive open lithium (n=78; serum levels 0.5–1.0 mEq/L) compared with lamotrigine (n=77; titrated to 400 mg/ day) administered for at least 1 year (for at least 3 and 5 years in 58% and 19%, respectively), had statistically similar prevention of both mood elevation and depressive episodes, but had more side effects with lithium (diarrhea NNH=4, tremor NNH=4, thirst NNH=5, and polyuria NNH=10), although two patients developed lamotrigine-related benign rash (NNH=39) (Licht et al. 2010). Despite efforts to avoid coadministering antipsychotics and antidepressants after the first 6 months, among patients followed for at least 5 years, only 6.9% (2/29) were maintained successfully with lithium or lamotrigine monotherapy.

In the BALANCE trial, patients ages 16 years and older with bipolar I disorder (29.4% taking antidepressants, 25.8% taking antipsychotics, and 5.5% taking other mood stabilizers) whose symptoms had not necessarily remitted after manic, mixed, or depressive episodes had a 4- to 8-week lithium plus divalproex tolerability run-in, followed by randomization to open (to patients and providers, but single-blind to raters) lithium (0.4–1.0 mEq/L, n=110), divalproex (750–1,250 mg/day, n=110), or lithium plus divalproex (n=110) for up to 24 months (Geddes et al. 2010). Lithium, divalproex, and lithium plus divalproex yielded recurrence rates of 59.1%, 69.1%, and 53.6%, respectively (Figure 4–4, left). Thus, lithium and lithium plus divalproex, compared with divalproex, both yielded significantly fewer recurrences (59.1% vs. 69.1%, NNT=10; and 53.6% vs. 69.1%, NNT=7, respectively). However, divalproex plus lithium compared with lithium yielded only nonsignificantly fewer recurrences (53.6% vs. 59.1%, NNT=19). Lithium, divalproex, and lithium plus divalproex yielded intolerability discontinuation rates of 5.5%, 1.8%, and 9.1%, respectively (Figure 4–4, right). Thus, intolerability discontinuation rates were only nonsignificantly more common with lithium than with divalproex monotherapy (5.5% vs. 1.8%, NNH=28) or with lithium plus divalproex than with lithium (9.1% vs. 5.5%, NNH=28), but were more common with lithium plus divalproex compared with divalproex (9.1% vs. 1.8%, NNH=14). The authors concluded that lithium and lithium plus divalproex were more effective than divalproex, but that the effectiveness of lithium plus divalproex compared with lithium could be neither established nor refuted.

In the LiTMUS study, participants were 283 patients with bipolar I disorder (76%) or bipolar II disorder (24%) and at least moderate mood symptoms randomly assigned either to single-blind (rater) moderate-dose lithium (median dosage=600 mg/day, mean serum lithium concentration = 0.47 mEq/L) plus OPT or to OPT without lithium for up to 6 months. The two groups had statistically similar numbers of medication changes and rates of sustained remission (Clinical Global Impressions [CGI] Scale Modified for Bipolar Illness Overall Level of Severity score of ≤2 for at least 2 months) of approximately 25%, and similar protocol discontinuation rates (17.7% vs. 14.8%, NNH=34), but a lower rate of SGA utilization (48.3% vs. 62.3%, NNH=–7.1, P=0.03) (Nierenberg et al. 2013).

In the Bipolar CHOICE study, 482 patients with bipolar I disorder (68%) or bipolar II disorder (32%) and at least moderate mood symp-

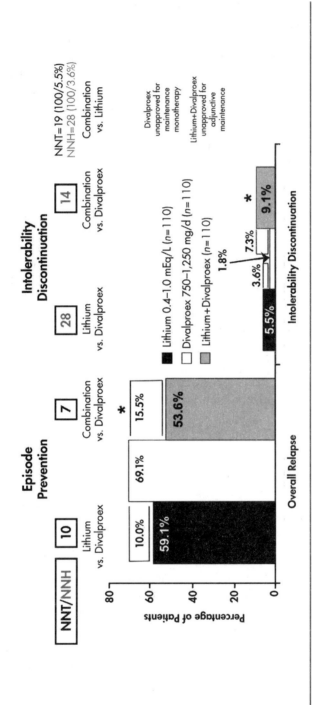

FIGURE 4–4. Bipolar Affective Disorder Lithium/Anticonvulsant Evaluation (BALANCE) study: numbers needed to treat, numbers needed to harm, relapse rates, and intolerability discontinuation rates.

Note. Single-blind, randomized prevention study assessing Li versus DVPX versus Li+DVPX for treating patients with bipolar I disorder after manic/mixed/depressive episodes. Patients were randomized after a 4- to 8-week Li+DVPX tolerability run-in. The primary outcome was time to intervention for any mood episode. Of the patients, 29.4% also took antidepressants, 25.8% also took antipsychotics, and 5.5% also took other mood stabilizers. DVPX=divalproex; Li=lithium.

*P<0.03 vs. divalproex.

Source. Data from Geddes et al. 2010.

toms were randomly assigned either to single-blind (rater) lithium (median dosage=900 mg/day, mean serum lithium concentration=0.6 mEq/L) plus APT or to quetiapine (median dosage=300 mg/day) plus APT for up to 6 months. Lithium plus OPT compared with OPT without lithium had statistically similar numbers of medication changes and benefit:harm ratios (on the CGI Efficacy Index), although those with more baseline mood elevation may have had marginally better mood outcome with quetiapine plus APT, whereas those with more anxiety may have had marginally fewer medication changes with lithium plus APT (Nierenberg et al. 2014). Moreover, side effects were marginally less problematic with lithium plus APT.

The following have been associated with lithium responsiveness: euphoric mania (Bowden et al. 1994), "classical" subtype of bipolar disorder (bipolar I without mood-incongruent delusions and without comorbidity) (Greil et al. 1998), an episode sequence of mania followed by depression followed by well interval (Maj et al. 1989), fewer prior episodes (Swann et al. 2000), complete recovery between episodes (Grof et al. 1993), a personal history of lithium response (Tondo et al. 1997), and a family history of bipolar disorder or lithium response (Maj et al. 1984).

In contrast, the following portend poorer responses to lithium: rapid cycling (Maj et al. 1998), dysphoric manic or mixed episodes (Bowden et al. 2005), having had at least three prior episodes (Swann et al. 2000), "nonclassical" subtype (bipolar II/not otherwise specified, mood-incongruent delusions, comorbidity) (Greil et al. 1998), an episode sequence of depression followed by mania followed by well interval (Maj et al. 1989), severe mania (Swann et al. 1986), secondary mania (Stoll et al. 1994), adolescent age (Strober et al. 1988), comorbid substance abuse (Pond et al. 1981), and a personal history of nonresponse to lithium (Bowden et al. 1994). Importantly, patients stabilized on lithium for extended periods of time occasionally become lithium resistant after discontinuing the agent and then suffering a mood episode recurrence (Post et al. 1992).

A conservative meta-analysis found only five strongly suggestive clinical markers of lithium prophylactic responsiveness (Kleindienst et al. 2005): better lithium responses in patients with 1) later onset (10 studies, 1,138 patients) and 2) episode sequence of mania then depression then well interval (7 studies, 904 patients), and poorer lithium responses in patients with 1) episode sequence of depression then mania then well interval (8 studies, 1,151 patients), 2) a continuous cycling pattern (the frequent absence of well intervals between episodes) (4 studies, 404 patients), and 3) more prior hospitalizations (4 studies, 677 patients).

Evidence continues to accumulate that lithium preventive treatment may decrease suicidality (suicide attempts and completed suicides). In a meta-analysis of 48 randomized controlled trials involving 6,674 patients with mood disorders, lithium was more effective than placebo in reducing suicide (odds ratio [OR] 0.13, 95% confidence interval [CI] 0.03–0.66) and death from any cause (OR 0.38, 95% CI 0.15–0.95), but not deliberate self-harm (Cipriani et al. 2013).

Taken together, the information presented in this subsection suggests that as of early 2015, lithium is an efficacious bipolar disorder preventive treatment but is somewhat less effective in preventing depression than mania. Clinicians and patients may deem tolerability of lithium inferior to that of lamotrigine but superior to that of SGAs. In clinical populations, there remains a major unmet need for very well-tolerated preventive treatments that adequately address the depressive component of bipolar disorder. Indeed, this tolerability issue may have contributed to lamotrigine overtaking lithium (and valproate) as the most prescribed mood stabilizer in the United States (Hooshmand et al. 2014).

Lamotrigine. In 2003, lamotrigine became the second medication approved by the FDA for bipolar disorder preventive treatment. As of early 2015, despite lacking an acute bipolar disorder indication (specifically, lacking an acute bipolar depression indication), lamotrigine was the most commonly prescribed mood stabilizer in America (Hooshmand et al. 2014).

In a pooled analysis of the lamotrigine bipolar disorder preventive treatment registration trials, compared with placebo, lamotrigine significantly delayed and significantly prevented (NNT=9; Figure 4–1, Table 4–1) overall relapse/recurrence, and significantly delayed but did not significantly prevent relapse/recurrence of depressive (NNT=15; Table 4–1) and manic/mixed (NNT=23; Table 4–1) episodes (Goodwin et al. 2004). In contrast, lithium significantly delayed and significantly prevented not only overall (NNT=7) but also manic/mixed (NNT=8) relapse/recurrence, but neither significantly delayed nor significantly prevented (NNT=49) depressive relapse/recurrence. Lamotrigine was generally well tolerated, including yielding no substantive somnolence or weight gain compared with placebo (Table 4–2). As noted in the previous subsection on lithium, lamotrigine compared with lithium yielded significantly less diarrhea (NNH=–9) and tremor (NNH=–10). Compared with placebo, lamotrigine had statistically similar rates not only of diarrhea and tremor but also of headache.

As noted in the previous subsection on lithium, in the DUAG-6 comparative effectiveness trial, lamotrigine compared with lithium for at least 1 year yielded comparable efficacy but better tolerability (Licht et al. 2010).

There are limited data regarding baseline markers of lamotrigine efficacy, which may in some ways overlap with and in other ways be complementary to baseline markers of lithium efficacy. In one study, for example, patients with poorer preventive responses to lamotrigine included patients who had index mixed episodes or who had experienced at least three depressions in the prior 2 years (Ketter et al. 2003); however, in another study lamotrigine response was associated with rapid cycling or having relatives with schizoaffective disorder, major depressive disorder, and panic attacks (Passmore et al. 2003).

In summary, lamotrigine is a bipolar disorder preventive treatment option with a novel profile, in that it is generally well tolerated and provides more robust depression prevention than mania prevention, although it lacks an acute bipolar disorder indication. Clinicians and patients may consider lamotrigine an attractive treatment option because of superior tolerability compared with SGAs and other mood stabilizers.

Second-Generation Antipsychotics

SGAs are commonly used in acute mania and are increasingly used for other aspects of the management of bipolar disorder. Indeed, as of early 2015, FDA bipolar disorder preventive treatment indications had been conferred upon three SGAs (olanzapine, aripiprazole, and risperidone LAI) as monotherapies (Figure 4–1, left) and four SGAs (quetiapine, risperidone LAI, ziprasidone, and aripiprazole) as adjunctive therapies (added to lithium/divalproex) (Figure 4–2).

Olanzapine (monotherapy). In 2004, olanzapine monotherapy became the third medication approved by the FDA for bipolar disorder preventive treatment. Although the olanzapine LAI formulation received FDA approval for the treatment of schizophrenia in 2009, as of early 2015, this medication lacked evidence of efficacy and safety/tolerability and had no FDA indication for bipolar disorder treatment.

Although olanzapine monotherapy yielded substantial efficacy, with an NNT for recurrence prevention compared with placebo of 3 (Figure 4–1, left; Tables 4–1 and 4–2), and more robust mania prevention (NNT = 5; Table 4–1) than depression prevention (NNT = 12; Table 4–1), these benefits were offset by substantial risks of weight gain/metabolic problems (Tohen et al. 2006). Detection of such harms was less sensitive when considering the NNH for at least 7% weight gain versus placebo during the controlled randomized phase of the bipolar disorder preventive treatment registration trial (NNH = 8; Table 4–2), compared with considering the sum of the rates of at least 7% weight gain for the controlled randomized phase and the uncontrolled prerandomization open stabilization phase (51.1% of patients; Table 4–2).

In summary, olanzapine monotherapy appears to provide more robust prevention of mania than of depression. Adverse effects (particularly weight gain/metabolic problems) with this agent can routinely be challenging, and clinicians and patients commonly deem this agent to have inferior tolerability not only compared with mood stabilizers but also compared with newer SGAs (e.g., aripiprazole and ziprasidone).

Aripiprazole (monotherapy).   In 2005, aripiprazole became the fourth medication (and second SGA) approved by the FDA for bipolar disorder preventive treatment in adults. In 2008, this indication was extended to include children and adolescents ages 10–17 years. As of early 2015, the aripiprazole LAI formulation lacked evidence of efficacy and safety/tolerability and had no FDA indication for bipolar disorder treatment.

Aripiprazole monotherapy yielded adequate efficacy with an NNT for recurrence prevention compared with placebo of 6 (Figure 4–1, left; Tables 4–1 and 4–2), more robust mania prevention (NNT=6; Table 4–1) than depression prevention (NNT=64; Table 4–1), and less risk of weight gain/metabolic problems than with olanzapine (Keck et al. 2006). However, detection of this harm appeared to be overly sensitive when considering the rate of at least 7% weight gain during the controlled randomized phase of the bipolar prevention registration trial (NNH=8; Table 4–2), although the absolute rate for this harm during this phase was only 12.5% (Table 4–2, blind medication harm rate). Unfortunately, the rate of at least 7% weight gain for the uncontrolled prerandomization open stabilization phase of the bipolar disorder preventive treatment registration trial was not published.

In summary, aripiprazole appears to provide more robust prevention of mania than of depression. Adverse effects with this agent may be less challenging than with older SGAs (e.g., olanzapine, quetiapine, risperidone) but more challenging than with mood stabilizers.

Risperidone long-acting injectable formulation (monotherapy).   In 2009, risperidone LAI formulation received approval for bipolar preventive monotherapy. Risperidone LAI monotherapy yielded adequate efficacy, with an NNT for recurrence prevention compared with placebo of 4 (Figure 4–1, left; Table 4–1), but with substantially more robust mania prevention (NNT=4; Table 4–1) than depression prevention (NNT=−26 [i.e., nonsignificantly worse than placebo]; Table 4–1). Also, compared with olanzapine, risperidone LAI had less risk of weight gain/metabolic problems, with an NNH for at least 7% weight gain compared with placebo of 12 (Table 4–2) (Quiroz et al. 2010). However, extrapyramidal symptoms (EPS) can occur with chronic risperidone LAI, albeit less often than with acute treatment with oral formulation.

In summary, risperidone LAI monotherapy appears to provide more robust prevention of mania than of depression (some clinicians opine that the medication may even increase the risk of depressive recurrence). Adverse effects (e.g., EPS, weight gain/metabolic problems) with this agent can be challenging, and clinicians and patients commonly deem this agent to have inferior tolerability compared not only with mood stabilizers but also with newer SGAs (e.g., aripiprazole and ziprasidone).

Quetiapine (adjunctive therapy). In 2008, quetiapine received an adjunctive (added to lithium or valproate) bipolar disorder preventive treatment indication (Suppes et al. 2009, 2013; Vieta et al. 2008). Adjunctive quetiapine yielded adequate efficacy, with an NNT for recurrence prevention compared with adjunctive placebo of 4 (Figure 4–2, Table 4–1), and ability to prevent not only mania (NNT=6; Table 4–1) but also depression (NNT=9; Table 4–1), as well as less risk of weight gain/metabolic problems (NNH=13; Table 4–2) than olanzapine (Suppes et al. 2013). However, quetiapine's utility can be routinely limited by somnolence/sedation, with the sum of the rates of these harms during the controlled randomized phase plus the uncontrolled prerandomization open stabilization phase of bipolar prevention registration trials being 30.4% (Table 4–2, legend footnote *c*) (Suppes et al. 2009; Vieta et al. 2008).

Adjunctive quetiapine (combined with lithium or divalproex) appears to be novel in that it may provide similarly robust prevention of mania and depression. However, somnolence/sedation may be challenging, and clinicians and patients may deem this agent to have inferior tolerability compared not only with mood stabilizers but also with newer SGAs such as aripiprazole and ziprasidone.

Risperidone long-acting injectable formulation (adjunctive therapy). In 2009, risperidone LAI formulation received approval for adjunctive (added to lithium or valproate) bipolar disorder preventive treatment. Risperidone LAI added to treatment as usual (TAU) (mostly lithium or valproate, but in some instances including lamotrigine, topiramate, antidepressants, and anxiolytics) yielded adequate efficacy, with an NNT for recurrence prevention compared with adjunctive placebo of 5 (Figure 4–2, Table 4–1), and with more robust mania prevention (NNT=7; Table 4–1) than depression prevention (NNT=16; Table 4–1). Also, compared with olanzapine, risperidone LAI plus TAU resulted in less risk of weight gain/metabolic problems but more risk of EPS and tremor (for the latter compared with placebo, NNH=7; Table 4–2) (Macfadden et al. 2009).

In summary, risperidone LAI adjunctive therapy appears to provide more robust prevention of mania than of depression. Adverse effects (e.g., EPS, tremor, and weight gain/metabolic problems) with this approach can be challenging, and clinicians and patients commonly deem risperidone LAI to have inferior tolerability compared not only with mood stabilizers but also with newer SGAs (e.g., aripiprazole and ziprasidone).

Ziprasidone (adjunctive therapy).   In 2009, adjunctive (added to lithium or valproate) ziprasidone was approved by the FDA for bipolar disorder preventive treatment. Adjunctive ziprasidone yielded adequate efficacy, with an NNT for recurrence prevention compared with adjunctive placebo of 8 (Figure 4–2, Table 4–1), and with more robust prevention of mania (NNT=10; Table 4–1) than depression (NNT=56; Table 4–1). Also, adjunctive ziprasidone had better longer-term tolerability than older SGAs, with only a limited risk of tremor (NNH=37; Table 4–2) during the controlled randomized phase, although akathisia was reported by 8.0% of patients during the uncontrolled prerandomization open stabilization phase (Bowden et al. 2010).

In summary, ziprasidone adjunctive therapy appears to provide more robust prevention of mania than of depression. Adverse effects during longer-term treatment with this agent are commonly less challenging than with older SGAs, although akathisia can be problematic during acute treatment. Clinicians and patients commonly deem this agent to have chronic tolerability that is superior to that of older SGAs (e.g., olanzapine, risperidone, and quetiapine) but inferior to that of mood stabilizers.

Aripiprazole (adjunctive therapy).   In 2011, adjunctive (added to lithium or valproate) aripiprazole was approved for bipolar disorder preventive treatment. Aripiprazole added to lithium or valproate yielded adequate efficacy, with an NNT for recurrence prevention compared with adjunctive placebo of 10 (Figure 4–2, Tables 4–1 and 4–2), more robust mania prevention (NNT=13; Table 4–1) than depression prevention (NNT=42; Table 4–1), and better tolerability than older SGAs, with only a limited risk of tremor (NNH=28; Table 4–2) (Marcus et al. 2011). However, in a similarly designed study, aripiprazole added to lamotrigine yielded inadequate bipolar disorder preventive efficacy but adequate safety/tolerability (Carlson et al. 2012).

In summary, adjunctive aripiprazole (combined with lithium or divalproex) appears to be more robust for preventing mania than for preventing depression. Adverse effects with adjunctive aripiprazole may be less problematic than with older SGAs. Although clinicians and patients may deem this agent to have superior tolerability compared with olanzapine, quetiapine, and risperidone, they may consider it more poorly tolerated than mood stabilizers.

Tier II: High-Priority Unapproved Bipolar Disorder Preventive Treatment Options

As noted in the Tier I section above, safety/tolerability limitations of some Tier I approved bipolar disorder preventive treatments, such as SGAs, may lead clinicians and patients to consider other options. One approach in assessing alternative treatments is to consider medications such as divalproex that have acute bipolar disorder indications, substantive familiarity, and/or evidence of efficacy in bipolar disorder preventive treatment. However, as of early 2015, divalproex lacked an FDA bipolar disorder preventive treatment indication. Although the pivotal divalproex monotherapy trial for bipolar disorder preventive treatment failed, apparently because of methodological limitations, divalproex has widespread familiarity and is ranked highly in multiple treatment guidelines (American Psychiatric Association 2002; Goodwin and Consensus Group of the British Association for Psychopharmacology 2009; Grunze et al. 2013; Keck et al. 2004; Suppes et al. 2005; Yatham et al. 2013). Indeed, several SGAs (i.e., quetiapine, risperidone LAI, aripiprazole, and ziprasidone) have FDA indications to be added to valproate (or lithium) for bipolar disorder preventive treatment.

Divalproex

Divalproex received FDA approval in 1994 for the monotherapy treatment of manic episodes associated with bipolar disorder. In 2005, an extended-release (ER) formulation of divalproex received a monotherapy indication for the treatment of acute manic and mixed episodes. However, as of early 2015, both divalproex formulations lacked a bipolar disorder preventive treatment indication.

In a multicenter, randomized, double-blind, placebo-controlled trial, divalproex yielded an NNT for recurrence prevention compared with adjunctive placebo of 8 (Figure 4–1, right; Tables 4–1 and 4–2), with the possibility of more robust depression prevention (NNT=11; Table 4–1) than mania prevention (NNT=22; Table 4–1). Although divalproex has been considered to have better tolerability than antipsychotics, it entailed a substantive risk of tremor (NNH=4; Table 4–2) (Bowden et al. 2000). In the BALANCE comparative effectiveness trial, divalproex appeared less effective than lithium for bipolar preventive treatment both as monotherapy and in combination with lithium (Geddes et al. 2010) (Figure 4–4). However, intolerability discontinuation rates were nonsignificantly less common with divalproex monotherapy than with lithium monotherapy (1.8% vs. 5.5%, NNH=–28) and significantly less common with divalproex monotherapy than with lithium plus divalproex (1.8% vs. 9.1%, NNH=–14) (Figure 4–4).

Baseline markers of divalproex compared with lithium response appear in some ways overlapping and in other ways complementary. Patients with poor responses to lithium may respond to divalproex, which can be effective in pure (Bowden et al. 1994), mixed (Freeman et al. 1992), or dysphoric (Swann et al. 1997) mania; in patients with at least three prior episodes (Swann et al. 2000); in adolescents (Papatheodorou and Kutcher 1993); in patients with rapid-cycling (Bowden et al. 1994) or secondary (Stoll et al. 1994) bipolar disorder, or bipolar disorder combined with concurrent substance abuse (Brady et al. 1995); and in patients whose symptoms were unresponsive to lithium or who cannot tolerate lithium (Bowden et al. 1994).

In summary, divalproex is a commonly used unapproved bipolar disorder preventive treatment option that may even yield more robust depression prevention than mania prevention. Clinicians and patients commonly deem this agent to have inferior tolerability compared with lamotrigine but superior tolerability compared with SGAs.

Quetiapine (Monotherapy)

Quetiapine was approved, in 2008, by the FDA for bipolar disorder preventive treatment as adjunct (added to lithium or valproate). However, in spite of publication in 2011 of controlled data supporting the use of quetiapine monotherapy in bipolar disorder preventive treatment (Weisler et al. 2011), as of early 2015 quetiapine monotherapy lacked FDA approval for this indication.

Quetiapine monotherapy yielded an NNT for recurrence prevention compared with adjunctive placebo of 4 (Figure 4–1, right; Tables 4–1 and 4–2), with ability to prevent not only mania (NNT=6; Table 4–1) but also depression (NNT=9; Table 4–1). The clinical utility of these benefits was limited, however, by a substantive risk of somnolence, seen in aggregate in 32.3% of patients during the controlled randomized phase and the uncontrolled prerandomization open stabilization phase, although the NNH for somnolence compared with adjunctive placebo during the controlled randomized phase was only 41 (Table 4–2, legend footnote a), and to a lesser extent by weight gain, seen in aggregate in 27.4% of patients during the controlled randomized phase and the uncontrolled prerandomization open stabilization phase, although the NNH for at least 7% weight gain compared with adjunctive placebo during the controlled randomized phase was only 13 (Table 4–2) (Weisler et al. 2011).

In summary, quetiapine monotherapy is a bipolar disorder preventive treatment option that may help prevent not only manic but also depressive recurrence. Quetiapine monotherapy is occasionally used, despite lacking an FDA indication for bipolar preventive treatment, although clinicians and patients commonly deem this agent to have inferior tolerability compared with mood stabilizers and newer SGAs (e.g., aripiprazole and ziprasidone).

Tier III—Intermediate-Priority Unapproved Bipolar Disorder Preventive Treatment Options

In this section we consider bipolar disorder preventive treatment options with more limited evidence of efficacy than the Tier I and Tier II treatments. These alternatives include the mood stabilizer carbamazepine, other SGAs (olanzapine plus fluoxetine combination [OFC], olanzapine [adjunctive to lithium or valproate], ziprasidone [monotherapy], lurasidone [monotherapy or adjunctive], asenapine [monotherapy], paliperidone [monotherapy], and clozapine [adjunctive]), adjunctive antidepressants, and adjunctive psychotherapy. Agents with proven efficacy and indications for acute mania (e.g., carbamazepine, ziprasidone, and asenapine monotherapy; adjunctive olanzapine) and acute bipolar depression (e.g., OFC, lurasidone) might ultimately prove to have utility in preventive treatment, but as of early 2015 the evidence supporting such use was insufficient for them to carry a high priority. In general, treatment guidelines do not consider these modalities to be first-line bipolar disorder preventive treatment interventions and instead list them as intermediate-priority options (American Psychiatric Association 2002; Goodwin and Consensus Group of the British Association for Psychopharmacology 2009; Grunze et al. 2013; Keck et al. 2004; Suppes et al. 2005; Yatham et al. 2013). However, some Tier III options have mitigating advantages, such as acute indications or tolerability, that might make them attractive for selected patients, and in certain circumstances some of these interventions may be considered early on (e.g., psychotherapy for pregnant women). For some of these treatments (e.g., adjunctive psychotherapy), advances in research, familiarity, and/or availability may ultimately be sufficient to merit their consideration for placement in higher tiers.

Carbamazepine

As of early 2015, the mood stabilizer carbamazepine, unlike the mood stabilizers lithium, lamotrigine, and divalproex, had less of an evidence base supporting its use in bipolar disorder preventive treatment. Also, unlike lithium and lamotrigine, carbamazepine lacked an FDA indication for bipolar disorder preventive treatment. Nevertheless, limited systematic data supported its consideration as an alternative treatment.

Limited data from a randomized controlled bipolar disorder preventive treatment comparative effectiveness study suggested that carbamazepine compared with lithium may be somewhat inferior overall (Greil et al. 1997), with the difference driven by marked inferiority of carbamazepine in patients with a "classical" subtype (bipolar I without mood-incongruent delusions and without comorbidity), which overshadowed a trend toward superiority in patients with a "nonclassical" subtype (bipolar II/ not otherwise specified, mood-incongruent delusions, comorbidity) (Greil et al. 1998). Other longer-term bipolar disorder treatment studies comparing effectiveness suggested that carbamazepine compared with lithium yielded similar overall outcome (Denicoff et al. 1997; Hartong et al. 2003; Okuma et al. 1981).

Clinical markers of carbamazepine response are similar in some respects to those for divalproex response, so that nonclassical (Greil et al. 1998), secondary (Himmelhoch and Garfinkel 1986), and lithium-unresponsive or -intolerant patients with bipolar disorder (Post et al. 1987) may respond to carbamazepine. However, findings have been less consistent with regard to the predictive value of a rapid-cycling pattern (Okuma 1993; Post et al. 1987), dysphoric mania (Lusznat et al. 1988; Post et al. 1989), and severe mania (Post et al. 1987; Small et al. 1991).

Adverse effects and drug interactions with carbamazepine can be challenging, but selected patients may experience adequate tolerability compared with the mood stabilizers lithium and divalproex, or compared with antipsychotics.

Other Second-Generation Antipsychotics

As of early 2015, the other SGAs OFC, olanzapine (adjunctive therapy), ziprasidone (monotherapy), lurasidone (monotherapy or adjunctive therapy), asenapine (monotherapy), paliperidone (monotherapy), and clozapine (adjunctive therapy) lacked FDA indications for bipolar disorder preventive treatment. Nevertheless, limited data suggest that on occasion at least some such agents may be worth considering as alternative bipolar disorder preventive treatments for patients with adequate acute efficacy and safety/tolerability, based on the hope that continuing these interventions might yield adequate longer-term preventive efficacy and safety/tolerability.

Olanzapine plus fluoxetine combination. Although a 24-week open-label extension of the OFC acute bipolar depression trial (Tohen et al. 2003a) provided some data regarding the potential safety/tolerability and efficacy of preventive OFC, the open, uncontrolled design constituted a serious limitation (Corya et al. 2006). Similarly, for a 25-week, multicenter, randomized, double-blind, head-to-head comparison of OFC and lamotrigine that extended a 7-week comparison of these agents in patients with acute bipolar depression (Brown et al. 2006), the lack of a placebo arm constituted a serious limitation (Brown et al. 2009). Thus, placebo-controlled trials are needed to establish the benefits and risks of OFC preventive treatment. However, safety/tolerability challenges such as weight gain/metabolic problems and sedation are expected to commonly limit OFC's utility, particularly in longer-term treatment.

Olanzapine (adjunctive therapy). In an 18-month, multicenter, randomized, double-blind, placebo-controlled trial, adjunctive (added to lithium or divalproex) olanzapine compared with adjunctive placebo yielded only a very limited (not statistically significant) recurrence prevention benefit (29.4% vs. 31.3% recurrence, NNT=55) but a much more robust harm for at least 7% weight gain (27% vs. 6%, NNH=5) (Tohen et al. 2004). Adverse effects such as weight gain/metabolic problems with olanzapine combined with mood stabilizers can be routinely challenging, and clinicians and patients commonly deem such combinations to have inferior safety/tolerability compared not only with two mood stabilizer combinations but also with combinations of newer SGAs (e.g., aripiprazole or ziprasidone) with mood stabilizers.

Ziprasidone (monotherapy). Controlled trials are necessary to assess the utility of ziprasidone monotherapy in the preventive treatment of bipolar disorder. Although ziprasidone initiation may be complex, with some patients experiencing substantial akathisia, the relative lack of weight gain/metabolic problems may make preventive ziprasidone worth considering for patients who have adequate acute efficacy and safety/tolerability with ziprasidone, and who fail to tolerate preventive treatment with other agents because of weight gain and/or metabolic problems.

Lurasidone (monotherapy or adjunctive therapy). In a 24-week open extension of the randomized controlled acute bipolar depression trials, lurasidone appeared to yield adequate safety/tolerability and efficacy (Ketter et al. 2014). However, as of early 2015, placebo-controlled data regarding the efficacy and safety/tolerability of lurasidone for bipolar disorder preventive treatment were lacking.

Asenapine (monotherapy). In a 40-week double-blind extension of randomized controlled acute mania trials, asenapine compared with olanzapine (there was no placebo control group) appeared to yield adequate safety/tolerability and efficacy. The NNH for at least 7% weight gain with asenapine compared with olanzapine was –7 (i.e., at least 7% weight gain was less common with asenapine than with olanzapine). However, as of early 2015, asenapine lacked placebo-controlled evidence of efficacy and safety/tolerability for bipolar disorder preventive treatment.

Paliperidone (monotherapy). Paliperidone (hydroxyrisperidone), the active metabolite of risperidone, is available in ER oral and LAI formulations. In a multicenter, randomized, double-blind, placebo-controlled trial, paliperidone ER compared with placebo yielded only limited mood episode prevention (NNT=13; Table 4–1, Table 4–2), driven by mania prevention (NNT=8; Table 4–1) rather than depression prevention (NNT = –17 [i.e., depressive recurrence was numerically more common with paliperidone ER than with placebo]; Table 4–1) (Berwaerts et al. 2012). Paliperidone ER, although fairly well tolerated, compared with placebo tended to yield greater somnolence (Table 4–2) and more EPS (Table 4–2, legend footnote *b*).

Paliperidone ER compared with placebo appeared to provide limited prevention of mania rather than depression (and may even have increased the risk of depressive recurrence) and entailed risks of adverse effects (e.g., EPS and somnolence). Hence, in the view of the FDA, paliperidone provided insufficient additional efficacy or safety/tolerability benefit over risperidone to merit an indication in patients with bipolar disorder. Although paliperidone LAI has more convenient dosing frequency (once monthly) than risperidone LAI (twice monthly), the absence of controlled data of efficacy and safety/tolerability in bipolar disorder preventive treatment makes off-label paliperidone LAI a low-priority option for patients with bipolar disorder.

Clozapine (adjunctive therapy). As of early 2015, there had been only one published controlled trial of clozapine adjunctive (added to TAU) longer-term administration in patients with treatment-resistant bipolar I disorder (Suppes et al. 1999). However, uncontrolled reports (for reviews, see Frye et al. 1998; Zarate et al. 1995) and one controlled acute mania study (Barbini et al. 1997) suggested that clozapine might have efficacy in bipolar disorder. It appears, therefore, that clozapine may have less therapeutic potential in depressive than in manic/mixed states. In view of the challenging adverse-effect profile of this agent, clozapine is usually held in reserve for patients with treatment-resistant illness.

Adjunctive Antidepressants

The use of adjunctive antidepressants, added to antimanic agents, in bipolar disorder preventive treatment is even more controversial than in the treatment of acute bipolar depression. These agents have been considered by some to be temporary adjuncts for administration during acute bipolar depression and to be best avoided in the longer term due to concerns about efficacy and tolerability (i.e., treatment-emergent affective switch). Indeed, a meta-analysis of seven controlled trials involving 350 patients with bipolar disorder (type I, type II, or not otherwise specified) (Amsterdam and Shults 2005; Ghaemi et al. 2005; Johnstone et al. 1990; Kane et al. 1982; Prien et al. 1973, 1984; Quitkin et al. 1981) indicated that adjunctive antidepressants only marginally enhanced depression prevention (NNT=10; Figure 4–5, left) while increasing the risk of manic recurrence (NNH=8; Figure 4–5, right) (Ghaemi et al. 2008).

Nevertheless, it may be that a minority of patients with bipolar disorder could benefit from preventive adjunctive antidepressants. In a naturalistic (i.e., not randomized) effectiveness study, only 34% (189/549) of Stanley Foundation Bipolar Network patients receiving adjunctive antidepressants for new-onset major depressive episodes continued these agents for at least 60 days (Altshuler et al. 2003). Among the 15% (84/549) who achieved durable remission (6 consecutive weeks with CGI Severity scores indicating no more than mild subsyndromal symptoms), continuing antidepressants for more than 6 months compared with less than 6 months was associated with a lower rate of depressive relapse (36% vs. 70%) and no increase in treatment-emergent affective switch. Thus, among the 15% of depressed patients with bipolar disorder who attained durable remission with antidepressants, continuing these agents for longer than 6 months had merit. Indeed, in its consensus report, the International Society for Bipolar Disorders Antidepressant Use in Bipolar Disorders Task Force stated that adjunctive antidepressants for bipolar preventive treatment were permissible if depressive relapse occurred after stopping antidepressants (Pacchiarotti et al. 2013).

In summary, preventive administration of adjunctive antidepressants in patients with bipolar disorder is controversial. In many instances, these agents may even have short-term efficacy and tolerability

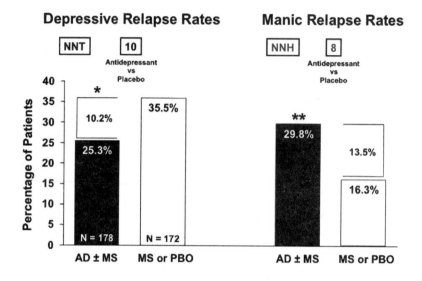

FIGURE 4–5.   Meta-analysis of controlled trials of adjunctive antidepressants in bipolar disorder preventive treatment: numbers needed to treat, number needed to harm, and depressive and manic recurrence rates.

Note.   Patients had bipolar I disorder, bipolar II disorder, or bipolar disorder not otherwise specified. AD=antidepressant; MS=mood stabilizer; NNH = number needed to harm; NNT=number needed to treat; PBO=placebo.

*P<0.05, **P<0.01 vs. placebo.

Source.   Data from Ghaemi et al. 2008.

problems that limit their utility. However, in the minority of patients who experience adequate acute relief of depression without treatment-emergent affective switch, continuing these agents in preventive therapy may be worth considering.

Adjunctive Psychotherapy for Bipolar Disorder

Adjunctive (added to pharmacotherapy) psychotherapies have been more thoroughly assessed for bipolar disorder preventive treatment than for acute bipolar depression (Geddes and Miklowitz 2013). Earlier studies assessed group psychoeducation (group PE), family focused therapy (FFT), cognitive-behavioral therapy (CBT), and interpersonal and social rhythm therapy (IPSRT); more recent research has begun to examine dialectical behavior therapy (DBT) (Goldstein et al. 2007) and mindfulness-based cognitive therapy (MBCT) (Perich et al. 2013). It is worth noting that adjunctive psychosocial interventions, several of which have demonstrated efficacy in acute bipolar depression but not in acute mania, might more robustly help prevent depression than mood elevation (Table 4–3), although more data are needed to definitively establish this polarity advantage.

Adjunctive group psychoeducation.   Group PE provides patients with information about bipolar disorder and its treatment (Colom et al. 2006). In an influential initial study, outpatients in remission undergoing standard pharmacological treatment were randomly assigned to receive adjunctive group PE or adjunctive nonstructured group meetings (both involving 21 weekly sessions). Group PE was associated with fewer mood episode recurrences (67% vs. 92%, NNT=4) (Colom et al. 2003), and preventive benefits persisted at 5-year follow-up (Colom et al. 2009).

Unfortunately, a subsequent study was less encouraging: adjunctive group PE compared with adjunctive (control) relaxation group (both administered in 16 twice-weekly sessions) did not lead to improvements in mood, functioning, or quality of life (de Barros Pellegrinelli et al. 2013). Limited efficacy could have been related to brevity of group PE intervention (only 16 sessions administered over 8 weeks) or to patients having more challenging illness. Indeed, this study, compared with the Colom et al. (2003) study, utilized 24% fewer sessions administered over 62% less time in a sample that was 28% older, with 68% longer bipolar illness duration, more prior episodes, and 83% shorter prior remission at entry. A post hoc analysis of the 2003 study revealed that the group PE lacked efficacy for time to recurrence in patients with more than seven prior episodes (Colom et al. 2010).

However, briefer-duration adjunctive group PE could provide substantive cost savings compared with longer-duration adjunctive individual CBT. Briefer (6-session) adjunctive group PE compared with longer (20-session) adjunctive individual CBT yielded statistically similar mood outcomes but required 70% fewer group (rather than individual) sessions, permitting an 85% lower per-patient psychotherapy cost (Parikh et al. 2012). Patients in this study had challenging later-stage illness that was comparable to that seen in the report by de Barros Pellegrinelli et al. (2013). Ultimately, even greater cost-effectiveness might be realized using adjunctive computerized PE, although such efforts are early in development (Proudfoot et al. 2012).

In summary, adjunctive group PE appears to yield mood benefits in bipolar disorder that can last up to 5 years, particularly with longer treatment regimens in patients with less challenging illness. Briefer adjunctive group PE may be more cost-effective than longer adjunctive individual CBT, although it is possible that adjunctive group PE may have less efficacy with a briefer format and/or in patients with more challenging illness.

Adjunctive family focused therapy. FFT involves family PE and training in communication and problem-solving (Miklowitz 2010). In a 2-year study, among 101 patients with bipolar disorder and recent syndromal mood episodes (86.1% manic/mixed, 13.9% depressed; 81.2% requiring hospitalization) who were not necessarily remitted at entry, adjunctive FFT (21 sessions over 9 months) compared with adjunctive crisis management (2 family sessions and follow-up crisis management) resulted in fewer relapses (35% vs. 54%, NNT=6) (Miklowitz et al. 2003).

Moreover, in another 2-year study conducted among 53 patients with bipolar I disorder who were recently hospitalized for mania and not necessarily remitted at entry, adjunctive FFT compared with adjunctive individual therapy (supportive, educational, and problem-focused), with both involving 21 sessions over 9 months, was associated with fewer hospitalizations and relapses (Rea et al. 2003). The benefit of FFT decreasing likelihood of hospitalization compared with individual therapy occurred in the posttreatment year (12% vs. 60%, NNT=3) but not during the first (active treatment) year (29% vs. 40%, NNT=10).

In summary, adjunctive FFT appears to yield mood benefits in bipolar disorder patients that can last up to 2 years, even in recently hospitalized individuals not necessarily remitted at entry and even compared with individual psychotherapy of similar intensity. Thus, when a family member is available for this type of intervention, FFT may be particularly useful in the aftermath of a patient's mood episode.

Adjunctive cognitive-behavioral therapy. CBT focuses on changing dysfunctional cognitions and maladaptive behaviors that increase vulnerability to mood episodes (Lam et al. 2010; Ramirez Basco and Rush 2005). Unfortunately, data regarding the efficacy of adjunctive CBT in patients with bipolar disorder have been variable.

An influential initial 1-year study of 103 interepisode bipolar disorder patients supported the efficacy of adjunctive cognitive therapy (CT) (12–18 sessions in first 6 months plus 2 booster sessions in following 6 months), which, compared with a no-adjunctive-psychotherapy control condition, yielded fewer mood episode recurrences (in 44% vs. 75%, NNT=4) and psychiatric hospitalizations (in 15% vs. 33%, NNT=6) (Lam et al. 2003). However, during the subsequent 18 months, mood episode recurrence rates were statistically similar in patients with and without prior adjunctive CT, raising the possibility that CT booster sessions may need to be continued beyond the first 6 months after acute CT for a longer-term benefit (Lam et al. 2005).

Scott et al. (2006) assessed CBT in 253 patients with highly recurrent or severe bipolar disorder, approximately two-thirds of whom had particularly challenging illness, either with a current mood episode (primarily depressive) or psychiatric comorbidity/high recurrence (at least 30 prior episodes). In this 18-month study, adjunctive CBT (22 sessions over 6 months, followed by 2 sessions in the next 6 months) did not improve mood outcomes compared with not receiving adjunctive psychotherapy. Further analysis, however, indicated that the CBT did improve mood outcomes in the subset of patients with fewer than 12 prior mood episodes.

Subsequent CBT studies in exclusively interepisode bipolar disorder patients were also less encouraging than Lam et al.'s (2003) report (Gomes et al. 2011; Zaretsky et al. 2008) or suggested that adjunctive CBT might result in mood outcomes comparable to those following other adjunctive psychotherapies (Meyer and Hautzinger 2012).

In summary, adjunctive individual (but not group) CBT may yield mood benefits in patients with bipolar disorder, although research suggests that beyond 1 year, booster sessions may need to be continued for a lasting benefit. CBT may be less effective in a group format, but it may be effective when conducted among interepisode patients with fewer prior mood episodes, although other psychotherapies such as supportive therapy may yield comparable mood benefits.

Adjunctive interpersonal and social rhythm therapy. IPSRT integrates PE, social rhythm therapy, and interpersonal psychotherapy components to stabilize daily routines, reduce interpersonal problems, and increase pharmacotherapy adherence (Frank 2005). In a paradigm of acute treatment followed by preventive treatment, IPSRT was compared with intensive clinical management (ICM, which included support/education regarding bipolar disorder, sleep, medications, and side effects) in four strategies: acute and preventive IPSRT, acute and preventive ICM, acute IPSRT followed by preventive ICM, or acute ICM followed by preventive IPSRT. In the acute phase, IPSRT and ICM yielded statistically similar times to remission and rates of remission (70% vs. 72%) (Frank et al. 2005). Among patients whose illness remitted, preventive IPSRT and preventive ICM (both administered every 2 weeks for 12 weeks, then monthly) yielded statistically similar mood outcomes, although patients who had previously received acute IPSRT rather than acute ICM had significantly longer time to recurrence and a numerically lower recurrence rate (41% vs. 46%, NNT=22) (Frank et al. 2005). The benefit of

IPSRT appeared to be mediated by increased stability of daily routines. Also, participants who changed treatment modality (i.e., from IPSRT to ICM or from ICM to IPSRT) had poorer outcomes compared with those who received the same treatment for stabilization and long-term prevention (Frank et al. 1999). In summary, IPSRT compared with ICM yielded generally similar acute and preventive outcomes, perhaps because of ICM being an effective active control intervention that entailed substantive PE and supportive therapy elements.

Adjunctive caregiver group psychoeducation (group PE and FFT components). In a 15-month study of 113 interepisode bipolar disorder patients (euthymic at least 3 months), providing live-in caregivers with group PE (12 weekly sessions) compared with no adjunctive intervention yielded a lower recurrence rate (42.1% vs. 66.1%, NNT=5) (Reinares et al. 2008). The preventive benefit was seen in patients with early-stage bipolar disorder (i.e., those capable of full symptomatic and functional recovery without psychiatric comorbidity) but not in patients with more advanced illness (Reinares et al. 2010).

Adjunctive group mindfulness-based cognitive therapy (mindfulness and CBT components). MBCT integrates mindfulness (maintaining nonjudgmental attention on the present moment) training with cognitive and behavioral elements of CBT (Sega et al. 2010). In a 1-year study in adults with interepisode bipolar disorder, 48 patients receiving adjunctive group MBCT compared with 47 receiving TAU did not have significantly different recurrence rate, time to recurrence, or mood symptoms, but did have greater relief of anxiety (Perich et al. 2013).

Adjunctive dialectical behavior therapy (group PE and DBT components). DBT strives to help individuals regulate their emotions (Van Dijk 2009) and has had encouraging preliminary studies (Goldstein et al. 2007; Van Dijk et al. 2013).

Adjunctive multimodal stress/mood symptom management group (group PE, CBT, DBT, and IPSRT components). Participation in an adjunctive multimodal (including elements of group PE, CBT, DBT, and IPSRT) stress/mood symptom management group (12 weekly sessions followed by 3 monthly booster sessions) compared with adjunctive telephone contact (12 weekly calls) yielded a lower recurrence rate (28.1% vs. 55.0%, NNT=4) (Castle et al. 2010).

Summary. Adjunctive psychosocial interventions can be a crucial component of preventive care for individuals with bipolar disorder. Unfortunately, access to therapists with training in these adjunctive psychotherapy modalities remains limited, hindering the dissemination of these valuable treatments, which thus remain in Tier III.

Adjunctive Psychosocial Interventions for Functional Impairment

In patients with bipolar disorder, mood disturbance can profoundly impair function, on occasion, even more during depression than during mood elevation (Rosa et al. 2010). Although functional impairment attenuates with resolution of mood episodes, even when patients are euthymic, functional impairment persists in excess of that seen in healthy individuals (Rosa et al. 2010), consistent with observations that functional recovery is more challenging to achieve than resolution of mood disturbance (Rosa et al. 2011; Tohen et al. 2000). Functional impairment is more severe in multiple-episode than in first-episode bipolar disorder patients (Reinares et al. 2013), consistent with the notion that functional impairment increases with number of episodes (Post 1992).

Thus, mechanisms of persistent functional impairment in interepisode bipolar disorder patients are of considerable interest. Because functional impairment may be related not only to mood symptoms but also to cognitive dysfunction (Martinez-Aran et al. 2007; Reinares et al. 2013), it appears feasible that subthreshold mood symptoms and/or cognitive dysfunction could contribute importantly to functional impairment in interepisode bipolar disorder patients (Goodwin et al. 2008). If that is the case, then interventions to relieve subthreshold mood symptoms and/or cognitive dysfunction could attenuate interepisode functional impairment. Accordingly, adjunctive psychosocial interventions targeting functional deficits in patients with bipolar disorder are beginning to emerge.

Adjunctive functional remediation group therapy. In a recent 21-week study of interepisode bipolar disorder patients (euthymic for at least 3 months) with moderate to severe functional impairment, 77 patients receiving adjunctive functional remediation group therapy (daily functioning training and cognition/problem-solving PE) had superior improvement in global psychosocial functioning compared with 80 receiving TAU (but not compared with 82 receiving group PE) (Torrent et al. 2013).

Adjunctive social cognition and interaction training. Social cognition (ability to understand environmental social information and predict others' behavior) is commonly impaired in bipolar disorder, even after recovery from mood episodes. A preliminary study of adjunctive social cognition and interaction training (added to TAU) was encouraging (Lahera et al. 2013).

Summary. Data are beginning to emerge regarding the utility of adjunctive psychosocial interventions in addressing functional impairment in patients with bipolar disorder, and this will likely be an important area of future research with substantial public health implications.

Tier IV: Novel Adjunctive Treatments

Tier IV includes novel adjunctive treatments—electroconvulsive therapy (ECT), vagus nerve stimulation (VNS), and transcranial magnetic stimulation (TMS) (Table 4–3)—that have even more limited evidence of efficacy than the treatments in Tiers II and III. In general, these modalities are considered to be low-priority interventions by treatment guidelines (American Psychiatric Association 2002; Goodwin and Consensus Group of the British Association for Psychopharmacology 2009; Grunze et al. 2013; Keck et al. 2004; Suppes et al. 2005; Yatham et al. 2013). Although insufficient data exist to determine the predominant polarity of benefits of these interventions, they are most often administered in hopes of relieving acute depression or preventing depressive recurrence. Acceptability, availability, and expense can substantially limit the utilization of these treatments. Nevertheless, some Tier IV options could prove attractive for carefully selected patients, after consideration of treatments in Tiers I–III (e.g., for patients resistant to or intolerant of Tier I–III treatments). For some Tier IV treatments, advances in research and increased availability and affordability may ultimately provide sufficient evidence to merit their consideration for placement in higher tiers.

Adjunctive Electroconvulsive Therapy

As reviewed by Vaidya et al. (2003), limited case reports and case series describe preventive ECT efficacy in mixed samples of bipolar and unipolar patients, although some patients may have better outcomes with mood stabilizer combinations than with preventive ECT (Jaffe et al. 1991).

Concerns based on case reports regarding the risks of delirium, seizures, and prolonged apnea resulted in recommendations that lithium not be combined with ECT (Small and Milstein 1990). Although subsequent larger case series reports suggested that the combination of lithium plus ECT may be safe and effective in certain clinical circumstances

(Dolenc and Rasmussen 2005), contrary reports of problems with the combination continued to occur (Sartorius et al. 2005).

As advocated in most treatment guidelines (American Psychiatric Association 2002; Goodwin and Consensus Group of the British Association for Psychopharmacology 2009; Grunze et al. 2013; Suppes et al. 2005; Yatham et al. 2013), preventive ECT is generally held in reserve for patients intolerant of or refractory to pharmacotherapy, because of the risk of interruption of function related to cognitive adverse effects, stigma, consent challenges, and logistical concerns such as coordination of care and aftercare.

Adjunctive Vagus Nerve Stimulation

VNS involves surgical implantation of an electronic device similar to a pacemaker with an electrode connecting it to the left vagus nerve, and delivering low-frequency, chronic, intermittent electrically pulsed signals to the left vagus nerve, yielding deep brain and limbic cortical stimulation. In 2005, VNS was approved by the FDA for the adjunctive long-term treatment of chronic or recurrent depression resistant to four or more antidepressants in adults. Given its invasiveness and expense, VNS is most often considered a longer-term option for patients with treatment-resistant depression.

In a meta-analysis of outpatient multicenter trials, adjunctive VNS (added to TAU) in 1,035 treatment-resistant depression patients compared with TAU without VNS in 425 patients yielded week-96 Montgomery-Åsberg Depression Rating Scale (MADRS) response rates of 32% and 14%, respectively (NNT=6) (Berry et al. 2013). Patients with VNS + TAU MADRS response at week 24 were more likely to have MADRS response at week 96. Interpretation of these data with respect to bipolar disorder preventive treatment is challenging, however, because only approximately 20% of the patients had bipolar disorder. Adjunctive VNS has been generally well tolerated, but treatment-emergent affective switch has occurred sporadically. Also, the cost and invasiveness of VNS and the relatively modest efficacy have raised cost-benefit concerns. Indeed, patients commonly find that their insurance companies deny reimbursement for VNS.

Adjunctive Transcranial Magnetic Stimulation

TMS strives to relieve depression by administration of nonconvulsive stimulation (with high frequency) or inhibition (with low frequency) of cerebral activity. TMS was approved by the FDA in late 2008 for the treatment of major depressive disorder (in adults with unsatisfactory improvement with one adequate antidepressant trial in their current episode), and in 2013 for the treatment of migraine headaches. TMS is well tolerated in most patients, although there is a slight risk of seizure. However, data regarding the utility of TMS in mood disorder maintenance treatment are only beginning to emerge (Connolly et al. 2012; Richieri et al. 2013). As of early 2015, TMS had not been approved by the FDA for the treatment of acute bipolar depression or bipolar disorder preventive treatment. Furthermore, utilization of TMS in patients with bipolar disorder has been limited by hesitation of third-party payers (including Medicare in most regions) to cover the cost of this expensive procedure.

■ Conclusion

The last decade has seen substantial expansion of bipolar disorder preventive treatment options, with the mood stabilizers lithium, lamotrigine, and divalproex being among the most commonly used agents. Lithium, despite no longer being the only FDA-approved bipolar disorder preventive treatment, remains an important option. Lamotrigine has FDA approval for bipolar disorder preventive treatment, addresses depressive more than mood elevation aspects of bipolar illness, and has generally good safety/tolerability, but lacks an FDA acute bipolar disorder indication. Divalproex, although lacking FDA approval for bipolar disorder preventive treatment (perhaps related to pivotal-trial methodological limitations), has an FDA acute mania indication, and at least some controlled data support longer-term safety/tolerability comparable to lithium. In contrast, carbamazepine, because of its having less compelling evidence of efficacy and greater complexity of treatment, is considered an alternative rather than a first-line bipolar disorder preventive treatment. Although five SGAs have FDA approval for bipolar disorder preventive treatment as monotherapy and/or adjunctive therapy, safety/tolerability concerns can limit their utility. The preventive administration of adjunctive antidepressants in patients with bipolar disorder is controversial and lacks FDA approval, but these agents commonly have adequate somatic safety/tolerability, and a minority of patients may benefit from this approach. An increasing amount of controlled data supports the use of adjunctive psychotherapy in bipolar disorder preventive treatment.

■ References

Ahlfors UG, Baastrup PC, Dencker SJ, et al: Flupenthixol decanoate in recurrent manic-depressive illness. A comparison with lithium. Acta Psychiatr Scand 64(3):226–237, 1981 7324992

Altshuler L, Suppes T, Black D, et al: Impact of antidepressant discontinuation after acute bipolar depression remission on rates of depressive relapse at 1-year follow-up. Am J Psychiatry 160(7):1252–1262, 2003 12832239

American Psychiatric Association: Practice guideline for the treatment of patients with bipolar disorder (revision). Am J Psychiatry 159(4)(Suppl):1–50, 2002 11958165

Amsterdam JD, Shults J: Fluoxetine monotherapy of bipolar type II and bipolar NOS major depression: a double-blind, placebo-substitution, continuation study. Int Clin Psychopharmacol 20(5):257–264, 2005 16096516

Baastrup PC, Poulsen JC, Schou M, et al: Prophylactic lithium: double blind discontinuation in manic-depressive and recurrent-depressive disorders. Lancet 2(7668):326–330, 1970 4194439

Baldessarini RJ, Tondo L, Floris G, et al: Reduced morbidity after gradual discontinuation of lithium treatment for bipolar I and II disorders: a replication study. Am J Psychiatry 154(4):551–553, 1997 9090345

Barbini B, Scherillo P, Benedetti F, et al: Response to clozapine in acute mania is more rapid than that of chlorpromazine. Int Clin Psychopharmacol 12(2):109–112, 1997 9219046

Bellaire W, Demish K, Stoll KD: Carbamazepine versus lithium in prophylaxis of recurrent affective disorder (abstract). Psychopharmacology (Berl) 96(Suppl):287, 1988

Berry SM, Broglio K, Bunker M, et al: A patient-level meta-analysis of studies evaluating vagus nerve stimulation therapy for treatment-resistant depression. Med Devices (Auckl) 6:17–35, 2013 23482508

Berwaerts J, Melkote R, Nuamah I, et al: A randomized, placebo- and active-controlled study of paliperidone extended-release as maintenance treatment in patients with bipolar I disorder after an acute manic or mixed episode. J Affect Disord 138(3):247–258, 2012 22377512

Bowden CL, Brugger AM, Swann AC, et al; The Depakote Mania Study Group: Efficacy of divalproex vs lithium and placebo in the treatment of mania. JAMA 271(12):918–924, 1994 8120960

Bowden CL, Calabrese JR, McElroy SL, et al; Divalproex Maintenance Study Group: A randomized, placebo-controlled 12-month trial of divalproex and lithium in treatment of outpatients with bipolar I disorder. Arch Gen Psychiatry 57(5):481–489, 2000 10807488

Bowden CL, Calabrese JR, Sachs G, et al; Lamictal 606 Study Group: A placebo-controlled 18-month trial of lamotrigine and lithium maintenance treatment in recently manic or hypomanic patients with bipolar I disorder. Arch Gen Psychiatry 60(4):392–400, 2003 12695317

Bowden CL, Collins MA, McElroy SL, et al: Relationship of mania symptomatology to maintenance treatment response with divalproex, lithium, or placebo. Neuropsychopharmacology 30(10):1932–1939, 2005 15956987

Bowden CL, Vieta E, Ice KS, et al: Ziprasidone plus a mood stabilizer in subjects with bipolar I disorder: a 6-month, randomized, placebo-controlled, double-blind trial. J Clin Psychiatry 71(2):130–137, 2010 20122373

Brady KT, Sonne SC, Anton R, et al: Valproate in the treatment of acute bipolar affective episodes complicated by substance abuse: a pilot study. J Clin Psychiatry 56(3):118–121, 1995 7883730

Brown EB, McElroy SL, Keck PE Jr, et al: A 7-week, randomized, double-blind trial of olanzapine/fluoxetine combination versus lamotrigine in the treatment of bipolar I depression. J Clin Psychiatry 67(7):1025–1033, 2006 16889444

Brown E, Dunner DL, McElroy SL, et al: Olanzapine/fluoxetine combination vs. lamotrigine in the 6-month treatment of bipolar I depression. Int J Neuropsychopharmacol 12(6):773–782, 2009 19079815

Calabrese JR, Bowden CL, Sachs G, et al; Lamictal 605 Study Group: A placebo-controlled 18-month trial of lamotrigine and lithium maintenance treatment in recently depressed patients with bipolar I disorder. J Clin Psychiatry 64(9):1013–1024, 2003 14628976

Carlson BX, Ketter TA, Sun W, et al: Aripiprazole in combination with lamotrigine for the long-term treatment of patients with bipolar I disorder (manic or mixed): a randomized, multicenter, double-blind study (CN138–392). Bipolar Disord 14(1):41–53, 2012 22329471

Castle D, White C, Chamberlain J, et al: Group-based psychosocial intervention for bipolar disorder: randomised controlled trial. Br J Psychiatry 196(5):383–388, 2010 20435965

Cipriani A, Hawton K, Stockton S, et al: Lithium in the prevention of suicide in mood disorders: updated systematic review and meta-analysis. BMJ 346:f3646, 2013 23814104

Citrome L, Ketter TA: Number needed to harm can be clinically useful: a response to Safer and Zito. J Nerv Ment Dis 201(11):1001–1002, 2013 24177490

Colom F, Vieta E, Martinez-Aran A, et al: A randomized trial on the efficacy of group psychoeducation in the prophylaxis of recurrences in bipolar patients whose disease is in remission. Arch Gen Psychiatry 60(4):402–407, 2003 12695318

Colom F, Vieta E, Scott J: Psychoeducation Manual for Bipolar Disorder. New York, Cambridge University Press, 2006

Colom F, Vieta E, Sánchez-Moreno J, et al: Group psychoeducation for stabilised bipolar disorders: 5-year outcome of a randomised clinical trial. Br J Psychiatry 194(3):260–265, 2009 19252157

Colom F, Reinares M, Pacchiarotti I, et al: Has number of previous episodes any effect on response to group psychoeducation in bipolar patients? A 5-year follow-up post hoc analysis. Acta Neuropsychiatr 22(2):50–53, 2010

Connolly KR, Helmer A, Cristancho MA, et al: Effectiveness of transcranial magnetic stimulation in clinical practice post-FDA approval in the United States: results observed with the first 100 consecutive cases of depression at an academic medical center. J Clin Psychiatry 73(4):e567–e573, 2012 22579164

Coppen A, Noguera R, Bailey J, et al: Prophylactic lithium in affective disorders. Controlled trial. Lancet 2(7719):275–279, 1971 4104974

Corya SA, Perlis RH, Keck PE Jr, et al: A 24-week open-label extension study of olanzapine-fluoxetine combination and olanzapine monotherapy in the treatment of bipolar depression. J Clin Psychiatry 67(5):798–806, 2006 16841630

Coxhead N, Silverstone T, Cookson J: Carbamazepine versus lithium in the prophylaxis of bipolar affective disorder. Acta Psychiatr Scand 85(2):114–118, 1992 1543034

Cundall RL, Brooks PW, Murray LG: A controlled evaluation of lithium prophylaxis in affective disorders. Psychol Med 2(3):308–311, 1972 4562449

de Barros Pellegrinelli K, de O Costa LF, Silval KI, et al: Efficacy of psychoeducation on symptomatic and functional recovery in bipolar disorder. Acta Psychiatr Scand 127(2):153–158, 2013 22943487

Denicoff KD, Smith-Jackson EE, Disney ER, et al: Comparative prophylactic efficacy of lithium, carbamazepine, and the combination in bipolar disorder. J Clin Psychiatry 58(11):470–478, 1997 9413412

Dolenc TJ, Rasmussen KG: The safety of electroconvulsive therapy and lithium in combination: a case series and review of the literature. J ECT 21(3):165–170, 2005 16127306

Dunner DL, Stallone F, Fieve RR: Lithium carbonate and affective disorders, V: a double-blind study of prophylaxis of depression in bipolar illness. Arch Gen Psychiatry 33(1):117–120, 1976 1108832

Fieve RR, Kumbaraci T, Dunner DL: Lithium prophylaxis of depression in bipolar I, bipolar II, and unipolar patients. Am J Psychiatry 133(8):925–929, 1976 782261

Frank E: Treating Bipolar Disorder: A Clinician's Guide to Interpersonal and Social Rhythm Therapy. New York, Guilford, 2005

Frank E, Swartz HA, Mallinger AG, et al: Adjunctive psychotherapy for bipolar disorder: effects of changing treatment modality. J Abnorm Psychol 108(4):579–587, 1999 10609422

Frank E, Kupfer DJ, Thase ME, et al: Two-year outcomes for interpersonal and social rhythm therapy in individuals with bipolar I disorder. Arch Gen Psychiatry 62(9):996–1004, 2005 16143731

Freeman TW, Clothier JL, Pazzaglia P, et al: A double-blind comparison of valproate and lithium in the treatment of acute mania. Am J Psychiatry 149(1):108–111, 1992 1728157

Frye MA, Ketter TA, Altshuler LL, et al: Clozapine in bipolar disorder: treatment implications for other atypical antipsychotics. J Affect Disord 48(2–3):91–104, 1998 9543198

Geddes JR, Miklowitz DJ: Treatment of bipolar disorder. Lancet 381(9878):1672–1682, 2013 23663953

Geddes JR, Goodwin GM, Rendell J, et al; BALANCE investigators and collaborators: Lithium plus valproate combination therapy versus monotherapy for relapse prevention in bipolar I disorder (BALANCE): a randomised open-label trial. Lancet 375(9712):385–395, 2010 20092882

Ghaemi SN, El-Mallakh RS, Baldassano CF, et al: Randomized clinical trial of efficacy and safety of long-term antidepressant use in bipolar disorder. Paper presented at the 6th International Conference on Bipolar Disorder, Pittsburgh, June 16–18, 2005

Ghaemi SN, Wingo AP, Filkowski MA, et al: Long-term antidepressant treatment in bipolar disorder: meta-analyses of benefits and risks. Acta Psychiatr Scand 118(5):347–356, 2008 18727689

Gitlin MJ, Swendsen J, Heller TL, et al: Relapse and impairment in bipolar disorder. Am J Psychiatry 152(11):1635–1640, 1995 7485627

Goldstein TR, Axelson DA, Birmaher B, et al: Dialectical behavior therapy for adolescents with bipolar disorder: a 1-year open trial. J Am Acad Child Adolesc Psychiatry 46(7):820–830, 2007 17581446

Gomes BC, Abreu LN, Brietzke E, et al: A randomized controlled trial of cognitive behavioral group therapy for bipolar disorder. Psychother Psychosom 80(3):144–150, 2011 21372622

Goodwin GM; Consensus Group of the British Association for Psychopharmacology: Evidence-based guidelines for treating bipolar disorder: revised second edition—recommendations from the British Association for Psychopharmacology. J Psychopharmacol 23(4):346–388, 2009 19329543

Goodwin GM, Bowden CL, Calabrese JR, et al: A pooled analysis of 2 placebo-controlled 18-month trials of lamotrigine and lithium maintenance in bipolar I disorder. J Clin Psychiatry 65(3):432–441, 2004 15096085

Goodwin GM, Martinez-Aran A, Glahn DC, et al: Cognitive impairment in bipolar disorder: neurodevelopment or neurodegeneration? An ECNP expert meeting report. Eur Neuropsychopharmacol 18(11):787–793, 2008 18725178

Greil W, Ludwig-Mayerhofer W, Erazo N, et al: Lithium versus carbamazepine in the maintenance treatment of bipolar disorders—a randomised study. J Affect Disord 43(2):151–161, 1997 9165384

Greil W, Kleindienst N, Erazo N, et al: Differential response to lithium and carbamazepine in the prophylaxis of bipolar disorder. J Clin Psychopharmacol 18(6):455–460, 1998 9864077

Grof P, Alda M, Grof E, et al: The challenge of predicting response to stabilising lithium treatment. The importance of patient selection. Br J Psychiatry Suppl (21):16–19, 1993 8217062

Grunze H, Vieta E, Goodwin GM, et al; WFSBP Task Force on Treatment Guidelines for Bipolar Disorders: The World Federation of Societies of Biological Psychiatry (WFSBP) guidelines for the biological treatment of bipolar disorders: update 2012 on the long-term treatment of bipolar disorder. World J Biol Psychiatry 14(3):154–219, 2013 23480132

Hartong EG, Moleman P, Hoogduin CA, et al; LitCar Group: Prophylactic efficacy of lithium versus carbamazepine in treatment-naive bipolar patients. J Clin Psychiatry 64(2):144–151, 2003 12633122

Himmelhoch JM, Garfinkel ME: Sources of lithium resistance in mixed mania. Psychopharmacol Bull 22(3):613–620, 1986 3797567

Hooshmand F, Miller S, Dore J, et al: Trends in pharmacotherapy in patients referred to a bipolar specialty clinic, 2000–2011. J Affect Disord 155:283–287, 2014 24314912

Hullin RP, McDonald R, Allsopp MN: Prophylactic lithium in recurrent affective disorders. Lancet 1(7759):1044–1046, 1972 4112185

Jaffe RL, Rives W, Dubin WR, et al: Problems in maintenance ECT in bipolar disorder: replacement by lithium and anticonvulsants. Convuls Ther 7(4):288–294, 1991 11941135

Johnstone EC, Owens DG, Lambert MT, et al: Combination tricyclic antidepressant and lithium maintenance medication in unipolar and bipolar depressed patients. J Affect Disord 20(4):225–233, 1990 2149728

Judd LL, Akiskal HS, Schettler PJ, et al: The long-term natural history of the weekly symptomatic status of bipolar I disorder. Arch Gen Psychiatry 59(6):530–537, 2002 12044195

Judd LL, Akiskal HS, Schettler PJ, et al: A prospective investigation of the natural history of the long-term weekly symptomatic status of bipolar II disorder. Arch Gen Psychiatry 60(3):261–269, 2003 12622659

Kane JM, Smith JM: Tardive dyskinesia: prevalence and risk factors, 1959 to 1979. Arch Gen Psychiatry 39(4):473–481, 1982 6121548

Kane JM, Quitkin FM, Rifkin A, et al: Lithium carbonate and imipramine in the prophylaxis of unipolar and bipolar II illness: a prospective, placebo-controlled comparison. Arch Gen Psychiatry 39(9):1065–1069, 1982 6810839

Keck PE, Perlis RH, Otto MW, et al: The expert consensus guideline series: medication treatment of bipolar disorder 2004. Postgrad Med Special Report 1–120, 2004

Keck PE Jr, Calabrese JR, McQuade RD, et al; Aripiprazole Study Group: A randomized, double-blind, placebo-controlled 26-week trial of aripiprazole in recently manic patients with bipolar I disorder. J Clin Psychiatry 67(4):626–637, 2006 16669728

Kessing LV, Hellmund G, Andersen PK: An observational nationwide register based cohort study on lamotrigine versus lithium in bipolar disorder. J Psychopharmacol 26(5):644–652, 2012 21948935

Ketter TA: Handbook of Diagnosis and Treatment of Bipolar Disorders. Washington, DC, American Psychiatric Publishing, 2010

Ketter TA, Calabrese JR: Stabilization of mood from below versus above baseline in bipolar disorder: a new nomenclature. J Clin Psychiatry 63(2):146–151, 2002 11874216

Ketter T, Bowden C, Suppes T, et al: Predictors of response to lithium and lamotrigine prophylaxis in bipolar I disorder. Program and abstracts of the Fifth International Conference on Bipolar Disorder, Pittsburgh, June 12–14, 2003

Ketter TA, Sarma K, Loebel A, et al: Lurasidone in bipolar I depression: A 24 week, open-label extension study. Paper presented at the 16th Annual Conference of the International Society for Bipolar Disorders., Seoul, South Korea, March 18–21, 2014

Kleindienst N, Engel R, Greil W: Which clinical factors predict response to prophylactic lithium? A systematic review for bipolar disorders. Bipolar Disord 7(5):404–417, 2005 16176433

Lahera G, Benito A, Montes JM, et al: Social cognition and interaction training (SCIT) for outpatients with bipolar disorder. J Affect Disord 146(1):132–136, 2013 22840617

Lam DH, Watkins ER, Hayward P, et al: A randomized controlled study of cognitive therapy for relapse prevention for bipolar affective disorder: outcome of the first year. Arch Gen Psychiatry 60(2):145–152, 2003 12578431

Lam DH, Hayward P, Watkins ER, et al: Relapse prevention in patients with bipolar disorder: cognitive therapy outcome after 2 years. Am J Psychiatry 162(2):324–329, 2005 15677598

Lam DH, Jones SH, Hayward P: Cognitive Therapy for Bipolar Disorder: A Therapist's Guide to Concepts, Methods, and Practice, 2nd Edition. Chichester, UK, Wiley-Blackwell, 2010

Lambert PA, Venaud G: Comparative study of valpromide versus lithium in treatment of affective disorders. Nervure 5:57–65, 1992

Licht RW, Nielsen JN, Gram LF, et al: Lamotrigine versus lithium as maintenance treatment in bipolar I disorder: an open, randomized effectiveness study mimicking clinical practice. The 6th trial of the Danish University Antidepressant Group (DUAG-6). Bipolar Disord 12(5):483–493, 2010 20712749

Lusznat RM, Murphy DP, Nunn CM: Carbamazepine vs lithium in the treatment and prophylaxis of mania. Br J Psychiatry 153:198–204, 1988 3151275

Macfadden W, Alphs L, Haskins JT, et al: A randomized, double-blind, placebo-controlled study of maintenance treatment with adjunctive risperidone long-acting therapy in patients with bipolar I disorder who relapse frequently. Bipolar Disord 11(8):827–839, 2009 19922552

Maj M, Del Vecchio M, Starace F, et al: Prediction of affective psychoses response to lithium prophylaxis. The role of socio-demographic, clinical, psychological and biological variables. Acta Psychiatr Scand 69(1):37–44, 1984 6422702

Maj M, Pirozzi R, Starace F: Previous pattern of course of the illness as a predictor of response to lithium prophylaxis in bipolar patients. J Affect Disord 17(3):237–241, 1989 2529291

Maj M, Pirozzi R, Magliano L, et al: Long-term outcome of lithium prophylaxis in bipolar disorder: a 5-year prospective study of 402 patients at a lithium clinic. Am J Psychiatry 155(1):30–35, 1998 9433335

Marcus R, Khan A, Rollin L, et al: Efficacy of aripiprazole adjunctive to lithium or valproate in the long-term treatment of patients with bipolar I disorder with an inadequate response to lithium or valproate monotherapy: a multicenter, double-blind, randomized study. Bipolar Disord 13(2):133–144, 2011 21443567

Martinez-Aran A, Vieta E, Torrent C, et al: Functional outcome in bipolar disorder: the role of clinical and cognitive factors. Bipolar Disord 9(1–2):103–113, 2007 17391354

Meyer TD, Hautzinger M: Cognitive behaviour therapy and supportive therapy for bipolar disorders: relapse rates for treatment period and 2-year follow-up. Psychol Med 42(7):1429–1439, 2012 22099722

Miklowitz DJ: Bipolar Disorder: A Family Focused Treatment Approach, 2nd Edition. New York, Guilford, 2010

Miklowitz DJ, George EL, Richards JA, et al: A randomized study of family focused psychoeducation and pharmacotherapy in the outpatient management of bipolar disorder. Arch Gen Psychiatry 60(9):904–912, 2003 12963672

Moncrieff J: Lithium revisited. A re-examination of the placebo-controlled trials of lithium prophylaxis in manic-depressive disorder. Br J Psychiatry 167(5):569–573, discussion 573–574, 1995 8564310

Nierenberg AA, Friedman ES, Bowden CL, et al: Lithium Treatment Moderate-dose Use Study (LiTMUS) for bipolar disorder: a randomized comparative effectiveness trial of optimized personalized treatment with and without lithium. Am J Psychiatry 170(1):102–110, 2013 23288387

Nierenberg AA, Sylvia LG, Leon AC, et al; Bipolar CHOICE Study Group: Clinical and Health Outcomes Initiative in Comparative Effectiveness for Bipolar Disorder (Bipolar CHOICE): a pragmatic trial of complex treatment for a complex disorder. Clin Trials 11(1):114–127, 2014 24346608

Okuma T: Effects of carbamazepine and lithium on affective disorders. Neuropsychobiology 27(3):138–145, 1993 8232828

Okuma T, Inanaga K, Otsuki S, et al: A preliminary double-blind study on the efficacy of carbamazepine in prophylaxis of manic-depressive illness. Psychopharmacology (Berl) 73(1):95–96, 1981 6785799

Pacchiarotti I, Bond DJ, Baldessarini RJ, et al: The International Society for Bipolar Disorders (ISBD) task force report on antidepressant use in bipolar disorders. Am J Psychiatry 170(11):1249–1262, 2013 24030475

Papatheodorou G, Kutcher SP: Divalproex sodium treatment in late adolescent and young adult acute mania. Psychopharmacol Bull 29(2):213–219, 1993 8290668

Parikh SV, Zaretsky A, Beaulieu S, et al: A randomized controlled trial of psychoeducation or cognitive-behavioral therapy in bipolar disorder: a Canadian Network for Mood and Anxiety Treatments (CANMAT) study [CME]. J Clin Psychiatry 73(6):803–810, 2012 22795205

Passmore MJ, Garnham J, Duffy A, et al: Phenotypic spectra of bipolar disorder in responders to lithium versus lamotrigine. Bipolar Disord 5(2):110–114, 2003 12680900

Perich T, Manicavasagar V, Mitchell PB, et al: A randomized controlled trial of mindfulness-based cognitive therapy for bipolar disorder. Acta Psychiatr Scand 127(5):333–343, 2013 23216045

Placidi GF, Lenzi A, Lazzerini F, et al: The comparative efficacy and safety of carbamazepine versus lithium: a randomized, double-blind 3-year trial in 83 patients. J Clin Psychiatry 47(10):490–494, 1986 3093468

Pond SM, Becker CE, Vandervoort R, et al: An evaluation of the effects of lithium in the treatment of chronic alcoholism: I, clinical results. Alcohol Clin Exp Res 5(2):247–251, 1981 7018305

Post RM: Transduction of psychosocial stress into the neurobiology of recurrent affective disorder. Am J Psychiatry 149(8):999–1010, 1992 1353322

Post RM, Uhde TW, Roy-Byrne PP, Joffe RT: Correlates of antimanic response to carbamazepine. Psychiatry Res 21(1):71–83, 1987 2885878

Post RM, Rubinow DR, Uhde TW, et al: Dysphoric mania. Clinical and biological correlates. Arch Gen Psychiatry 46(4):353–358, 1989 2930331

Post RM, Leverich GS, Altshuler L, et al: Lithium-discontinuation-induced refractoriness: preliminary observations. Am J Psychiatry 149(12):1727–1729, 1992 1443252

Prien RF, Caffey EM Jr, Klett CJ: Prophylactic efficacy of lithium carbonate in manic-depressive illness. Report of the Veterans Administration and National Institute of Mental Health collaborative study group. Arch Gen Psychiatry 28(3):337–341, 1973 4569674

Prien RF, Kupfer DJ, Mansky PA, et al: Drug therapy in the prevention of recurrences in unipolar and bipolar affective disorders. Report of the NIMH Collaborative Study Group comparing lithium carbonate, imipramine, and a lithium carbonate-imipramine combination. Arch Gen Psychiatry 41(11):1096–1104, 1984 6437366

Proudfoot J, Parker G, Manicavasagar V, et al: Effects of adjunctive peer support on perceptions of illness control and understanding in an online psychoeducation program for bipolar disorder: a randomised controlled trial. J Affect Disord 142(1–3):98–105, 2012 22858215

Quiroz JA, Yatham LN, Palumbo JM, et al: Risperidone long-acting injectable monotherapy in the maintenance treatment of bipolar I disorder. Biol Psychiatry 68(2):156–162, 2010 20227682

Quitkin FM, Kane J, Rifkin A, et al: Prophylactic lithium carbonate with and without imipramine for bipolar 1 patients. A double-blind study. Arch Gen Psychiatry 38(8):902–907, 1981 6789793

Ramirez Basco M, Rush A: Cognitive-Behavioral Therapy for Bipolar Disorders, 2nd Edition. New York, Guilford, 2005

Rea MM, Tompson MC, Miklowitz DJ, et al: Family focused treatment versus individual treatment for bipolar disorder: results of a randomized clinical trial. J Consult Clin Psychol 71(3):482–492, 2003 12795572

Reinares M, Colom F, Sánchez-Moreno J, et al: Impact of caregiver group psychoeducation on the course and outcome of bipolar patients in remission: a randomized controlled trial. Bipolar Disord 10(4):511–519, 2008 18452447

Reinares M, Colom F, Rosa AR, et al: The impact of staging bipolar disorder on treatment outcome of family psychoeducation. J Affect Disord 123(1–3):81–86, 2010 19853922

Reinares M, Papachristou E, Harvey P, et al: Towards a clinical staging for bipolar disorder: defining patient subtypes based on functional outcome. J Affect Disord 144(1–2):65–71, 2013 22862890

Richieri R, Guedj E, Michel P, et al: Maintenance transcranial magnetic stimulation reduces depression relapse: a propensity-adjusted analysis. J Affect Disord 151(1):129–135, 2013 23790811

Rosa AR, Reinares M, Michalak EE, et al: Functional impairment and disability across mood states in bipolar disorder. Value Health 13(8):984–988, 2010 20667057

Rosa AR, Reinares M, Amann B, et al: Six-month functional outcome of a bipolar disorder cohort in the context of a specialized-care program. Bipolar Disord 13(7–8):679–686, 2011 22085481

Sachs G, Bowden C, Calabrese JR, et al: Effects of lamotrigine and lithium on body weight during maintenance treatment of bipolar I disorder. Bipolar Disord 8(2):175–181, 2006 16542188

Safer DJ, Zito JM: Number needed to harm: its limitations in psychotropic drug safety research. J Nerv Ment Dis 201(8):714–718, 2013 23896857

Sartorius A, Wolf J, Henn FA: Lithium and ECT—concurrent use still demands attention: three case reports. World J Biol Psychiatry 6(2):121–124, 2005 16156485

Scott J, Paykel E, Morriss R, et al: Cognitive-behavioural therapy for severe and recurrent bipolar disorders: randomised controlled trial. Br J Psychiatry 188:313–320, 2006 16582056

Sega ZV, Williams JMG, Teasdale JD: Mindfulness-Based Cognitive Therapy for Depression, 2nd Edition. New York, Guilford, 2010

Small JG, Milstein V: Lithium interactions: lithium and electroconvulsive therapy. J Clin Psychopharmacol 10(5):346–350, 1990 2258451

Small JG, Klapper MH, Milstein V, et al: Carbamazepine compared with lithium in the treatment of mania. Arch Gen Psychiatry 48(10):915–921, 1991 1929761

Stallone F, Shelley E, Mendlewicz J, et al: The use of lithium in affective disorders: 3, a double-blind study of prophylaxis in bipolar illness. Am J Psychiatry 130(9):1006–1010, 1973 4580439

Stoll AL, Banov M, Kolbrener M, et al: Neurologic factors predict a favorable valproate response in bipolar and schizoaffective disorders. J Clin Psychopharmacol 14(5):311–313, 1994 7806685

Strober M, Morrell W, Burroughs J, et al: A family study of bipolar I disorder in adolescence. Early onset of symptoms linked to increased familial loading and lithium resistance. J Affect Disord 15(3):255–268, 1988 2975298

Suppes T, Webb A, Paul B, et al: Clinical outcome in a randomized 1-year trial of clozapine versus treatment as usual for patients with treatment-resistant illness and a history of mania. Am J Psychiatry 156(8):1164–1169, 1999 10450255

Suppes T, Dennehy EB, Hirschfeld RM, et al; Texas Consensus Conference Panel on Medication Treatment of Bipolar Disorder: The Texas implementation of medication algorithms: update to the algorithms for treatment of bipolar I disorder. J Clin Psychiatry 66(7):870–886, 2005 16013903

Suppes T, Vieta E, Liu S, et al; Trial 127 Investigators: Maintenance treatment for patients with bipolar I disorder: results from a North American study of quetiapine in combination with lithium or divalproex (trial 127). Am J Psychiatry 166(4):476–488, 2009 19289454

Suppes T, Vieta E, Gustafsson U, et al: Maintenance treatment with quetiapine when combined with either lithium or divalproex in bipolar I disorder: analysis of two large randomized, placebo-controlled trials. Depress Anxiety 30(11):1089–1098, 2013 23761037

Swann AC, Secunda SK, Katz MM, et al: Lithium treatment of mania: clinical characteristics, specificity of symptom change, and outcome. Psychiatry Res 18(2):127–141, 1986 3725997

Swann AC, Bowden CL, Morris D, et al: Depression during mania. Treatment response to lithium or divalproex. Arch Gen Psychiatry 54(1):37–42, 1997 9006398

Swann AC, Bowden CL, Calabrese JR, et al: Mania: differential effects of previous depressive and manic episodes on response to treatment. Acta Psychiatr Scand 101(6):444–451, 2000 10868467

Tohen M, Hennen J, Zarate CM Jr, et al: Two-year syndromal and functional recovery in 219 cases of first-episode major affective disorder with psychotic features. Am J Psychiatry 157(2):220–228, 2000 10671390

Tohen M, Vieta E, Calabrese J, et al: Efficacy of olanzapine and olanzapine-fluoxetine combination in the treatment of bipolar I depression. Arch Gen Psychiatry 60(11):1079–1088, 2003a 14609883

Tohen M, Zarate CA Jr, Hennen J, et al: The McLean-Harvard First-Episode Mania Study: prediction of recovery and first recurrence. Am J Psychiatry 160(12):2099–2107, 2003b 14638578

Tohen M, Chengappa KN, Suppes T, et al: Relapse prevention in bipolar I disorder: 18-month comparison of olanzapine plus mood stabiliser v. mood stabiliser alone. Br J Psychiatry 184:337–345, 2004 15056579

Tohen M, Calabrese JR, Sachs GS, et al: Randomized, placebo-controlled trial of olanzapine as maintenance therapy in patients with bipolar I disorder responding to acute treatment with olanzapine. Am J Psychiatry 163(2):247–256, 2006 16449478

Tondo L, Baldessarini RJ, Floris G, Rudas N: Effectiveness of restarting lithium treatment after its discontinuation in bipolar I and bipolar II disorders. Am J Psychiatry 154(4):548–550, 1997 9090344

Torrent C, Bonnin CdelM, Martínez-Arán A, et al: Efficacy of functional remediation in bipolar disorder: a multicenter randomized controlled study. Am J Psychiatry 170(8):852–859, 2013 23511717

Vaidya NA, Mahableshwarkar AR, Shahid R: Continuation and maintenance ECT in treatment-resistant bipolar disorder. J ECT 19(1):10–16, 2003 12621271

Van Dijk S: The Dialectical Behavior Therapy Skills Workbook for Bipolar Disorder: Using DBT to Regain Control of Your Emotions and Your Life. Oakland, CA, New Harbinger Publications, 2009

Van Dijk S, Jeffrey J, Katz MR: A randomized, controlled, pilot study of dialectical behavior therapy skills in a psychoeducational group for individuals with bipolar disorder. J Affect Disord 145(3):386–393, 2013 22858264

Vieta E, Suppes T, Eggens I, et al: Efficacy and safety of quetiapine in combination with lithium or divalproex for maintenance of patients with bipolar I disorder (international trial 126). J Affect Disord 109(3):251–263, 2008 18579216

Vieta E, Berk M, Wang W, et al: Predominant previous polarity as an outcome predictor in a controlled treatment trial for depression in bipolar I disorder patients. J Affect Disord 119(1–3):22–27, 2009 19324419

Watkins SE, Callender K, Thomas DR, et al: The effect of carbamazepine and lithium on remission from affective illness. Br J Psychiatry 150:180–182, 1987 3115347

Weisler RH, Nolen WA, Neijber A, et al; Trial 144 Study Investigators: Continuation of quetiapine versus switching to placebo or lithium for maintenance treatment of bipolar I disorder (Trial 144: a randomized controlled study). J Clin Psychiatry 72(11):1452–1464, 2011 22054050

Yatham LN, Kennedy SH, Parikh SV, et al: Canadian Network for Mood and Anxiety Treatments (CANMAT) and International Society for Bipolar Disorders (ISBD) collaborative update of CANMAT guidelines for the management of patients with bipolar disorder: update 2013. Bipolar Disord 15(1):1–44, 2013 23237061

Zarate CA Jr, Tohen M, Baldessarini RJ: Clozapine in severe mood disorders. J Clin Psychiatry 56(9):411–417, 1995 7665540

Zaretsky A, Lancee W, Miller C, et al: Is cognitive-behavioural therapy more effective than psychoeducation in bipolar disorder? Can J Psychiatry 53(7):441–448, 2008 18674402

5 Treatment of Pediatric Bipolar Disorder

Terence A. Ketter, M.D.
Kiki D. Chang, M.D.
Manpreet K. Singh, M.D., M.S.

Bipolar disorder onset prior to age 18 years has been reported by up to over two-thirds of American adults with bipolar disorder (Perlis et al. 2009), and the diagnosis of bipolar disorder in youths in the United States is on the rise (Merikangas et al. 2012). Pediatric (and early-onset) bipolar disorder is associated with multiple unfavorable illness characteristics, including poorer mood outcomes, co-occurring substance use disorders, increased risk of suicide attempt/self-injury, poor psychosocial outcome, and academic problems (McClellan et al. 2007; Singh and Chang 2007). Importantly, the clinical presentations, treatment responses, and side effects differ in youths compared with adults with bipolar disorder. Consequently, the management of bipolar disorder in younger individuals has to be tailored to address these considerations. This chapter describes advances in the specialized knowledge necessary to provide optimized treatment for children and adolescents with bipolar disorder.

Because of differences in pediatric bipolar disorder presentations in youths compared with adults, including more mixed/rapid-cycling symptoms and more chronic/continuous courses in the younger group, the clinical diagnosis of bipolar disorder in youths can be challenging (Chang 2009a, 2009b, 2010; Cosgrove et al. 2013; Ketter 2010). Diagnostic challenges may contribute to varying epidemiological reports of the prevalence of pediatric bipolar disorder. For example, one study reported an alarming rise in diagnosis of bipolar disorder in a community sample of youths in the United States; in this group, outpatient pediatric bipolar disorder office visits increased approximately 40-fold over less than a decade (from 1994–1995 to 2002–2003) (Moreno et al. 2007). In contrast, a more recent meta-analysis of 12 epidemiological community sample studies enrolling over 16,000 youths suggested that only 1.8%

had bipolar spectrum disorders (Van Meter et al. 2011). An even more recent American epidemiological study found that there had been a nearly twofold increase in the rate of adolescent mania (Merikangas et al. 2012). Importantly, this increase in pediatric bipolar diagnosis has been accompanied by a marked increase in antipsychotic administration to youths (Olfson et al. 2010). Taken together, these studies raise the worrisome possibilities of an increase in clinical overdiagnosis of pediatric bipolar spectrum disorder and undue administration of potentially harmful medications (e.g., antipsychotics) to youths in the United States.

Interestingly, the recent dramatic increase in diagnosis of pediatric bipolar disorder in the United States has not been seen internationally. European compared with American studies have reported later retrospectively recalled bipolar disorder onset ages (Weissman et al. 1996), which may indicate that more American youths have already fully developed bipolar disorder. Furthermore, diagnostic delays and misdiagnosis may also explain low prevalence rates outside of the United States (Soutullo et al. 2009). It has been theorized that the relatively less frequent use of stimulants and antidepressants in youths in Europe may account for less "creation" of pediatric bipolar disorder (Reichart and Nolen 2004), although the notion that such treatments can "create" pediatric bipolar disorder has been challenged (Goldsmith et al. 2011). Finally, there may be important methodological differences in the epidemiological studies that report rates of pediatric bipolar disorder in international settings, such as differences in the definition of bipolar disorder between the *International Classification of Diseases*, 10th Revision (ICD-10), and DSM-IV-TR (Soutullo et al. 2005). There is also a relative lack of data on incidence and prevalence of bipolar disorder among international youths, perhaps due to different levels of recognition or clinician biases against the diagnosis.

The bipolar spectrum concept has been proposed as a dimensional approach to mood disorders (ranging from bipolar I disorder to bipolar II disorder to bipolar disorder not otherwise specified [NOS] to unipolar major depressive disorder) that could help avoid overdiagnosis of unipolar major depressive disorder. This overdiagnosis of major depressive disorder may be at the expense of underdiagnosis of bipolar disorder, and the consequent administration of antidepressants may fail to relieve bipolar depression and/or destabilize mood. Misdiagnosed individuals may be better served by prescription of the different agents used in the treatment of bipolar disorder (Akiskal and Pinto 1999). In recent years, however, the bipolar spectrum concept has become particularly controversial in youths (for whom some clinicians have also included depression with family history of bipolar disorder and even attention-deficit/hyperactivity disorder with family history of bipolar disorder in the spectrum) because of concerns that it may lead practitioners to overdiagnose pediatric bipolar disorder in marginal cases and then increase use of agents such as antipsychotics with substantially more side effects than antidepressants (Parens et al. 2010). Youths with severe mood dysregulation have attracted particular attention for being at risk for overdiagnosis with pediatric bipolar disorder; this is a problem that, according to some (e.g., Leibenluft 2011), could be mitigated by the introduction of disruptive mood dysregulation disorder (DMDD).

Therefore, in DSM-5 (American Psychiatric Association 2013), bipolar I disorder and bipolar II disorder criteria for youths are similar to those for adults, but the diagnosis for DMDD was added to the depressive disorders section (see Box 5–1) to address concerns that pediatric bipolar spectrum disorder was increasingly overdiagnosed. DMDD was developed to address the possible overdiagnosis of pediatric bipolar spectrum disorder by identifying children with significant impairment due to mood dysregulation who do not meet full criteria for pediatric bipolar I disorder or bipolar II disorder.

Box 5–1.   DSM-5 Diagnostic Criteria for Disruptive Mood Dysregulation Disorder

---

296.99 (F34.8)

A. Severe recurrent temper outbursts manifested verbally (e.g., verbal rages) and/or behaviorally (e.g., physical aggression toward people or property) that are grossly out of proportion in intensity or duration to the situation or provocation.

B. The temper outbursts are inconsistent with developmental level.

C. The temper outbursts occur, on average, three or more times per week.

D. The mood between temper outbursts is persistently irritable or angry most of the day, nearly every day, and is observable by others (e.g., parents, teachers, peers).

E. Criteria A–D have been present for 12 or more months. Throughout that time, the individual has not had a period lasting 3 or more consecutive months without all of the symptoms in Criteria A–D.

F. Criteria A and D are present in at least two of three settings (i.e., at home, at school, with peers) and are severe in at least one of these.

G. The diagnosis should not be made for the first time before age 6 years or after age 18 years.

H. By history or observation, the age at onset of Criteria A–E is before 10 years.

I. There has never been a distinct period lasting more than 1 day during which the full symptom criteria, except duration, for a manic or hypomanic episode have been met.

Note: Developmentally appropriate mood elevation, such as occurs in the context of a highly positive event or its anticipation, should not be considered as a symptom of mania or hypomania.

J. The behaviors do not occur exclusively during an episode of major depressive disorder and are not better explained by another mental disorder (e.g., autism spectrum disorder, posttraumatic stress disorder, separation anxiety disorder, persistent depressive disorder [dysthymia]).

Note: This diagnosis cannot coexist with oppositional defiant disorder, intermittent explosive disorder, or bipolar disorder, though it can coexist with others, including major depressive disorder, attention-deficit/hyperactivity disorder, conduct disorder, and substance use disorders. Individuals whose symptoms meet criteria for both disruptive mood dysregulation disorder and oppositional defiant disorder should only be given the diagnosis of disruptive mood dysregulation disorder. If an individual has ever experienced a manic or hypomanic episode, the diagnosis of disruptive mood dysregulation disorder should not be assigned.

K. The symptoms are not attributable to the physiological effects of a substance or to another medical or neurological condition.

Source. Reprinted from the *Diagnostic and Statistical Manual of Mental Disorders*, 5th Edition. Arlington, VA, American Psychiatric Association, 2013. Used with permission. Copyright © 2013 American Psychiatric Association.

Bipolar disorder is differentiated from DMDD in that the former involves discrete manic and major depressive episodes (rather than severe episodic and chronic irritability), may or may not involve temper outbursts (rather than requiring temper outbursts), can be diagnosed at any age (rather than only at ages 6–18 years), has peak onset in late teens to early 20s (rather than requiring onset before age 10 years), and can entail psychosis (rather than not being associated with psychosis). Unlike bipolar disorder, DMDD can be accompanied by major depressive disorder, whereas like bipolar disorder, it can be accompanied by substance use, anxiety, conduct, and attention-deficit/hyperactivity disorders.

DMDD is a controversial new DSM-5 diagnosis that may address overdiagnosis of pediatric bipolar spectrum disorder. Proponents of DMDD contend that it may identify youths differing importantly from those with pediatric bipolar I disorder and bipolar II disorder in that they are at increased risk for unipolar depressive and anxiety disorders (rather than bipolar disorder) and lack high rates of familial bipolar disorder (Leibenluft 2011). Furthermore, by focusing on pediatric irritability,

DMDD draws attention to an important and common, yet relatively understudied phenomenon that treatment of individuals with DMDD may be more safely addressed with psychotherapies and/or medications other than antipsychotics, such as stimulants and antidepressants. In contrast, critics of DMDD contend that the diagnosis may not be able to be delimited from other already-defined pediatric psychiatric disorders, such as oppositional defiant disorder and conduct disorder; has limited diagnostic stability; and is not associated with current, future-onset, or parental history of mood or anxiety disorders (Axelson et al. 2012). If this criticism is correct, then DMDD could be diagnosed in individuals currently diagnosed with "milder" disorders (e.g., obsessive-compulsive disorder, conduct disorder, and intermittent explosive disorder) and could be invoked in a fashion similar to pediatric bipolar spectrum disorder to aggressively medicate "difficult children" with medications with substantial side-effect risks, such as antipsychotics. Thus, because there are no data regarding diagnosis and treatment of youths with DMDD, it would be unclear how this new diagnosis would aid in management of these children.

■ Pediatric Bipolar Spectrum Disorder Longitudinal Course

The stability of pediatric bipolar spectrum disorders over time provides an important rationale for accurate early identification and treatment. Longitudinal course was assessed in a 4-year multicenter study of 413 youths (mean age at entry=12.6 years) with bipolar spectrum disorder (59% bipolar I disorder, 7% bipolar II disorder, and 34% bipolar disorder NOS) (Birmaher et al. 2006). At entry, 27% of patients had manic/hypomanic, 17% had mixed, 14% had depressive, and 42% had not otherwise specified mood states. Over time, syndromal and subsyndromal mood symptoms were more pervasive than euthymia, and depressive symptoms were more pervasive than mood elevation symptoms (Figure 5–1), with 40% of participants having syndromal or subsyndromal symptoms for three-quarters of the follow-up period. Although over 80% of the patients recovered from their index episode, almost two-thirds had syndromal (particularly depressive) episode recurrence. In almost 40% of the patients with bipolar disorder NOS, the diagnosis converted to bipolar I disorder or bipolar II disorder. Early onset, bipolar disorder NOS diagnosis, long illness duration, low socioeconomic status, and family history of mood disorders were associated with poorer outcomes. Thus,

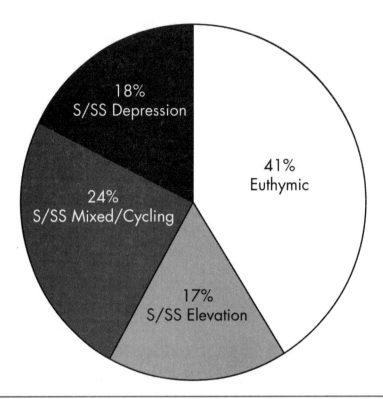

FIGURE 5–1. Four-year longitudinal course in 413 children and adolescents with bipolar disorder.

Note. Percentages indicate percentages of weeks that subjects had different mood states. Over time, syndromal and subsyndromal (S/SS) mood symptoms were more pervasive than euthymia, and depressive symptoms were more pervasive than mood elevation symptoms. Mean age at entry was 12.6 years.

Source. Data from Birmaher et al. 2006.

youths with bipolar spectrum disorders have persistent and progressive symptoms over time that rarely resolve spontaneously.

■ Treatment of Pediatric Bipolar Disorder

Because of the pervasiveness of mood symptoms and the efficacy and safety/tolerability limitations of pharmacotherapy, children and adolescents with bipolar disorder require a multifaceted treatment approach, including a combination of pharmacotherapy, psychotherapy (including individual, group, and family therapy), and educational interventions (ensuring that educational settings are appropriate, both for educational and for therapeutic purposes) (Singh et al. 2010). Thus, a multimodal treatment approach combining pharmacological agents and psychosocial interventions is needed, with the goals of improving symptoms, providing psychoeducation about bipolar disorder, and promoting treatment adherence for relapse prevention and attenuation of long-term illness complications (Madaan and Chang 2007). Clinicians need to advocate prevention, early intervention, and biopsychosocial treatments that promote healthy growth and development for all children affected by bipolar disorder, in any cultural context. This section provides a summary of recent advances in the treatment of pediatric bipolar disorder that may help to enhance outcomes.

Important developments in the last decade regarding the pharmacotherapy of pediatric bipolar disorder include approval by the U.S. Food and Drug Administration (FDA) of risperidone (Haas et al. 2009), aripiprazole (Findling et al. 2009), and olanzapine (Tohen et al. 2007) monotherapy for the treatment of pediatric acute manic and mixed episodes, and of quetiapine immediate-release formulation monotherapy for the treatment of pediatric acute manic episodes (Pathak et al. 2013), raising the number of pediatric acute mania monotherapy indications to five (Table 5–1). In addition, in the last decade aripiprazole has been approved as adjunctive therapy (added to lithium or valproate) for pediatric acute manic and mixed episodes, and as monotherapy for pediatric bipolar maintenance treatment. The latter approval raised the number of pediatric bipolar maintenance treatment indications to two (Table 5–1). Finally, in 2014, the olanzapine plus fluoxetine combination became the first treatment approved for pediatric bipolar depression (down to age 10) (Table 5–1).

Treatment of Pediatric Acute Manic and Mixed Episodes

Although lithium has long had a pediatric acute mania indication, only limited controlled data support lithium's use in pediatric acute mania (Geller et al. 1998; Kafantaris et al. 2003). More efficacy data are needed, because lithium therapy can yield adverse effects of particular concern in youths, such as neurotoxicity (tremor, ataxia) (Silva et al. 1992), weight gain (Chengappa et al. 2002), acne (Chan et al. 2000), and enuresis (Silva et al. 1992). Also, although some uncontrolled divalproex data were en-

TABLE 5–1. U.S. Food and Drug Administration–approved pediatric bipolar disorder treatments, with years of initial pediatric bipolar disorder approvals

Acute mania	Bipolar depression	Bipolar maintenance
1970, Lithium[a(e)]	2014, Olanzapine + fluoxetine[b]	1974, Lithium[a(e)]
2007, Risperidone[b]		2008, Aripiprazole[b(e)]
2008, Aripiprazole[b,*(e)]		
2009, Quetiapine[b]		
2009, Olanzapine[c]		

*Adjunctive therapy (as well as monotherapy).
[a]Ages ≥12 to 17.
[b]Ages 10 to 17.
[c]Ages 13 to 17.
[(e)]Indication extrapolated from adult data.

couraging (Papatheodorou et al. 1995; Redden et al. 2009; Wagner et al. 2002), in a controlled trial divalproex extended-release formulation was no better than placebo in the treatment of pediatric acute mania (Wagner et al. 2009). Divalproex-related sedation (Herranz et al. 1982), weight gain (Chengappa et al. 2002), vomiting (Herranz et al. 1982), and polycystic ovarian syndrome (Rasgon 2004) are of particular concern in pediatric bipolar disorder.

Only limited open data support the use of carbamazepine in pediatric acute mania (Joshi et al. 2010), and this agent has been associated with side effects such as somnolence (Ginsberg 2006), rash (Joshi et al. 2010; Konishi et al. 1993; Pellock 1987), and blood dyscrasias (Konishi et al. 1993; Pellock 1987). There are also limited controlled data suggesting that oxcarbazepine (in children but not in adolescents) (Wagner et al. 2006) and topiramate in youths (DelBello et al. 2005) may have utility in the treatment of acute manic and mixed episodes; however, the primary results from these studies found that these agents were no better than placebo for treating youths with bipolar disorder.

Multicenter, randomized, double-blind, placebo-controlled trials have robustly supported the efficacy of several second-generation antipsychotics (SGAs) in pediatric acute mania, with numbers needed to treat (NNTs) for response compared with placebo ranging between 3 and 4 (Figure 5–2) (Singh et al. 2010). Five SGAs have been efficacious in multicenter, randomized, double-blind, placebo-controlled pediatric acute mania studies, with single-digit NNTs comparable to those seen in adult studies. The age range in these studies was 10–17 years, except in the olanzapine study, in which the age range was 13–17 years. Response rates were based on last observation carried forward analyses, except in the ziprasidone study, in which rates were based on the less stringent observed cases analysis. As of early 2015, olanzapine, risperidone, and aripiprazole monotherapy had FDA approval for the treatment of pediatric acute manic and mixed episodes; quetiapine immediate-release formulation was approved for the treatment of pediatric acute manic (but not mixed) episodes; and ziprasidone (perhaps, in part, due to clinical trial methodological limitations) lacked FDA approval for the treatment of pediatric acute manic and mixed episodes despite positive placebo-controlled data in this regard (Findling et al. 2013a).

Importantly, although olanzapine monotherapy yielded a favorable (single-digit) NNT for pediatric acute mania response compared with placebo of 4, it also yielded a very unfavorable (even lower single-digit) NNH for at least 7% weight gain compared with placebo of 3 (Figure 5–3) (Tohen et al. 2007). Similarly, although quetiapine immediate-release formulation monotherapy yielded a favorable (single-digit) NNT for pediatric acute mania response compared with placebo of 4, this was accompanied by unfavorable (single-digit) NNHs for somnolence, dizziness, and at least 7% weight gain compared with placebo of 5, 7, and 9, respectively (Pathak et al. 2013). In addition, although risperidone monotherapy yielded a favorable (single-digit) NNT for pediatric acute mania response compared with placebo of 3, it also yielded unfavorable (single-digit) NNHs for somnolence and fatigue compared with placebo of 4 and 5, respectively, and these were accompanied by an only somewhat less unfavorable (low double-digit) NNH for at least 7% weight gain compared with placebo of 15 (Haas et al. 2009). In contrast, aripiprazole monotherapy yielded a favorable (single-digit) NNT for pediatric acute mania response compared with placebo of 4, which although accompanied by unfavorable (single-digit) NNHs for somnolence and fatigue compared with placebo of 4 and 5, respectively, was also accompanied by a favorable (double-digit) NNH for at least 7% weight gain compared with placebo of 29 (Findling et al. 2009). Finally, ziprasidone monotherapy yielded a favorable (single-digit) NNT for pediatric acute mania response compared with placebo of 4 (DelBello et al. 2008), which although accompanied by unfavorable (single-digit) NNHs for sedation and dizziness compared with placebo of 4 and 7, respectively, was also accompanied by a favorable (double-digit) NNH for at least 7% weight gain compared with placebo of 32 (Findling et al. 2013a).

Thus, although SGAs were similarly efficacious in pediatric acute mania, with favorable (single-digit) NNTs for response compared with pla-

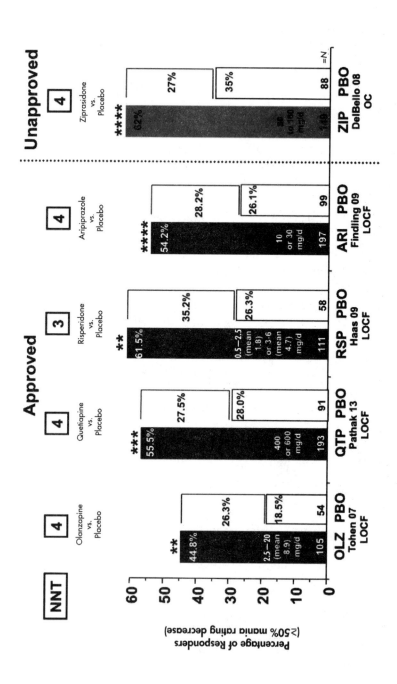

FIGURE 5–2. Benefits of second-generation antipsychotics for pediatric acute mania.

Note. Five second-generation antipsychotics—olanzapine (Tohen et al. 2007), quetiapine (Pathak et al. 2013), risperidone (Haas et al. 2009), aripiprazole (Findling et al. 2009), and ziprasidone (DelBello et al. 2008)—have been efficacious in pediatric acute mania studies, with single-digit numbers needed to treat for response compared with placebo, similar to those seen in adult studies (see Chapter 3, "Treatment of Acute Manic and Mixed Episodes"). ARI=aripiprazole; LOCF=last observation carried forward; NNT=number needed to treat; OC=observed cases; OLZ=olanzapine; PBO=placebo; QTP=quetiapine; RSP=risperidone; ZIP=ziprasidone.

**P<0.01, ***P<0.001, ****P<0.0001 vs. placebo.

Source. Adapted from Ketter TA: *Handbook of Diagnosis and Treatment of Bipolar Disorders.* Washington, DC, American Psychiatric Publishing, 2010. Copyright 2010, American Psychiatric Publishing. Used with permission.

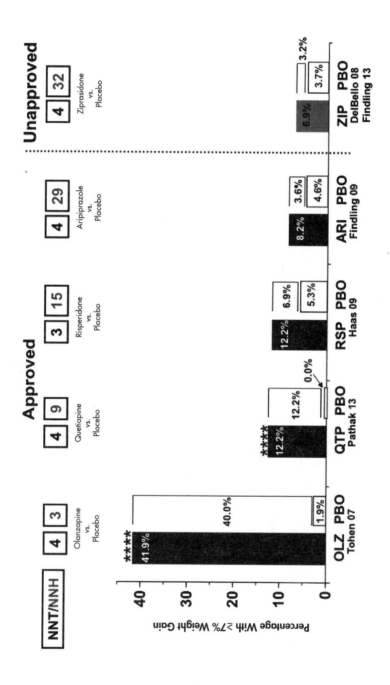

FIGURE 5–3. Benefit and harm (at least 7% weight gain) of second-generation antipsychotics for pediatric acute mania.

Note. Among second-generation antipsychotics, older agents (olanzapine [Tohen et al. 2007], quetiapine [Pathak et al. 2013], and risperidone [Haas et al. 2009]) more commonly yielded weight gain than newer agents (aripiprazole [Findling et al. 2009] and ziprasidone [Del Bello et al. 2008; Findling et al. 2013a]). ARI=aripiprazole; NNH=number needed to harm; NNT=number needed to treat; OLZ = olanzapine; PBO=placebo; QTP=quetiapine; RSP=risperidone; ZIP=ziprasidone.

****$P < 0.0001$ vs. placebo.

Source. Adapted from Ketter TA: *Handbook of Diagnosis and Treatment of Bipolar Disorders.* Washington, DC, American Psychiatric Publishing, 2010. Copyright 2010, American Psychiatric Publishing. Used with permission.

cebo ranging from 3 to 4, they all yielded at least one unfavorable (single-digit) NNH, making the likelihood of benefit and harm comparable. However, these SGAs entailed markedly different weight gain risks, with olanzapine being particularly problematic, as it was more likely to yield at least 7% weight gain (NNH=3) than response (NNT=4) compared with placebo (Figure 5–3). Quetiapine was also problematic (NNH=9), and risperidone was only somewhat less problematic (NNH=15), although aripiprazole and ziprasidone were clearly less problematic (NNHs of 29 and 32, respectively) with respect to weight gain risk.

Weight gain is commonly accompanied by medical complications such as diabetes and dyslipidemia, and this is particularly problematic in youths. One review of randomized controlled acute mania studies found that SGAs caused more weight gain than did mood stabilizers in youths but not in adults (Correll et al. 2010). Indeed, in one American study, over 17,000 adolescents with schizophrenia or bipolar disorder treated with antipsychotics, compared with more than 180,000 adolescents in the general population, had significantly higher risks of developing diabetes (hazard ratio 1.8) and dyslipidemia (hazard ratio 1.7) (Enger et al. 2013). Hence, if youths are treated with SGAs, it is crucial that clinicians and caregivers be aware of potential endocrine and metabolic adverse effects of these agents and that they use careful patient selection, agents with potentially lesser risk for such adverse events, healthy lifestyle counseling, and close health monitoring to enhance safety/tolerability (Correll and Carlson 2006). The risks of weight gain and metabolic complications in youths administered SGAs have been sufficiently concerning that researchers have conducted controlled studies to demonstrate the benefits of adjunctive metformin to attenuate such risks (Klein et al. 2006).

Limited data are available comparing the risks and benefits of different treatment options for pediatric acute manic/mixed episodes. However, in a multi-site, 8-week, randomized trial in 279 medication-naïve youths with acute manic/mixed episodes, risperidone (mean dosage = 2.6 mg/day) was more efficacious than lithium (mean level=1.1 mEq/L) or divalproex (mean level=114 µg/mL), yielding response rates of 68.5%, 35.6%, and 24.0%, respectively (Geller et al. 2012). The NNTs for response with risperidone were 4 and 5 compared with lithium and divalproex, respectively. However, risperidone yielded greater weight and prolactin increases, whereas lithium increased thyrotropin levels. Hence, the NNHs for new-onset weight gain with risperidone were 5 and 6 compared with lithium and divalproex, respectively. Therefore, risperidone compared with lithium and divalproex was comparably likely to yield benefit (response) and harm (weight gain).

Finally, a U.K. government-funded review found that although aripiprazole yielded less weight gain than olanzapine and quetiapine, and less prolactin increase than olanzapine, quetiapine, and risperidone, there was not robust enough evidence to recommend a preferential place for aripiprazole within the pediatric acute mania treatment pathway (Uttley et al. 2013).

Treatment of Pediatric Acute Bipolar Depression

In bipolar youths, as in adults, depressive compared with manic symptoms are more pervasive (Figure 5–1). Indeed, during a 4-year follow-up, more than 400 pediatric patients with bipolar spectrum disorders were more likely to relapse into depressive or mixed episodes than manic episodes (Birmaher et al. 2009). Moreover, pediatric mixed depression (which may be more severe than pure depression) is common, perhaps related in part to the pervasiveness of irritability in pediatric depression (Stringaris et al. 2012). Importantly, pediatric bipolar depression, compared with mania, may be more deleterious to youths' psychosocial functioning and quality of life (Van Meter et al. 2013). In this subsection, we describe recent advances in the treatment of pediatric acute bipolar depression, with lithium, lamotrigine, the olanzapine plus fluoxetine combination, and adjunctive psychotherapy being particularly noteworthy treatment options.

In spite of the pervasiveness of depression in pediatric bipolar disorder, only one treatment (the olanzapine plus fluoxetine combination) has FDA approval for pediatric acute bipolar depression, and this modality has substantial safety/tolerability limitations (Table 5–1). Lithium is considered a foundational treatment for adult bipolar disorder, because of lithium's well-established efficacy and safety/tolerability in adult bipolar maintenance and acute mania treatment, as well as its potential utility in adult acute bipolar depression (Nivoli et al. 2010). Given that lithium has FDA approval for pediatric bipolar maintenance treatment and pediatric acute mania, lithium's potential utility in pediatric acute bipolar depression is of considerable interest. Unfortunately, there have been relatively few controlled studies assessing lithium's efficacy and safety/tolerability in pediatric acute bipolar depression (Washburn et al. 2011). An open-label study in 27 adolescents with bipolar I disorder found that lithium yielded a 48% Children's Depression Rating Scale, Revised (CDRS-R) response rate, suggesting that lithium's effectiveness in pediatric acute bipolar depression should be assessed in larger placebo-controlled studies (Patel et al. 2006).

In addition, lamotrigine in pediatric acute bipolar depression is of considerable interest because of its established efficacy and safety/tolerability in adult bipolar maintenance treatment as well as its potential utility in adult acute bipolar depression. Although lamotrigine is commonly not associated with problematic somnolence or weight gain, lamotrigine-related rash may be more common in youths than adults (Guberman et al. 1999). Once again, there is a need for controlled studies assessing lamotrigine's efficacy and safety/tolerability in pediatric acute bipolar depression. A study of open lamotrigine adjunctive or monotherapy in 20 adolescents with acute bipolar depression was encouraging, finding a 63% CDRS-R response rate, good tolerability, and minimal weight gain (Chang et al. 2006), indicating the need for larger placebo-controlled studies to assess the efficacy and safety/tolerability of lamotrigine in pediatric acute bipolar depression.

There are limited controlled data regarding the efficacy and safety/tolerability of SGAs for pediatric acute bipolar depression (Singh et al. 2010). In view of the very substantial risks of weight gain and metabolic problems with olanzapine in patients with pediatric acute mania (Tohen et al. 2007), the clinical utility of olanzapine and the olanzapine plus fluoxetine combination in pediatric acute bipolar depression is expected to be limited. Indeed, although a recent 255-patient study demonstrated that the olanzapine plus fluoxetine combination had sufficient efficacy to become the first FDA-approved treatment for pediatric (ages 10–17) bipolar I depression (Table 5–1), with a CDRS-R response ($\geq$50% improvement) rate of 78.2% compared with 59.2% with placebo (NNT=6), it was even more robustly associated with $\geq$7% weight gain (52% vs. 4% with placebo, NNH=3) (Detke et al. 2015). In contrast, assessment of the potential role of quetiapine in pediatric acute bipolar depression is of considerable interest, given its demonstrated efficacy in pediatric acute mania; its efficacy in adult acute bipolar depression, acute mania, and bipolar preventive treatment, as described in Chapters 2, 3, and 4, respectively, in this volume; and its somewhat less prohibitive safety/tolerability profile (at least compared with olanzapine) in pediatric acute mania (Figure 5–3) (Pathak et al. 2013). To date, however, the only published controlled trial of quetiapine in pediatric bipolar depression found that among 32 adolescents with acute bipolar I depression, quetiapine monotherapy yielded a CDRS-R response ($\geq$50% improvement) rate of 71%, although this was not significantly better than that with placebo (67%; NNT=25) (DelBello et al. 2009). Also, quetiapine therapy was associated with dizziness, gastrointestinal-related adverse events, and increased triglycerides. Clearly, additional controlled studies are needed of quetiapine in larger samples of patients with pediatric acute bipolar depression. Finally, in view of lurasidone's demonstrated efficacy and safety/tolerability in adult acute bipolar depression (described in Chapter 2, "Treatment of Acute Bipolar Depression"), the potential role of lurasidone in pediatric acute bipolar depression needs to be assessed in controlled trials.

Insufficient systematic data have been reported in pediatric acute bipolar depression, as in adult acute bipolar depression, to assess the efficacy and safety/tolerability of antidepressants. Indeed, data continue to suggest that although antidepressants may relieve pediatric bipolar depression in some patients, they can yield suicidality in others (Hammad et al. 2006). Also, in patients with bipolar disorder, antidepressants can be associated with a treatment-emergent affective switch more often in youths than in adults (Baumer et al. 2006; Faedda et al. 2004; Goldsmith et al. 2011). Accordingly, the American Academy of Child and Adolescent Psychiatry practice parameters have long recommended use of antidepressants only in conjunction with antimanic or mood-stabilizing agents (McClellan and Werry 1997).

In the United States, following the FDA's stipulation that the prescribing information of all antidepressants include a boxed warning of the risk of increased suicidality in children, adolescents, and young adults, prescriptions for antidepressants decreased but the suicide rate increased (Gibbons et al. 2007). A similar finding was noted in the Netherlands (Gibbons et al. 2007). More international research in pediatric mood disorders in general, and pediatric bipolar disorder in particular, is clearly needed to address these important issues.

In view of the various concerns, it continues to be recommended that other options, such as lithium, lamotrigine, quetiapine, and psychotherapy, be considered prior to antidepressants when treating pediatric acute bipolar depression (Cosgrove et al. 2013).

Although a small, open-label trial suggested that omega-3 fatty acid monotherapy might help relieve manic symptoms in patients with pediatric bipolar disorder (Wozniak et al. 2007), in a small, randomized, placebo-controlled trial, adjunctive omega-3 fatty acid did not yield manic or depressive symptom improvement in children and adolescents with bipolar I or bipolar II disorder (Gracious et al. 2010). However, omega-3 fatty acids have recently been shown to be beneficial for youths with major depressive disorder resistant to selective serotonin reuptake inhibitors (McNamara et al. 2014), and a meta-analysis pooling data from 291 individuals found strong evidence that adult bipolar depressive symptoms may be ameliorated by adjunctive omega-3 fatty acids (Sarris et al. 2012). There is a lack of controlled trials of electroconvulsive therapy (ECT) in pediatric acute bipolar depression. Indeed, because of the acceptability and adverse-effect limitations of ECT, experts recommend considering ECT only when other options have proved ineffective (Kowatch et al. 2005). In contrast, there is hope that repetitive transcranial magnetic stimulation, because of its noninvasiveness, may ultimately prove useful in pediatric acute bipolar depression (Croarkin et al. 2011).

In view of the substantial efficacy and safety/tolerability limitations of somatic therapies for pediatric acute bipolar depression, it is not surprising that considerable efforts have been made to develop a variety of adjunctive psychotherapeutic treatments. In pediatric as in adult patients with bipolar disorder, there is more evidence supporting such interventions as preventive treatments than as interventions for acute bipolar depression. Unfortunately, the data supporting psychosocial interventions for pediatric acute bipolar depression are very limited. For example, in a 12-week uncontrolled open trial in 26 children (ages 6–12 years) with pediatric bipolar spectrum disorder (39% bipolar I disorder, 4% bipolar II disorder, 46% bipolar disorder NOS, 11% diagnosis not coded but presumed bipolar disorder) and current mood symptoms, group child- and family-focused cognitive-behavioral therapy (CFF-CBT), administered in 12 weekly group sessions, appeared feasible and acceptable, and significantly decreased acute manic but not depressive symptoms (West et al. 2009). Although benefits with respect to relieving acute depressive symptoms remain to be established, it is hoped that CFF-CBT could yield other benefits in pediatric bipolar disorder, such as enhancing access to better treatment and positive perceptions of parental messages. Also, in a 20-week uncontrolled open trial in 12 adolescents with bipolar spectrum disorder who were currently depressed ($n=8$), manic ($n=3$), or recovered ($n=1$), adjunctive interpersonal and social rhythm therapy for adolescents (IPSRT-A) appeared feasible and acceptable, and was associated with mood improvement from baseline (Hlastala et al. 2010). In a 6-week uncontrolled open trial in 11 children (ages 8.0–11.5 years) with depressive, anxiety, or suicidal ideation symptoms (diagnoses not specified), a dialectical behavior therapy (DBT) skills group demonstrated feasibility and possible ($P<0.05$ on paired one-tailed t tests) benefits in decreasing depressive and suicidal ideation symptoms (Perepletchikova et al. 2011). Family focused therapy (FFT) has had more data supporting its use for adolescents with bipolar disorder. For example, a randomized, controlled trial in 58 youths with bipolar I disorder found that those in the FFT condition, compared with those in a comparison condition, recovered from depressive symptoms faster and spent less time in depressive episodes over 2 years (Miklowitz et al. 2008).

Pediatric Bipolar Preventive Treatment

Despite having FDA indications, only limited data support the use of lithium (Findling et al. 2013c) and aripiprazole (Findling et al. 2012, 2013b) for pediatric bipolar preventive treatment. Furthermore, the mood-stabilizing anticonvulsants divalproex (Redden et al. 2009), lamotrigine (Pavuluri et al. 2009), and carbamazepine (Joshi et al. 2010) have only very limited data supporting their use as pediatric bipolar preventive treatments, and in fact these anticonvulsants all lack any FDA treatment indication for pediatric bipolar disorder. Although olanzapine, quetiapine, and risperidone do have pediatric acute mania indications (Haas et al. 2009; Pathak et al. 2013; Tohen et al. 2007), their substantial acute safety/tolerability limitations make them challenging options for pediatric bipolar maintenance treatment for relapse prevention. Ziprasidone, although entailing less severe safety/tolerability challenges than olanzapine, quetiapine, and risperidone, lacks any FDA indication for pediatric bipolar disorder and has only limited data supporting its use in pediatric bipolar preventive treatment (Findling et al. 2013a).

For pediatric bipolar preventive treatment, as for the treatment of pediatric acute bipolar depression, the efficacy and safety/tolerability limitations of somatic therapies make adjunctive psychotherapies important treatment options. However, the data supporting psychosocial interventions for pediatric acute bipolar depression are limited. In an 18-month randomized trial in 165 children ages 8–12 years with mood disorders (70% bipolar spectrum disorder, 30% unipolar depression) and on average moderate baseline mood symptoms, adjunctive group multifamily psychoeducational psychotherapy (MF-PEP), administered in eight weekly sessions, yielded better mood outcome than did wait-list control (Fristad et al. 2009).

Also, in a 2-year randomized trial in 58 adolescents with bipolar spectrum disorder (66% with bipolar I disorder, 10% with bipolar II disorder, and 24% with bipolar disorder NOS) who had been ill for a minimum of 1 week in the prior 3 months (31% syndromal depression, 26% syndromal mood elevation, 43% with subthreshold mood disturbance), adjunctive family focused therapy for adolescents (FFT-A), administered in 21 sessions over 9 months, compared with an adjunctive education control condition, which involved three relapse prevention sessions, yielded statistically similar overall recovery and recurrence rates (pooled rates of 91.4% and 49.1%, respectively) and times to overall recovery and recurrence, but faster recovery from depression (10.2 vs. 14.1 weeks) and decreased time with syndromal depression (on average 3.3 weeks vs. 5.0 weeks) (Miklowitz et al. 2008).

Family focused therapy adapted for youths at high risk for bipolar disorder (FFT-HR) is also a promising preventive strategy to reduce the probability of developing bipolar I or II disorder among genetically vulnerable youths who have mood symptoms but have not yet developed bipolar I or II disorder (Miklowitz et al. 2011). In a 1-year open-label treatment development trial, youths at risk for bipolar disorder showed significant improvements in depression, hypomania, and psychosocial functioning with FFT-HR (Miklowitz et al. 2011). A subsequent randomized study examined the effects of 4-month FFT-HR on the 1-year course of mood symptoms in youths at high familial risk for bipolar disorder, compared with an education control condition (one or two family sessions), and found that youths in FFT-HR had more rapid recovery from their initial mood symptoms, more weeks in remission, and a more favorable trajectory of mania severity over 1 year than did youths in the education control condition (Miklowitz et al. 2013). However, in a study with 2 years of follow-up, among 145 adolescents with bipolar I or II disorder and a depressive, manic or hypomanic, or mixed episode in the prior 3 months, adding three weekly enhanced-care (family psychoeducation) sessions versus adding 21 sessions of FFT over 9 months yielded similar time to recovery/recurrence and proportion of weeks ill, although secondary analysis indicated that FFT might be associated with less severe manic symptoms during the second year (Miklowitz et al. 2014).

In a 1-year uncontrolled open study in 10 adolescents with bipolar spectrum disorder (7 with bipolar I disorder, 2 with bipolar II disorder, and 1 with bipolar disorder NOS) and a syndromal mood episode in the prior 3 months, adjunctive DBT (individual therapy and family skills group administered in alternating fashion, weekly for 3 months, then monthly for 9 months) appeared feasible and acceptable and yielded significant improvements in depressive symptoms, emotional dysregulation, suicidality, and self-harming behaviors (Goldstein et al. 2007). Also, in a 1-year uncontrolled open study in 12 adolescents (83% with borderline personality disorder), DBT (individual therapy and family skills group weekly for 16–24 weeks) appeared feasible and prevented suicidal behavior and reduced self-injurious behavior (Fleischhaker et al. 2011).

■ Conclusion

Recognition and treatment of pediatric bipolar disorder remain major clinical challenges. Age-specific presentations and differential treatment

TABLE 5–2. Medication safety/tolerability challenges in pediatric bipolar disorder

Lithium	Neurotoxicity (tremor, ataxia) (Silva et al. 1992), weight gain (Chengappa et al. 2002), acne (Chan et al. 2000), enuresis (Silva et al. 1992)
Divalproex	Sedation (Herranz et al. 1982), weight gain (Chengappa et al. 2002), vomiting (Herranz et al. 1982), polycystic ovarian syndrome (Rasgon 2004)
Carbamazepine	Somnolence (Ginsberg 2006), rash (Joshi et al. 2010; Konishi et al. 1993; Pellock 1987), blood dyscrasia (Konishi et al. 1993; Pellock 1987)
Lamotrigine	Rash (Guberman et al. 1999)
Antidepressants	Suicidality (Hammad et al. 2006), treatment-emergent affective switch (Faedda et al. 2004)
Benzodiazepines	Disinhibition, cognitive impairment, depression (Bond 1998; Hawkridge and Stein 1998)
Second-generation antipsychotics	Somnolence and weight gain/metabolic problems (Correll et al. 2010)

responses make the diagnosis and management particularly complex. Moreover, certain medications entail distinct safety and tolerability challenges when administered to youths in general, and specifically to those with bipolar disorder (Table 5–2). Efficacy must be balanced with the safety and tolerability of an agent to aid in optimizing treatment selection. Lithium administration is limited by the risks of neurotoxicity (tremor, ataxia) (Silva et al. 1992), weight gain (Chengappa et al. 2002), acne (Chan et al. 2000), and enuresis (Silva et al. 1992). Divalproex can yield sedation (Herranz et al. 1982), weight gain (Chengappa et al. 2002), vomiting (Herranz et al. 1982), and polycystic ovarian syndrome (Rasgon 2004). Carbamazepine can cause somnolence (Ginsberg 2006), rash (Joshi et al. 2010; Konishi et al. 1993; Pellock 1987), and blood dyscrasias (Konishi et al. 1993; Pellock 1987). Although lithium, divalproex, carbamazepine, topiramate, and gabapentin considered collectively (but not SGAs, stimulants, or antidepressants considered as categories) may cause cognitive impairment in this population, few studies have used neuropsychological tests to assess youths with bipolar disorder before and after treatment with psychotropic agents (Henin et al. 2009). Youths compared with adults appear to be at greater risk for rash with lamotrigine (Guberman et al. 1999), but more recent data are lacking in this regard. Antidepressants appear to be more likely to yield suicidality in youths (Hammad et al. 2006) and treatment-emergent affective switch in pediatric bipolar disorder (Faedda et al. 2004). Benzodiazepines, which can be useful adjuncts in adults, have abuse potential and entail increased risks of disinhibition, cognitive impairment, and depression in youths (Bond 1998; Hawkridge and Stein 1998). Finally, SGA-related somnolence and weight gain/metabolic problems are of particular concern in youths (Correll et al. 2010), but SGAs have been proven to be effective in the treatment of acute mania and mixed states in children and adolescents with bipolar disorder (Singh et al. 2010).

Somatic therapies in pediatric bipolar disorder clearly require additional studies that will be critical to determine the acute and long-term efficacy and tolerability of these interventions across different mood states. Meanwhile, because of the debilitating nature of bipolar disorder in children and adolescents, psychotropic agents continue to be first-line treatments for many individuals. Given the safety/tolerability problems and efficacy limitations of these therapies, however, the risks and benefits of using psychotropics in this population need to be carefully weighed on an individual basis.

Furthermore, given the unique developmental state of youths with bipolar disorder, multimodal treatment approaches, combining psychopharmacological, psychosocial, and educational interventions, are needed. Early identification and implementation of comprehensive treatment regimens can help achieve the goal of preventing symptom chronicity and associated complications in children and adolescents with bipolar disorder.

■ References

Akiskal HS, Pinto O: The evolving bipolar spectrum: prototypes I, II, III, and IV. Psychiatr Clin North Am 22(3):517–534, vii, 1999 10550853

American Psychiatric Association: Diagnostic and Statistical Manual of Mental Disorders, 5th Edition. Washington, DC, American Psychiatric Association, 2013

Axelson D, Findling RL, Fristad MA, et al: Examining the proposed disruptive mood dysregulation disorder diagnosis in children in the Longitudinal Assessment of Manic Symptoms study. J Clin Psychiatry 73(10):1342–1350, 2012 23140653

Baumer FM, Howe M, Gallelli K, et al: A pilot study of antidepressant-induced mania in pediatric bipolar disorder: characteristics, risk factors, and the serotonin transporter gene. Biol Psychiatry 60(9):1005–1012, 2006 16945343

Birmaher B, Axelson D, Strober M, et al: Clinical course of children and adolescents with bipolar spectrum disorders. Arch Gen Psychiatry 63(2):175–183, 2006 16461861

Birmaher B, Axelson D, Goldstein B, et al: Four-year longitudinal course of children and adolescents with bipolar spectrum disorders: the Course and Outcome of Bipolar Youth (COBY) study. Am J Psychiatry 166(7):795–804, 2009 19448190

Bond AJ: Drug-induced behavioural disinhibition. Incidence, mechanisms and therapeutic implications. CNS Drugs 9(1):41–57, 1998

Chan HH, Wing Y, Su R, et al: A control study of the cutaneous side effects of chronic lithium therapy. J Affect Disord 57(1–3):107–113, 2000 10708822

Chang K, Saxena K, Howe M: An open-label study of lamotrigine adjunct or monotherapy for the treatment of adolescents with bipolar depression. J Am Acad Child Adolesc Psychiatry 45(3):298–304, 2006 16540814

Chang K: Challenges in the diagnosis and treatment of pediatric bipolar depression. Dialogues Clin Neurosci 11(1):73–80, 2009a 19432389

Chang KD: Diagnosing bipolar disorder in children and adolescents. J Clin Psychiatry 70(11):e41, 2009b 20031089

Chang KD: Course and impact of bipolar disorder in young patients. J Clin Psychiatry 71(2):e05, 2010 20193644

Chengappa KN, Chalasani L, Brar JS, et al: Changes in body weight and body mass index among psychiatric patients receiving lithium, valproate, or topiramate: an open-label, nonrandomized chart review. Clin Ther 24(10):1576–1584, 2002 12462287

Correll CU, Carlson HE: Endocrine and metabolic adverse effects of psychotropic medications in children and adolescents. J Am Acad Child Adolesc Psychiatry 45(7):771–791, 2006 16832314

Correll CU, Sheridan EM, DelBello MP: Antipsychotic and mood stabilizer efficacy and tolerability in pediatric and adult patients with bipolar I mania: a comparative analysis of acute, randomized, placebo-controlled trials. Bipolar Disord 12(2):116–141, 2010 20402706

Cosgrove VE, Roybal D, Chang KD: Bipolar depression in pediatric populations: epidemiology and management. Paediatr Drugs 15(2):83–91, 2013 23529869

Croarkin PE, Wall CA, Lee J: Applications of transcranial magnetic stimulation (TMS) in child and adolescent psychiatry. Int Rev Psychiatry 23(5):445–453, 2011 22200134

DelBello MP, Findling RL, Kushner S, et al: A pilot controlled trial of topiramate for mania in children and adolescents with bipolar disorder. J Am Acad Child Adolesc Psychiatry 44(6):539–547, 2005 15908836

DelBello MP, Findling RL, Wang PP, et al: Safety and efficacy of ziprasidone in pediatric bipolar disorder. Paper presented at the 55th Annual Convention and Scientific Program of the Society of Biological Psychiatry, Washington, DC, May 1–3, 2008

DelBello MP, Chang K, Welge JA, et al: A double-blind, placebo-controlled pilot study of quetiapine for depressed adolescents with bipolar disorder. Bipolar Disord 11(5):483–493, 2009 19624387

Detke HC, DelBello MP, Landry J, et al: Olanzapine/fluoxetine combination in children and adolescents with bipolar I depression: a randomized, double-blind, placebo-controlled trial. J Am Acad Child Adol Psychiatry 54(3):217–224, 2015 25721187

Enger C, Jones ME, Kryzhanovskaya L, et al: Risk of developing diabetes and dyslipidemia among adolescents with bipolar disorder or schizophrenia. Int J Adolesc Med Health 25(1):3–11, 2013 23337048

Faedda GL, Baldessarini RJ, Glovinsky IP, et al: Treatment-emergent mania in pediatric bipolar disorder: a retrospective case review. J Affect Disord 82(1):149–158, 2004 15465590

Findling RL, Nyilas M, Forbes RA, et al: Acute treatment of pediatric bipolar I disorder, manic or mixed episode, with aripiprazole: a randomized, double-blind, placebo-controlled study. J Clin Psychiatry 70(10):1441–1451, 2009 19906348

Findling RL, Youngstrom EA, McNamara NK, et al: Double-blind, randomized, placebo-controlled long-term maintenance study of aripiprazole in children with bipolar disorder. J Clin Psychiatry 73(1):57–63, 2012 22152402

Findling RL, Cavus I, Pappadopulos E, et al: Efficacy, long-term safety, and tolerability of ziprasidone in children and adolescents with bipolar disorder. J Child Adolesc Psychopharmacol 23(8):545–557, 2013a 24111980

Findling RL, Correll CU, Nyilas M, et al: Aripiprazole for the treatment of pediatric bipolar I disorder: a 30-week, randomized, placebo-controlled study. Bipolar Disord 15(2):138–149, 2013b 23437959

Findling RL, Kafantaris V, Pavuluri M, et al: Post-acute effectiveness of lithium in pediatric bipolar I disorder. J Child Adolesc Psychopharmacol 23(2):80–90, 2013c 23510444

Fleischhaker C, Böhme R, Sixt B, et al: Dialectical Behavioral Therapy for Adolescents (DBT-A): a clinical trial for patients with suicidal and self-injurious behavior and borderline symptoms with a one-year follow-up. Child Adolesc Psychiatry Ment Health 5(1):3, 2011 21276211

Fristad MA, Verducci JS, Walters K, et al: Impact of multifamily psychoeducational psychotherapy in treating children aged 8 to 12 years with mood disorders. Arch Gen Psychiatry 66(9):1013–1021, 2009 19736358

Geller B, Cooper TB, Sun K, et al: Double-blind and placebo-controlled study of lithium for adolescent bipolar disorders with secondary substance dependency. J Am Acad Child Adolesc Psychiatry 37(2):171–178, 1998 9473913

Geller B, Luby JL, Joshi P, et al: A randomized controlled trial of risperidone, lithium, or divalproex sodium for initial treatment of bipolar I disorder, manic or mixed phase, in children and adolescents. Arch Gen Psychiatry 69(5):515–528, 2012 22213771

Gibbons RD, Brown CH, Hur K, et al: Early evidence on the effects of regulators' suicidality warnings on SSRI prescriptions and suicide in children and adolescents. Am J Psychiatry 164(9):1356–1363, 2007 17728420

Ginsberg LD: Carbamazepine extended-release capsules: a retrospective review of its use in children and adolescents. Ann Clin Psychiatry 18(Suppl 1):3–7, 2006 16754405

Goldsmith M, Singh M, Chang K: Antidepressants and psychostimulants in pediatric populations: is there an association with mania? Paediatr Drugs 13(4):225–243, 2011 21692547

Goldstein TR, Axelson DA, Birmaher B, et al: Dialectical behavior therapy for adolescents with bipolar disorder: a 1-year open trial. J Am Acad Child Adolesc Psychiatry 46(7):820–830, 2007 17581446

Gracious BL, Chirieac MC, Costescu S, et al: Randomized, placebo-controlled trial of flax oil in pediatric bipolar disorder. Bipolar Disord 12(2):142–154, 2010 20402707

Guberman AH, Besag FM, Brodie MJ, et al: Lamotrigine-associated rash: risk/benefit considerations in adults and children. Epilepsia 40(7):985–991, 1999 10403224

Haas M, Delbello MP, Pandina G, et al: Risperidone for the treatment of acute mania in children and adolescents with bipolar disorder: a randomized, double-blind, placebo-controlled study. Bipolar Disord 11(7):687–700, 2009 19839994

Hammad TA, Laughren T, Racoosin J: Suicidality in pediatric patients treated with antidepressant drugs. Arch Gen Psychiatry 63(3):332–339, 2006 16520440

Hawkridge SM, Stein DJ: A risk-benefit assessment of pharmacotherapy for anxiety disorders in children and adolescents. Drug Saf 19(4):283–297, 1998 9804443

Henin A, Mick E, Biederman J, et al: Is psychopharmacologic treatment associated with neuropsychological deficits in bipolar youth? J Clin Psychiatry 70(8):1178–1185, 2009 19573494

Herranz JL, Arteaga R, Armijo JA: Side effects of sodium valproate in monotherapy controlled by plasma levels: a study in 88 pediatric patients. Epilepsia 23(2):203–214, 1982 6804224

Hlastala SA, Kotler JS, McClellan JM, et al: Interpersonal and social rhythm therapy for adolescents with bipolar disorder: treatment development and results from an open trial. Depress Anxiety 27(5):457–464, 2010 20186968

Joshi G, Wozniak J, Mick E, et al: A prospective open-label trial of extended-release carbamazepine monotherapy in children with bipolar disorder. J Child Adolesc Psychopharmacol 20(1):7–14, 2010 20166791

Kafantaris V, Coletti D, Dicker R, et al: Lithium treatment of acute mania in adolescents: a large open trial. J Am Acad Child Adolesc Psychiatry 42(9):1038–1045, 2003 12960703

Ketter TA: Handbook of Diagnosis and Treatment of Bipolar Disorders. Washington, DC, American Psychiatric Publishing, 2010

Klein DJ, Cottingham EM, Sorter M, et al: A randomized, double-blind, placebo-controlled trial of metformin treatment of weight gain associated with initiation of atypical antipsychotic therapy in children and adolescents. Am J Psychiatry 163(12):2072–2079, 2006 17151157

Konishi T, Naganuma Y, Hongo K, et al: Carbamazepine-induced skin rash in children with epilepsy. Eur J Pediatr 152(7):605–608, 1993 8354323

Kowatch RA, Fristad M, Birmaher B, et al; Child Psychiatric Workgroup on Bipolar Disorder: Treatment guidelines for children and adolescents with bipolar disorder. J Am Acad Child Adolesc Psychiatry 44(3):213–235, 2005 15725966

Leibenluft E: Severe mood dysregulation, irritability, and the diagnostic boundaries of bipolar disorder in youths. Am J Psychiatry 168(2):129–142, 2011 21123313

Madaan V, Chang KD: Pharmacotherapeutic strategies for pediatric bipolar disorder. Expert Opin Pharmacother 8(12):1801–1819, 2007 17696785

McClellan J, Werry J; American Academy of Child and Adolescent Psychiatry: Practice parameters for the assessment and treatment of children and adolescents with bipolar disorder. J Am Acad Child Adolesc Psychiatry 36(10)(Suppl):157S–176S, 1997 9432516

McClellan J, Kowatch R, Findling RL; Work Group on Quality Issues: Practice parameter for the assessment and treatment of children and adolescents with bipolar disorder. J Am Acad Child Adolesc Psychiatry 46(1):107–125, 2007 17195735

McNamara RK, Strimpfel J, Jandacek R, et al: Detection and treatment of long-chain omega-3 fatty acid deficiency in adolescents with SSRI-resistant major depressive disorder. PharmaNutrition 2(2):38–46, 2014

Merikangas KR, Cui L, Kattan G, et al: Mania with and without depression in a community sample of US adolescents. Arch Gen Psychiatry 69(9):943–951, 2012 22566563

Miklowitz DJ, Axelson DA, Birmaher B, et al: Family focused treatment for adolescents with bipolar disorder: results of a 2-year randomized trial. Arch Gen Psychiatry 65(9):1053–1061, 2008 18762591

Miklowitz DJ, Chang KD, Taylor DO, et al: Early psychosocial intervention for youth at risk for bipolar I or II disorder: a one-year treatment development trial. Bipolar Disord 13(1):67–75, 2011 21320254

Miklowitz DJ, Schneck CD, Singh MK, et al: Early intervention for symptomatic youth at risk for bipolar disorder: a randomized trial of family focused therapy. J Am Acad Child Adolesc Psychiatry 52(2):121–131, 2013 23357439

Miklowitz DJ, Schneck CD, George EL, et al: Pharmacotherapy and family focused treatment for adolescents with bipolar I and II disorders: a 2-year randomized trial. Am J Psychiatry 171(6):658–667, 2014 24626789

Moreno C, Laje G, Blanco C, et al: National trends in the outpatient diagnosis and treatment of bipolar disorder in youth. Arch Gen Psychiatry 64(9):1032–1039, 2007 17768268

Nivoli AM, Murru A, Vieta E: Lithium: still a cornerstone in the long-term treatment in bipolar disorder? Neuropsychobiology 62(1):27–35, 2010 20453532

Olfson M, Crystal S, Huang C, et al: Trends in antipsychotic drug use by very young, privately insured children. J Am Acad Child Adolesc Psychiatry 49(1):13–23, 2010 20215922

Papatheodorou G, Kutcher SP, Katic M, et al: The efficacy and safety of divalproex sodium in the treatment of acute mania in adolescents and young adults: an open clinical trial. J Clin Psychopharmacol 15(2):110–116, 1995 7782483

Parens E, Johnston J, Carlson GA: Pediatric mental health care dysfunction disorder? N Engl J Med 362(20):1853–1855, 2010 20484395

Patel NC, DelBello MP, Bryan HS, et al: Open-label lithium for the treatment of adolescents with bipolar depression. J Am Acad Child Adolesc Psychiatry 45(3):289–297, 2006 16540813

Pathak S, Findling RL, Earley WR, et al: Efficacy and safety of quetiapine in children and adolescents with mania associated with bipolar I disorder: a 3-week, double-blind, placebo-controlled trial. J Clin Psychiatry 74(1):e100–e109, 2013 23419231

Pavuluri MN, Henry DB, Moss M, et al: Effectiveness of lamotrigine in maintaining symptom control in pediatric bipolar disorder. J Child Adolesc Psychopharmacol 19(1):75–82, 2009 19232025

Pellock JM: Carbamazepine side effects in children and adults. Epilepsia 28(Suppl 3):S64–S70, 1987 2961558

Perepletchikova F, Axelrod SR, Kaufman J, et al: Adapting dialectical behaviour therapy for children: towards a new research agenda for paediatric suicidal and non-suicidal self-injurious behaviours. Child Adolesc Ment Health 16(2):116–121, 2011 21643467

Perlis RH, Dennehy EB, Miklowitz DJ, et al: Retrospective age at onset of bipolar disorder and outcome during two-year follow-up: results from the STEP-BD study. Bipolar Disord 11(4):391–400, 2009 19500092

Rasgon N: The relationship between polycystic ovary syndrome and antiepileptic drugs: a review of the evidence. J Clin Psychopharmacol 24(3):322–334, 2004 15118487

Redden L, DelBello M, Wagner KD, et al; Depakote ER Pediatric Mania Group: Long-term safety of divalproex sodium extended-release in children and adolescents with bipolar I disorder. J Child Adolesc Psychopharmacol 19(1):83–89, 2009 19232026

Reichart CG, Nolen WA: Earlier onset of bipolar disorder in children by antidepressants or stimulants? An hypothesis. J Affect Disord 78(1):81–84, 2004 14672801

Sarris J, Mischoulon D, Schweitzer I: Omega-3 for bipolar disorder: meta-analyses of use in mania and bipolar depression. J Clin Psychiatry 73(1):81–86, 2012 21903025

Silva RR, Campbell M, Golden RR, et al: Side effects associated with lithium and placebo administration in aggressive children. Psychopharmacol Bull 28(3):319–326, 1992 1480737

Singh MK, Chang K: The impact of bipolar disorder on selected areas of pediatric development: a research update. Pediatric Health 1(2):199–215, 2007

Singh MK, Ketter TA, Chang KD: Atypical antipsychotics for acute manic and mixed episodes in children and adolescents with bipolar disorder: efficacy and tolerability. Drugs 70(4):433–442, 2010 20205485

Soutullo CA, Chang KD, Díez-Suárez A, et al: Bipolar disorder in children and adolescents: international perspective on epidemiology and phenomenology. Bipolar Disord 7(6):497–506, 2005 16403175

Soutullo CA, Escamilla-Canales I, Wozniak J, et al: Pediatric bipolar disorder in a Spanish sample: features before and at the time of diagnosis. J Affect Disord 118(1–3):39–47, 2009 19285348

Stringaris A, Zavos H, Leibenluft E, et al: Adolescent irritability: phenotypic associations and genetic links with depressed mood. Am J Psychiatry 169(1):47–54, 2012 22193524

Tohen M, Kryzhanovskaya L, Carlson G, et al: Olanzapine versus placebo in the treatment of adolescents with bipolar mania. Am J Psychiatry 164(10):1547–1556, 2007 17898346

Uttley L, Kearns B, Ren S, Stevenson M: Aripiprazole for the treatment and prevention of acute manic and mixed episodes in bipolar I disorder in children and adolescents: a NICE single technology appraisal. Pharmacoeconomics 31(11):981–990, 2013 24092620

Van Meter AR, Moreira AL, Youngstrom EA: Meta-analysis of epidemiologic studies of pediatric bipolar disorder. J Clin Psychiatry 72(9):1250–1256, 2011 21672501

Van Meter AR, Henry DB, West AE: What goes up must come down: the burden of bipolar depression in youth. J Affect Disord 150(3):1048–1054, 2013 23768529

Wagner KD, Weller EB, Carlson GA, et al: An open-label trial of divalproex in children and adolescents with bipolar disorder. J Am Acad Child Adolesc Psychiatry 41(10):1224–1230, 2002 12364844

Wagner KD, Kowatch RA, Emslie GJ, et al: A double-blind, randomized, placebo-controlled trial of oxcarbazepine in the treatment of bipolar disorder in children and adolescents. Am J Psychiatry 163(7):1179–1186, 2006 16816222

Wagner KD, Redden L, Kowatch RA, et al: A double-blind, randomized, placebo-controlled trial of divalproex extended-release in the treatment of bipolar disorder in children and adolescents. J Am Acad Child Adolesc Psychiatry 48(5):519–532, 2009 19325497

Washburn JJ, West AE, Heil JA: Treatment of pediatric bipolar disorder: a review. Minerva Psichiatr 52(1):21–35, 2011 21822352

Weissman MM, Bland RC, Canino GJ, et al: Cross-national epidemiology of major depression and bipolar disorder. JAMA 276(4):293–299, 1996 8656541

West AE, Jacobs RH, Westerholm R, et al: Child and family focused cognitive-behavioral therapy for pediatric bipolar disorder: pilot study of group treatment format. J Can Acad Child Adolesc Psychiatry 18(3):239–246, 2009 19718425

Wozniak J, Biederman J, Mick E, et al: Omega-3 fatty acid monotherapy for pediatric bipolar disorder: a prospective open-label trial. Eur Neuropsychopharmacol 17(6–7):440–447, 2007 17258897

6 Treatment of Women With Bipolar Disorder

Terence A. Ketter, M.D.
Natalie L. Rasgon, M.D., Ph.D.
Mytilee Vemuri, M.D., M.B.A.

Although the prevalence of bipolar disorder is equal in males and females, the clinical presentations, treatment responses, and side effects in women differ substantively from those in men, and therefore the management of bipolar disorder in women entails application of at times complex gender-specific information in order to enhance outcomes (Burt and Rasgon 2004). Accordingly, in this chapter, we describe advances in the specialized knowledge necessary to provide optimized treatment for women with bipolar disorder.

As described in detail in the chapter "Management of Bipolar Disorders in Women" (Zappert and Rasgon 2010) in *Handbook of Diagnosis and Treatment of Bipolar Disorders* (Ketter 2010), there is an overrepresentation of women compared with men with bipolar disorder who have DSM-IV-TR (American Psychiatric Association 2000) depressive and mixed episodes, bipolar II disorder subtype, rapid-cycling course, comorbid anxiety and thyroid disorders, and antidepressant treatment-emergent affective switch (Altshuler et al. 2010). In this section, we review noteworthy recent advances in the treatment of bipolar disorder in women.

Arguably, the most important recent development in psychiatric diagnosis with respect to women with bipolar disorder was the status change for premenstrual dysphoric disorder (PMDD) in DSM-5 in 2013 (American Psychiatric Association 2013), which superseded DSM-IV-TR. Specifically, PMDD has been moved from DSM-IV-TR Appendix B, "Criteria Sets and Axes Provided for Further Study," to the depressive disorders section in the main body of DSM-5 (Box 6–1). This change was based on research indicating that PMDD is a specific and treatment-responsive form of depressive disorder that entails cyclic severe lability, depression, irritability, and/or anxiety that begin sometime after ovulation and remit within a few days of menses onset (Epperson et al. 2012).

Box 6–1. DSM-5 Criteria for Premenstrual Dysphoric Disorder

625.4 (N94.3)

A. In the majority of menstrual cycles, at least five symptoms must be present in the final week before the onset of menses, start to *improve* within a few days after the onset of menses, and become *minimal* or absent in the week postmenses.
B. One (or more) of the following symptoms must be present:
   1. Marked affective lability (e.g., mood swings; feeling suddenly sad or tearful, or increased sensitivity to rejection).
   2. Marked irritability or anger or increased interpersonal conflicts.
   3. Marked depressed mood, feelings of hopelessness, or self-deprecating thoughts.
   4. Marked anxiety, tension, and/or feelings of being keyed up or on edge.
C. One (or more) of the following symptoms must additionally be present, to reach a total of *five* symptoms when combined with symptoms from Criterion B above.
   1. Decreased interest in usual activities (e.g., work, school, friends, hobbies).
   2. Subjective difficulty in concentration.
   3. Lethargy, easy fatigability, or marked lack of energy.
   4. Marked change in appetite; overeating; or specific food cravings.
   5. Hypersomnia or insomnia.
   6. A sense of being overwhelmed or out of control.
   7. Physical symptoms such as breast tenderness or swelling, joint or muscle pain, a sensation of "bloating," or weight gain.

Note: The symptoms in Criteria A–C must have been met for most menstrual cycles that occurred in the preceding year.

D. The symptoms are associated with clinically significant distress or interference with work, school, usual social activities, or relationships with others (e.g., avoidance of social activities; decreased productivity and efficiency at work, school, or home).
E. The disturbance is not merely an exacerbation of the symptoms of another disorder, such as major depressive disorder, panic disorder, persistent depressive disorder (dysthymia), or a personality disorder (although it may co-occur with any of these disorders).
F. Criterion A should be confirmed by prospective daily ratings during at least two symptomatic cycles. (**Note:** The diagnosis may be made provisionally prior to this confirmation.)

G. The symptoms are not attributable to the physiological effects of a substance (e.g., a drug of abuse, a medication, other treatment) or another
medical condition (e.g., hyperthyroidism).

Approximately 2% of women have PMDD (Gehlert et al. 2009), which
may have a heritability as high as 50% (Kendler et al. 1998) and by definition can occur only between menarche and menopause. Unipolar major
depressive disorder is the disorder most frequently reported prior to
the diagnosis of PMDD (Pearlstein et al. 1990). Women with mood disorders commonly report having PMDD, although menstrual cycle symptom entrainment is often *not* confirmed with prospective charting (Dias
et al. 2011; Payne et al. 2007); in such cases, affective worsening in the
premenstrual phase that fails to consistently remit after menses is better
considered premenstrual exacerbation of mood disorder than PMDD
(Hartlage et al. 2004). Premenstrual exacerbation is reported in 65% of
women with bipolar disorder and has substantive clinical implications.
For example, in a 1-year longitudinal study of 293 women with bipolar
disorder, retrospectively self-reported premenstrual mood exacerbation
was associated with earlier and more frequent prospectively observed
emergent syndromal/subsyndromal mood (especially depressive) symptoms and with more retrospectively reported but not prospectively observed rapid cycling (Dias et al. 2011).

Although the PMDD criteria overlap with those of recurrent major
depressive episodes (MDEs), there are several important differences:
1) PMDD is menstrually entrained, occurring prior to onset of most menses and requiring confirmation by prospective daily ratings for at least
two symptomatic cycles; 2) PMDD episodes have briefer duration than
the 2-week MDE minimum; 3) core (essential) PMDD symptoms include
not only depressed (like adult MDE) or irritable (like pediatric MDE)
mood, but also anxiety or affective lability; and 4) additional PMDD symptoms, unlike those for MDEs, do *not* include psychomotor disturbance
or suicidality.

Another DSM-5 change with implications for women with bipolar
disorder is the removal of the DSM-IV-TR mixed episode, which required simultaneously meeting full criteria for both manic and depressive episodes. In DSM-5, the "with mixed features" specifier has been
added and can be applied to manic episodes when sufficient depressive
symptoms are present or to MDEs when sufficient hypomanic or sub-

threshold manic symptoms are present. Because PMDD diagnostic criteria overlap those of MDE and because they include at least one feature of hypomania/mania (irritability), PMDD may prove difficult to distinguish from MDE with mixed features. In these cases, a careful history and prospective rating of mood symptoms to distinguish the presence and exclusivity of menstrual entrainment can be essential to making the correct diagnosis.

PMDD is distinguished from premenstrual syndrome, with the latter being less severe and lacking the PMDD requirements of affective symptom(s) and clinically significant distress/functional impairment. PMDD differs from dysmenorrhea, with the latter defined as painful menses but lacking the requirement of PMDD core or additional affective symptoms, and beginning with (rather than prior to) onset of menses. Women taking oral contraceptives, compared with those not taking such contraceptives, may have similar, fewer, or more premenstrual complaints. If premenstrual dysphoric symptoms commence after exogenous hormone initiation and remit with discontinuation, this presentation is consistent with substance/medication-induced depressive disorder rather than PMDD.

The U.S Food and Drug Administration (FDA) has approved five treatments for PMDD, which are listed in Table 6–1. Additional approaches that may yield benefit in PMDD include acupuncture; nutriceuticals, such as L-tryptophan and vitamin B_6; and lifestyle modifications, such as getting regular exercise, having a balanced diet, and limiting alcohol and caffeine ingestion. When conservative treatments are not sufficient, medical menopause (gonadotropin-releasing hormone agonists) or surgical menopause (oophorectomy) with add-back estrogen/progestin may even merit consideration (Cunningham et al. 2009).

Data regarding treatment of premenstrual exacerbation of bipolar disorder are limited, but such treatment commonly involves aggressively treating the underlying bipolar disorder (Becker et al. 2004; Karadag et al. 2004). However, such efforts may prove complex, because some bipolar disorder treatments may have important gender-specific adverse effects, such as menstrual abnormalities and polycystic ovarian syndrome (Burt and Rasgon 2004; Rasgon 2004; Rasgon et al. 2000, 2005). There are limited data regarding use of the PMDD interventions (described in the preceding paragraphs) for premenstrual exacerbation of bipolar disorder. Oral contraceptives may have mood-stabilizing effects on women with bipolar disorder (Rasgon et al. 2003). However, concerns have been raised regarding the use of antidepressants in such circumstances (Dias et al. 2011).

TABLE 6–1.   U.S. Food and Drug Administration–approved
treatments for premenstrual dysphoric disorder

Selective serotonin reuptake inhibitors

Fluoxetine (Sarafem)

Sertraline (Zoloft)

Paroxetine CR (Paxil CR)

Low-dose birth control pills

Drospirenone/ethinyl estradiol (Yaz, Gianvi)

Drospirenone/ethinyl estradiol + levomefolate calcium (Beyaz)

Note.   CR = controlled release.

■ Phases of the Female Reproductive Cycle and Mood Disorder Symptom Risk

The risk of mood symptoms varies substantially across the female reproductive cycle. Although prior to puberty boys compared with girls may have greater risk of depression (Douglas and Scott 2014), starting with menarche, females are at increased risk of mood symptoms (particularly depression), with this being more evident during the luteal phase than during the follicular phase of the menstrual cycle (Freeman et al. 2002). As noted in the introduction of this chapter, one important way these symptoms can manifest in women with bipolar disorder is by premenstrual exacerbation of their mood problems (Dias et al. 2011). Although pregnancy appears neutral with respect to risk of mood symptoms (Viguera et al. 2000), the postpartum period represents arguably the time of greatest risk for exacerbation of mood problems in women's lives, with this being particularly the case in women with bipolar disorder (Freeman et al. 2002). Emerging data suggest that depressive symptoms can worsen in women with bipolar disorder during the menopausal transition (Marsh et al. 2009), although postmenopausal women and similarly aged men appear to be at comparable risk for mood symptoms. Therefore, it has been hypothesized that times with specific female hormonal changes (e.g., during puberty, before menstruation, following childbirth, during the menopausal transition) represent increased risk periods for affective symptoms. Because only some women undergoing such hormonal changes experience significant mood symptom exacerbation, it is theorized that only a subset of women are vulnerable to mood symptoms with female hormonal changes (Soares and Frey 2010).

■ Bipolar Disorder During Pregnancy

Although pregnancy can be psychologically and biologically stressful, it does not appear to markedly affect the risk of mood symptoms in women with bipolar disorder when considered collectively. Thus, although during pregnancy mood stabilizer discontinuation (particularly if abrupt) can increase the risk of recurrence of a syndromal mood episode approximately twofold, this increased risk is of a magnitude similar to that encountered after discontinuing lithium in nonpregnant women (Viguera et al. 2007b). Consideration for treatment of depression during pregnancy should account for the high risk of bipolar conversion in early postpartum, especially among depressed women not receiving antidepressants during pregnancy (Sharma et al. 2014). Optimal decisions regarding whether or not to discontinue psychotropic medications during pregnancy in women with bipolar disorder require careful personalized assessments of the risks of discontinuing (e.g., mood episode recurrence during pregnancy or postpartum) compared with continuing (e.g., teratogenicity, perinatal complications, neurobehavioral sequelae) such agents (Burt and Rasgon 2004).

Management guidelines for women with bipolar disorder contemplating pregnancy include commencing comprehensive prenatal counseling at least 3 months before conception, using folate supplementation, avoiding psychotropic medication (particularly during the first trimester) if clinically feasible, gradually rather than abruptly discontinuing psychotropics, and increasing psychosocial and clinical supports (Burt and Rasgon 2004). Also, if pharmacotherapy is administered, recommendations include using minimal effective dose (preferably monotherapy), avoiding changing effective medications unless there is a significant clinical or safety advantage, and increasing frequency of clinical monitoring as indicated (American Academy of Pediatrics Committee on Drugs 2000; Burt and Rasgon 2004). In some cases, electroconvulsive therapy (ECT) may be a reasonable option given its low risk of teratogenicity, side effects, and complications (Yonkers et al. 2004).

The FDA has traditionally defined the following use-in-pregnancy risk ratings for teratogenicity with medications[1]:

A. Evidence of no risk (based on controlled human data)
B. No evidence of risk (based on negative or absent animal and/or human data)
C. No evidence of no risk (risk cannot be ruled out, based on positive animal and lack of human data)
D. Evidence of risk (based on animal and/or lack of human data, although benefits may outweigh risk)
X. Contraindicated in pregnancy

Most mood stabilizers are rated pregnancy category D, with the exception of lamotrigine, which is rated pregnancy category C (Galbally et al. 2010). Compared with other anticonvulsants, divalproex (pregnancy category D) has been associated with higher rates of congenital malformation, ranging from 6.2% to 13.3% (the latter being more than fourfold the population 2%–3% rate); these malformations include neural tube, cardiac, and cranial defects and are more likely with maternal divalproex dosages over 800 mg/day (Tomson and Battino 2009; Wyszynski et al. 2005). Divalproex perinatal complications have included vitamin K deficiency, heart decelerations, abnormal tone, and growth retardation (Yonkers et al. 2004), whereas divalproex neurobehavioral sequelae may include lower intelligence quotient scores, with cognitive problems in offspring being more likely with maternal divalproex dosages over 800 mg/day (Meador et al. 2009).

Lithium (pregnancy category D) has been associated with congenital malformation rates ranging from 2.8% prospectively assessed to 11% retrospectively assessed (Cohen et al. 1994; Yacobi and Ornoy 2008). Fetal echocardiography is recommended at approximately 16 weeks because of the risk of Ebstein's (cardiac) anomaly, which may occur at a rate up to 20 times that of the population rate but which has an absolute risk of only 0.1% (Cohen et al. 1994). During pregnancy, lithium doses may need to be divided to maintain stable serum levels, and monthly serum lithium concentrations may be necessary because of increased glomerular filtration rate and plasma volume. The postpartum risk of

---

[1]In late 2014, the FDA decided to do away with letter-based pregnancy categories in favor of a text-based descriptive approach. Although this change was planned to take effect in June 2015, in this chapter we present the FDA's still current (as of early 2015) letter-based pregnancy categories.

lithium toxicity (Newport et al. 2005) may be mitigated by discontinuation of lithium 24–48 hours prior to delivery. Lithium perinatal complications may include higher birth weight, "floppy baby" syndrome (cyanosis and hypotonicity), neonatal hypothyroidism, and nephrogenic diabetes (Yonkers et al. 2004). The risk of neurobehavioral sequelae with lithium exposure in utero appears to be low in small, retrospective studies (Schou 1976; van der Lugt et al. 2012).

Lamotrigine (pregnancy category C) has been associated with congenital malformation rates ranging from 1.9% to 4.6%, with such malformations including cleft lip and/or palate, and risk is greater with maternal lamotrigine dosages over 200 mg/day (Cunnington et al. 2011; Tomson and Battino 2009) or over 300 mg/day (Tomson et al. 2011). Because lamotrigine and certain other antiepileptic drugs have antifolate effects, and folate deficiency, which can occur during pregnancy, has been associated with neural tube defects, supplementation with folate 5 mg/day is suggested (Galbally et al. 2011). Lamotrigine clearance increases through gestational week 32, so higher doses may be needed as pregnancy progresses, whereas plasma concentrations can increase postpartum and may need to be checked in the first 2 weeks after delivery. There are insufficient data regarding the risks of neurobehavioral sequelae with lamotrigine, although these appear to be less marked than with divalproex (Meador et al. 2009).

Carbamazepine (pregnancy category D) has been associated with congenital malformation rates ranging from 2.6% to 6.3%, with such malformations including neural tube, cardiac, and cranial defects (Campbell et al. 2014; Tomson and Battino 2009; Vajda et al. 2012). Carbamazepine perinatal complications have included vitamin K deficiency (Yonkers et al. 2004). Neurobehavioral sequelae with carbamazepine may include cognitive deficits, although these appear to be less marked than with divalproex (Meador et al. 2009).

Most second-generation antipsychotics are pregnancy category C, with the exceptions being clozapine and lurasidone, which are pregnancy category B. Although second-generation compared with first-generation antipsychotics may have better-demonstrated efficacy in bipolar disorder and entail fewer extrapyramidal symptoms, there are fewer data regarding their comparative safety/tolerability during pregnancy. The older second-generation antipsychotics clozapine (pregnancy category B), olanzapine (pregnancy category C), risperidone (pregnancy category C), and quetiapine (pregnancy category C) have congenital malformation rates ranging from 0.9% to 4.1% (McKenna et al. 2005; Reis and Källén 2008). Placental passage may be highest for olanzapine and haloperidol, intermediate for risperidone, and lowest for quetiapine

(Newport et al. 2007). Perinatal complications have included maternal gestational diabetes, large offspring for gestational age, and neonatal extrapyramidal symptoms (Reis and Källén 2008). In contrast, there are insufficient data regarding safety/tolerability during pregnancy of the newer second-generation antipsychotics aripiprazole (pregnancy category C), ziprasidone (pregnancy category C), asenapine (pregnancy category C), and lurasidone (pregnancy category B).

Most antidepressants are pregnancy category C, with the exception of paroxetine, which has been associated with risk of cardiac defects (2% with vs. 1% without exposure) and therefore is pregnancy category D (Udechuku et al. 2010). The true magnitude of risk from in utero exposure to antidepressants is controversial (Alwan et al. 2007; Bérard et al. 2007; Greene 2007; Källén and Otterblad Olausson 2007; Louik et al. 2007). Although antidepressant exposure has been associated with fetal growth changes, shorter gestation, short-term neonatal irritability, and neurobehavioral changes, ascribing causality is challenging because these problems are also related to depressive symptoms (Yonkers et al. 2009). Additionally, it has been noted that fetal malformations reported with first-trimester antidepressant exposure lack a specific pattern of defects ascribable to individual medications or classes of agents (Yonkers et al. 2009). Although late-gestational selective serotonin reuptake inhibitor (SSRI) exposure has been associated with transitory neonatal signs and a low risk of persistent pulmonary hypertension in the newborn (Yonkers et al. 2009), duration rather than timing of gestational SSRI exposure may be crucial with respect to the risks of neonatal respiratory distress, lower birth weight, and reduced gestational age (Oberlander et al. 2008a). In women with bipolar disorder, the additional risks of antidepressant inefficacy and treatment-emergent affective switch need to be integrated into the complex assessment of potential benefits and harms of utilizing such agents during pregnancy.

Benzodiazepines have been associated with cleft palate (at a rate of 80% over the general population risk, but still only in 1 in 10,000 births), as well as rare musculoskeletal and cardiovascular abnormalities, so their use in pregnant women requires careful assessment of potential benefits and risks, and using agents with the longest safety records as monotherapy at the lowest effective dosage for the shortest possible duration is recommended (Dolovich et al. 1998; Iqbal et al. 2002; Wikner et al. 2007; Yonkers et al. 2004). Indeed, combining benzodiazepines with SSRIs may increase the risk of congenital heart disease (Oberlander et al. 2008b). Risks with benzodiazepines and hypnotic benzodiazepine receptor agonists such as zolpidem may be comparable, and risks may include preterm birth, low birth weight, and a 24% increase in major congenital malformation risk with early pregnancy exposure (Wikner et al. 2007).

ECT does not entail prohibitive fetal risks and can be effective with adequate tolerability; however, because of feasibility and acceptability limitations, it is commonly held in reserve for refractory or urgent cases. Nevertheless, some providers opine that this modality ought to be invoked more liberally in pregnant women with bipolar disorder who are experiencing syndromal mood episodes.

■ Bipolar Disorder During Postpartum

The postpartum period may represent the time of greatest risk for mood problems in women's lives, with this being particularly the case in women with bipolar disorder (Freeman et al. 2002; Kendell et al. 1987; Yonkers et al. 2011). Women with first psychiatric contacts (for any disorder other than bipolar disorder) occurring in the first postpartum month, compared with women with first contacts that are not related to childbirth, may be more than threefold as likely (in 14% vs. 4%) to develop bipolar disorder over the following 15 years (Munk-Olsen et al. 2012). Other predictors of bipolar outcome include postpartum depression, psychosis, and/or psychiatric hospitalization, as well as having a father with bipolar disorder (Munk-Olsen et al. 2012).

Thus, more severe postpartum psychiatric problems appear to entail increased risk of bipolar outcome (Sit et al. 2006). Although the population risk for postpartum psychosis is only 1 in 500, this risk rises to 1 in 7 if there is a personal prior history of postpartum psychosis, and to 50%–75% in women with bipolar disorder and a prior personal or family history of postpartum psychosis (Jones and Craddock 2001; Kendell et al. 1987; Yonkers et al. 2004). Most women with postpartum psychosis appear to have bipolar disorder (Kendell et al. 1987), and for as many as one-third of mothers with bipolar disorder, their index episode may entail postpartum psychosis (Hunt and Silverstone 1995).

Postpartum mood episodes appear to be more common in women with bipolar disorder who are medication-free compared with taking medication during their pregnancy (Maina et al. 2014). For example, the risk of a post-lithium-discontinuation emergent mood episode rises markedly postpartum compared with during pregnancy or nonpregnant state

(Viguera et al. 2000). Serious consequences of postpartum mood and psychotic disorders can include psychiatric hospitalization, suicide attempt, completed suicide, and (rarely) infanticide (Sit et al. 2006; Spinelli 2009). Fortunately, starting mood stabilizers within 48 hours postpartum may decrease the risk of postpartum relapse (Cohen et al. 1995). Of interest, postpartum mania has been described in male partners of new mothers and is hypothesized to be related to sleep loss in men as well as in women (Stevens et al. 2014).

Treatment recommendations for postpartum mood episodes in women with bipolar disorder are similar to those for nonpostpartum mood episodes, taking into account medication compatibility with breastfeeding (Kelly and Sharma 2010). Thus, mood stabilizers and second-generation antipsychotics are commonly used, with ECT typically held in reserve for refractory or urgent cases. Substantial measures need to be employed to minimize sleep disruption, including mobilizing additional supports for overnight infant care, such as invoking the aid of the patient's spouse, family, or social network, or possibly night nurses, as well as in some instances specific pharmacotherapy. More severe postpartum episodes (i.e., postpartum psychosis) require aggressive multimodal interventions. For example, in such instances, to attenuate risk of harm to the infant, it is crucial to supervise mother-infant interactions until all symptoms of psychosis have resolved (Spinelli 2009).

Although breastfeeding has multiple advantages for mother-infant bonding and infant health, it also commonly entails sleep deprivation, which may undermine mood stability. Although all medications pass to the child through breast milk, most do so to a lesser extent than through the placenta. Infant serum levels, considered as a percentage of maternal serum levels, vary substantially, with estimates ranging from 6% to 65% for carbamazepine, 33% to 50% for lithium, and 23% to 33% for lamotrigine, but only 1% to 10% for valproate, and less than 5% for second-generation antipsychotics (American Academy of Pediatrics Committee on Drugs 2001; Gentile 2006).

Perceptions of risks for at least some psychotropics appear to be evolving over time. For example, although older guidelines are conservative with respect to the risk of infant exposure to lithium (American Academy of Pediatrics Committee on Drugs 2001), more recent data suggest that this risk may be less problematic (11%–56% infant:maternal serum concentration ratio, but with adequate infant tolerability) and thus may merit reconsideration (Viguera et al. 2007a). Moreover, for lamotrigine, although the rate of excretion into milk may not be excessive, lamotrigine milk:infant plasma ratios appear to be highly variable (Newport et al. 2008). Finally, a recent study failed to demonstrate deleterious effects of breastfeeding during carbamazepine, lamotrigine, phenytoin, or valproate therapy on cognitive outcomes in 3-year-old children previously exposed in utero (Meador et al. 2010). For some women, forgoing breastfeeding may be an acceptable approach to avoiding the at-times variably perceived risks of breastfeeding while taking psychotropic medications. If breastfeeding is attempted while the woman is taking medication, it is crucial to closely monitor the infant, with a low threshold for cessation or suspension of breastfeeding should problems arise (Llewellyn et al. 1998).

■ Conclusion

Gender-specific complex psychiatric presentations and differential treatment responses make the diagnosis and treatment of bipolar disorder in women challenging. Also, certain medications entail distinctive safety/ tolerability problems when administered to women in general and to those with bipolar disorder in particular (Table 6–2). Divalproex administration is limited by the risks of teratogenicity (Koren et al. 2006; Wyszynski et al. 2005) and polycystic ovarian syndrome (Rasgon 2004). In addition, lithium-induced thyroid problems are of particular concern in women (Bauer et al. 2014; Özerdem et al. 2014). Moreover, carbamazepine is a potent enzyme inducer that can yield inefficacy for multiple other medications, including hormonal contraceptives (Davis et al. 2011). Although lamotrigine's rate of excretion into milk may not be excessive, lamotrigine milk:infant plasma ratios appear to be highly variable (Newport et al. 2008). Second-generation antipsychotic–related weight gain/metabolic problems are of particular concern in women (Andersen et al. 2005; Baskaran et al. 2014). The antidepressant paroxetine has been associated with cardiac malformations (Wurst et al. 2010). Finally, the hypnotic zolpidem has lower clearance in women, increasing the risk of somnolence (Physicians' Desk Reference 2014).

To enhance outcomes in women with bipolar disorder, knowledge of female-specific illness characteristics, including increased risks of depressive, mixed, and rapid-cycling presentations, as well as phases of the female reproductive cycle entailing greater risk of mood symptoms (e.g., prior to menses and postpartum), must be combined with skillful assessment of the risks and benefits of interventions (including the risks of in utero or breast milk medication exposure for offspring).

TABLE 6–2. **Medication safety/tolerability challenges in women with bipolar disorder**

Divalproex	Teratogenicity (Koren et al. 2006; Wyszynski et al. 2005) Polycystic ovarian syndrome (Rasgon 2004)
Lithium	Thyroid problems (Bauer et al. 2014; Özerdem et al. 2014)
Carbamazepine	Contraceptive inefficacy (Davis et al. 2011)
Lamotrigine	Variable milk:infant plasma ratios (Newport et al. 2008)
Second-generation antipsychotics	Weight gain/metabolic problems (Andersen et al. 2005; Baskaran et al. 2014)
Antidepressants	Cardiac teratogenicity with paroxetine (Wurst et al. 2010)
Anxiolytics/hypnotics	Somnolence (with zolpidem) (Physicians' Desk Reference 2014)

■ References

Altshuler LL, Kupka RW, Hellemann G, et al: Gender and depressive symptoms in 711 patients with bipolar disorder evaluated prospectively in the Stanley Foundation bipolar treatment outcome network. Am J Psychiatry 167(6):708–715, 2010 20231325

Alwan et al. 2007 S, Reefhuis J, Rasmussen SA, et al; National Birth Defects Prevention Study: Use of selective serotonin-reuptake inhibitors in pregnancy and the risk of birth defects. N Engl J Med 356(26):2684–2692, 2007 17596602

American Academy of Pediatrics Committee on Drugs: Use of psychoactive medication during pregnancy and possible effects on the fetus and newborn. Pediatrics 105(4 Pt 1):880–887, 2000 10742343

American Academy of Pediatrics Committee on Drugs: Transfer of drugs and other chemicals into human milk. Pediatrics 108(3):776–789, 2001 11533352

American Psychiatric Association: Diagnostic and Statistical Manual of Mental Disorders, 4th Edition, Text Revision. Washington, DC, American Psychiatric Association, 2000

American Psychiatric Association: Diagnostic and Statistical Manual of Mental Disorders, 5th Edition. Washington, DC, American Psychiatric Association, 2013

Andersen SW, Clemow DB, Corya SA: Long-term weight gain in patients treated with open-label olanzapine in combination with fluoxetine for major depressive disorder. J Clin Psychiatry 66(11):1468–1476, 2005 16420086

Baskaran A, Cha DS, Powell AM, et al: Sex differences in rates of obesity in bipolar disorder: postulated mechanisms. Bipolar Disord 16(1):83–92, 2014 24467470

Bauer M, Glenn T, Pilhatsch M, et al: Gender differences in thyroid system function: relevance to bipolar disorder and its treatment. Bipolar Disord 16(1):58–71, 2014 24245529

Becker OV, Rasgon NL, Marsh WK, et al: Lamotrigine therapy in treatment-resistant menstrually related rapid cycling bipolar disorder: a case report. Bipolar Disord 6(5):435–439, 2004 15383138

Bérard A, Ramos E, Rey E, et al: First trimester exposure to paroxetine and risk of cardiac malformations in infants: the importance of dosage. Birth Defects Res B Dev Reprod Toxicol 80(1):18–27, 2007 17187388

Burt VK, Rasgon N: Special considerations in treating bipolar disorder in women. Bipolar Disord 6(1):2–13, 2004 14996136

Campbell E, Kennedy F, Russell A, et al: Malformation risks of antiepileptic drug monotherapies in pregnancy: updated results from the UK and Ireland Epilepsy and Pregnancy Registers. J Neurol Neurosurg Psychiatry 85(9):1029–1034, 2014 24444855

Cohen LS, Friedman JM, Jefferson JW, et al: A reevaluation of risk of in utero exposure to lithium. JAMA 271(2):146–150, 1994 8031346

Cohen LS, Sichel DA, Robertson LM, et al: Postpartum prophylaxis for women with bipolar disorder. Am J Psychiatry 152(11):1641–1645, 1995 7485628

Cunningham J, Yonkers KA, O'Brien S, et al: Update on research and treatment of premenstrual dysphoric disorder. Harv Rev Psychiatry 17(2):120–137, 2009 19373620

Cunnington MC, Weil JG, Messenheimer JA, et al: Final results from 18 years of the International Lamotrigine Pregnancy Registry. Neurology 76(21):1817–1823, 2011 21606453

Davis AR, Westhoff CL, Stanczyk FZ: Carbamazepine coadministration with an oral contraceptive: effects on steroid pharmacokinetics, ovulation, and bleeding. Epilepsia 52(2):243–247, 2011 21204827

Dias RS, Lafer B, Russo C, et al: Longitudinal follow-up of bipolar disorder in women with premenstrual exacerbation: findings from STEP-BD. Am J Psychiatry 168(4):386–394, 2011 21324951

Dolovich LR, Addis A, Vaillancourt JM, et al: Benzodiazepine use in pregnancy and major malformations or oral cleft: meta-analysis of cohort and case-control studies. BMJ 317(7162):839–843, 1998 9748174

Douglas J, Scott J: A systematic review of gender-specific rates of unipolar and bipolar disorders in community studies of pre-pubertal children. Bipolar Disord 16(1):5–15, 2014 24305108

Epperson CN, Steiner M, Hartlage SA, et al: Premenstrual dysphoric disorder: evidence for a new category for DSM-5. Am J Psychiatry 169(5):465–475, 2012 22764360

Freeman MP, Smith KW, Freeman SA, et al: The impact of reproductive events on the course of bipolar disorder in women. J Clin Psychiatry 63(4):284–287, 2002 12004800

Galbally M, Roberts M, Buist A, et al; Perinatal Psychotropic Review Group: Mood stabilizers in pregnancy: a systematic review. Aust NZ J Psychiatry 44(11):967–977, 2010 21034180

Galbally M, Snellen M, Lewis AJ: A review of the use of psychotropic medication in pregnancy. Curr Opin Obstet Gynecol 23(6):408–414, 2011 21897237

Gehlert S, Song IH, Chang CH, et al: The prevalence of premenstrual dysphoric disorder in a randomly selected group of urban and rural women. Psychol Med 39(1):129–136, 2009 18366818

Gentile S: Prophylactic treatment of bipolar disorder in pregnancy and breast-feeding: focus on emerging mood stabilizers. Bipolar Disord 8(3):207–220, 2006 16696822

Greene MF: Teratogenicity of SSRIs—serious concern or much ado about little? N Engl J Med 356(26):2732–2733, 2007 17596609

Hartlage SA, Brandenburg DL, Kravitz HM: Premenstrual exacerbation of depressive disorders in a community-based sample in the United States. Psychosom Med 66(5):698–706, 2004 15385694

Hunt N, Silverstone T: Does puerperal illness distinguish a subgroup of bipolar patients? J Affect Disord 34(2):101–107, 1995 7665801

Iqbal MM, Sobhan T, Ryals T: Effects of commonly used benzodiazepines on the fetus, the neonate, and the nursing infant. Psychiatr Serv 53(1):39–49, 2002 11773648

Jones I, Craddock N: Familiality of the puerperal trigger in bipolar disorder: results of a family study. Am J Psychiatry 158(6):913–917, 2001 11384899

Källén BA, Otterblad Olausson P: Maternal use of selective serotonin re-uptake inhibitors in early pregnancy and infant congenital malformations. Birth Defects Res A Clin Mol Teratol 79(4):301–308, 2007 17216624

Karadag F, Akdeniz F, Erten E, et al: Menstrually related symptom changes in women with treatment-responsive bipolar disorder. Bipolar Disord 6(3):253–259, 2004 15117404

Kelly E, Sharma V: Diagnosis and treatment of postpartum bipolar depression. Expert Rev Neurother 10(7):1045–1051, 2010 20586688

Kendell RE, Chalmers JC, Platz C: Epidemiology of puerperal psychoses. Br J Psychiatry 150:662–673, 1987 3651704

Kendler KS, Karkowski LM, Corey LA, et al: Longitudinal population-based twin study of retrospectively reported premenstrual symptoms and lifetime major depression. Am J Psychiatry 155(9):1234–1240, 1998 9734548

Ketter TA: Handbook of Diagnosis and Treatment of Bipolar Disorders. Washington, DC, American Psychiatric Publishing, 2010

Koren G, Nava-Ocampo AA, Moretti ME, et al: Major malformations with valproic acid. Can Fam Physician 52:441–442, 444, 447, 2006 16639967

Llewellyn A, Stowe ZN, Strader JR Jr: The use of lithium and management of women with bipolar disorder during pregnancy and lactation. J Clin Psychiatry 59(Suppl 6):57–64, discussion 65, 1998 9674938

Louik C, Lin AE, Werler MM, et al: First-trimester use of selective serotonin-reuptake inhibitors and the risk of birth defects. N Engl J Med 356(26):2675–2683, 2007 17596601

Maina G, Rosso G, Aguglia A, et al: Recurrence rates of bipolar disorder during the postpartum period: a study on 276 medication-free Italian women. Arch Womens Ment Health Jan 22, 2014 [Epub ahead of print]

Marsh WK, Ketter TA, Rasgon NL: Increased depressive symptoms in menopausal age women with bipolar disorder: age and gender comparison. J Psychiatr Res 43(8):798–802, 2009 19155021

McKenna K, Koren G, Tetelbaum M, et al: Pregnancy outcome of women using atypical antipsychotic drugs: a prospective comparative study. J Clin Psychiatry 66(4):444–449, quiz 546, 2005 15816786

Meador KJ, Baker GA, Browning N, et al; NEAD Study Group: Cognitive function at 3 years of age after fetal exposure to antiepileptic drugs. N Engl J Med 360(16):1597–1605, 2009 19369666

Meador KJ, Baker GA, Browning N, et al; NEAD Study Group: Effects of breastfeeding in children of women taking antiepileptic drugs. Neurology 75(22):1954–1960, 2010 21106960

Munk-Olsen T, Laursen TM, Meltzer-Brody S, et al: Psychiatric disorders with postpartum onset: possible early manifestations of bipolar affective disorders. Arch Gen Psychiatry 69(4):428–434, 2012 22147807

Newport DJ, Viguera AC, Beach AJ, et al: Lithium placental passage and obstetrical outcome: implications for clinical management during late pregnancy. Am J Psychiatry 162(11):2162–2170, 2005 16263858

Newport DJ, Calamaras MR, DeVane CL, et al: Atypical antipsychotic administration during late pregnancy: placental passage and obstetrical outcomes. Am J Psychiatry 164(8):1214–1220, 2007 17671284

Newport DJ, Pennell PB, Calamaras MR, et al: Lamotrigine in breast milk and nursing infants: determination of exposure. Pediatrics 122(1):e223–e231, 2008 18591203

Oberlander TF, Warburton W, Misri S, et al: Effects of timing and duration of gestational exposure to serotonin reuptake inhibitor antidepressants: population-based study. Br J Psychiatry 192(5):338–343, 2008a 18450656

Oberlander TF, Warburton W, Misri S, et al: Major congenital malformations following prenatal exposure to serotonin reuptake inhibitors and benzodiazepines using population-based health data. Birth Defects Res B Dev Reprod Toxicol 83(1):68–76, 2008b 18293409

Özerdem A, Tunca Z, Çımrın D, et al: Female vulnerability for thyroid function abnormality in bipolar disorder: role of lithium treatment. Bipolar Disord 16(1):72–82, 2014 24330379

Payne JL, Roy PS, Murphy-Eberenz K, et al: Reproductive cycle-associated mood symptoms in women with major depression and bipolar disorder. J Affect Disord 99(1–3):221–229, 2007 17011632

Pearlstein TB, Frank E, Rivera-Tovar A, et al: Prevalence of axis I and axis II disorders in women with late luteal phase dysphoric disorder. J Affect Disord 20(2):129–134, 1990 2148327

Physicians' Desk Reference 2015, 69th Edition. Montvale, NJ, PDR Network, 2014

Rasgon N: The relationship between polycystic ovary syndrome and antiepileptic drugs: a review of the evidence. J Clin Psychopharmacol 24(3):322–334, 2004 15118487

Rasgon NL, Altshuler LL, Gudeman D, et al: Medication status and polycystic ovary syndrome in women with bipolar disorder: a preliminary report. J Clin Psychiatry 61(3):173–178, 2000 10817101

Rasgon N, Bauer M, Glenn T, et al: Menstrual cycle related mood changes in women with bipolar disorder. Bipolar Disord 5(1):48–52, 2003 12656938

Rasgon NL, Altshuler LL, Fairbanks L, et al: Reproductive function and risk for PCOS in women treated for bipolar disorder. Bipolar Disord 7(3):246–259, 2005 15898962

Reis M, Källén B: Maternal use of antipsychotics in early pregnancy and delivery outcome. J Clin Psychopharmacol 28(3):279–288, 2008 18480684

Schou M: What happened later to the lithium babies? A follow-up study of children born without malformations. Acta Psychiatr Scand 54(3):193–197, 1976 970196

Sharma V, Xie B, Campbell MK, et al: A prospective study of diagnostic conversion of major depressive disorder to bipolar disorder in pregnancy and postpartum. Bipolar Disord 16(1):16–21, 2014 24127853

Sit D, Rothschild AJ, Wisner KL: A review of postpartum psychosis. J Womens Health (Larchmt) 15(4):352–368, 2006 16724884

Soares CN, Frey BN: Challenges and opportunities to manage depression during the menopausal transition and beyond. Psychiatr Clin North Am 33(2):295–308, 2010 20385338

Spinelli MG: Postpartum psychosis: detection of risk and management. Am J Psychiatry 166(4):405–408, 2009 19339365

Stevens AW, Geerling B, Kupka RW: Postpartum mania in a man with bipolar disorder: case report and a review of the role of sleep loss. Bipolar Disord 16(1):93–96, 2014 24467471

Tomson T, Battino D: Teratogenic effects of antiepileptic medications. Neurol Clin 27(4):993–1002, 2009 19853219

Tomson T, Battino D, Bonizzoni E, et al; EURAP study group: Dose-dependent risk of malformations with antiepileptic drugs: an analysis of data from the EURAP epilepsy and pregnancy registry. Lancet Neurol 10(7):609–617, 2011 21652013

Udechuku A, Nguyen T, Hill R, Szego K: Antidepressants in pregnancy: a systematic review. Aust N Z J Psychiatry 44(11):978–996, 2010 21034181

Vajda FJ, Graham J, Roten A, et al: Teratogenicity of the newer antiepileptic drugs—the Australian experience. J Clin Neurosci 19(1):57–59, 2012 22104350

van der Lugt NM, van de Maat JS, van Kamp IL, et al: Fetal, neonatal and developmental outcomes of lithium-exposed pregnancies. Early Hum Dev 88(6):375–378, 2012 22000820

Viguera AC, Nonacs R, Cohen LS, et al: Risk of recurrence of bipolar disorder in pregnant and nonpregnant women after discontinuing lithium maintenance. Am J Psychiatry 157(2):179–184, 2000 10671384

Viguera AC, Newport DJ, Ritchie J, et al: Lithium in breast milk and nursing infants: clinical implications. Am J Psychiatry 164(2):342–345, 2007a 17267800

Viguera AC, Whitfield T, Baldessarini RJ, et al: Risk of recurrence in women with bipolar disorder during pregnancy: prospective study of mood stabilizer discontinuation. Am J Psychiatry 164(12):1817–1824; quiz 1923, 2007b

Wikner BN, Stiller CO, Bergman U, et al: Use of benzodiazepines and benzodiazepine receptor agonists during pregnancy: neonatal outcome and congenital malformations. Pharmacoepidemiol Drug Saf 16(11):1203–1210, 2007 17894421

Wurst KE, Poole C, Ephross SA, Olshan AF: First trimester paroxetine use and the prevalence of congenital, specifically cardiac, defects: a meta-analysis of epidemiological studies. Birth Defects Res A Clin Mol Teratol 88(3):159–170, 2010 19739149

Wyszynski DF, Nambisan M, Surve T, et al; Antiepileptic Drug Pregnancy Registry: Increased rate of major malformations in offspring exposed to valproate during pregnancy. Neurology 64(6):961–965, 2005 15781808

Yacobi S, Ornoy A: Is lithium a real teratogen? What can we conclude from the prospective versus retrospective studies? A review. Isr J Psychiatry Relat Sci 45(2):95–106, 2008 18982835

Yonkers KA, Wisner KL, Stowe Z, et al: Management of bipolar disorder during pregnancy and the postpartum period. Am J Psychiatry 161(4):608–620, 2004 15056503

Yonkers KA, Wisner KL, Stewart DE, et al: The management of depression during pregnancy: a report from the American Psychiatric Association and the American College of Obstetricians and Gynecologists. Obstet Gynecol 114(3):703–713, 2009 19701065

Yonkers KA, Vigod S, Ross LE: Diagnosis, pathophysiology, and management of mood disorders in pregnant and postpartum women. Obstet Gynecol 117(4):961–977, 2011 21422871

Zappert LN, Rasgon NL: Management of bipolar disorder in women, in Handbook of Diagnosis and Treatment of Bipolar Disorders. Edited by Ketter TA. Washington, DC, American Psychiatric Publishing, 2010

7 Treatment of Older Adults With Bipolar Disorder

Terence A. Ketter, M.D.
John O. Brooks III, Ph.D., M.D.

Older adults, commonly defined as those 60 years and older, constitute an important subgroup of individuals with bipolar disorder because of the substantial human and economic resources necessary to address their complex psychiatric and medical problems. Age-specific clinical presentations, treatment response, and side-effect concerns can make the diagnosis and treatment of bipolar disorder and comorbid psychiatric and medical problems in older adults challenging. In this chapter, we describe advances in the specialized knowledge necessary to provide optimized treatment of bipolar disorder in older adults.

Although estimates of bipolar disorder prevalence in older adults in the community tend to be lower than those in younger adults, ranging between 0.5% (Hirschfeld et al. 2003) and 1% (Kessler et al. 2005), in clinical settings bipolar disorder prevalence in older adults rises more than 10-fold, to 8% (Yassa et al. 1988) to 17% (Depp et al. 2005). For example, in the Systematic Treatment Enhancement Program for Bipolar Disorder (STEP-BD) study, 246 of 3,615 patients (6.8%) were at least age 60 (Al Jurdi et al. 2008). The need for better management of bipolar disorder in aging adults will increase as the American population ages.

Approximately half of older adults with bipolar disorder have an index major depressive episode and then have a mood elevation episode on average 15 years later (Shulman et al. 1992). Most older adults with bipolar disorder have earlier onset of illness (i.e., onset at age <50 years) (Dols et al. 2014; Sajatovic et al. 2005a), although a minority of older adults experience later-onset bipolar disorder (i.e., onset at age≥50 years) (Sajatovic et al. 2005a). Although later-onset bipolar disorder may manifest more cognitive impairment (Schouws et al. 2009), it is associated with lower per capita rates of psychiatric service utilization (Sajatovic et al. 2005a). Indeed, the combined effects of delayed treatment, aging, and repeated mood episodes in earlier-onset bipolar disorder may be associated with worsening of disease state. For example, in the European Mania

217

in Bipolar Longitudinal Evaluation of Medication (EMBLEM) observational study, among older (age >60 years) patients, 323 with earlier-onset compared with 141 with later-onset bipolar disorder had slower recovery and longer hospital stays (Oostervink et al. 2009).

Although genetic influences are probably less in older than in younger patients with bipolar disorder, over half of older adults with bipolar disorder have a first-degree relative with mood disorder (Shulman et al. 1992). Genetic vulnerability interacts with stress, and bipolar disorder in older adults is associated with substantial medical burden (Dols et al. 2014; Gildengers et al. 2008; Lala and Sajatovic 2012). Although individuals with longer illness duration (Post 1992) may be less reactive to psychosocial stress (i.e., more spontaneous), a common phenomenon in older adults with bipolar disorder is for stressful life events to precede syndromal mood episodes (Beyer et al. 2008).

There may be synergy between recurrent mood episodes and adverse effects of aging (particularly with respect to cognitive decline) (Cacilhas et al. 2009; Elshahawi et al. 2011; Gildengers et al. 2013a; Lewandowski et al. 2013; Schouws et al. 2010), with opinions varying with regard to the extent to which this synergy is mediated by increased vascular burden in older adults with bipolar disorder (Gildengers et al. 2010; Schouws et al. 2009). Common medical comorbidities such as cardiovascular disease, diabetes, hypertension, hyperlipidemia, and obesity likely contribute to unfavorable bipolar illness course and high rates of service utilization (Bartels et al. 2000; Sajatovic et al. 1996). Indeed, mania secondary to neurological, endocrine, and other medical problems is relatively common in older compared with younger adults (Krauthammer and Klerman 1978).

Perhaps not surprisingly, compared with younger adults, older adults with bipolar disorder appear to have substantially higher psychiatric service utilization, with psychiatric hospitalizations that are nearly twice as long and expensive and four times as likely to result in discharge to an institution. Increased psychiatric service utilization may be related to the threefold higher risk of complex medical comorbidities (Brown 2001). Cognitive deficits may occur in over half of older adults with bipolar disorder (Aprahamian et al. 2014; Gildengers et al. 2004). Older adults with mood disorders have a greater risk of developing dementia than do those with other psychiatric or medical disorders (Kessing and Nilsson 2003; Kessing et al. 1999), and the risk of dementia increases with the number of prior syndromal mood episodes (Kessing and Andersen 2004).

The comorbidity rate of anxiety disorder, which is high in younger individuals with bipolar disorder, may be relatively low in older adults with bipolar disorder (Dols et al. 2014; Lala and Sajatovic 2012; Sajatovic and Kales 2006). Also, there is evidence that older adults with bipolar disorder use substances marginally less often than do younger adults with bipolar disorder (7.0% vs. 8.3% current prevalence) (Depp et al. 2005). However, among older patients with bipolar disorder and dementia, comorbid alcohol abuse/dependence is associated with a greater risk of inpatient hospitalization (Brooks et al. 2006).

Diagnosing and treating bipolar disorder in older adults is complex because of the patients' distinctive psychiatric presentations. Older compared with younger adults with bipolar disorder may present more often with severe depression, psychotic symptoms, and mania or hypomania (Kessing 2006), as well as a rapid-cycling course and more complex psychotropic regimens (Oostervink et al. 2009). In older adults with bipolar disorder, incomplete response in acute manic/mixed episodes is common (Himmelhoch et al. 1980; Van der Velde 1970), as are relapses (Dhingra and Rabins 1991; Shulman et al. 1992; Tohen et al. 1994).

Medical comorbidities in older adults present a variety of challenges to treatment, especially in terms of increased health care needs, medication interactions, and even the impact of bipolar disorder (especially with respect to cognitive impairment). For example, coronary artery disease is more prevalent among patients with bipolar disorder, with diagnosis usually being at a younger age, than among patients with major depressive disorder (Goldstein et al. 2009). Adults with bipolar disorder commonly have neurological, endocrine/metabolic (including being overweight or obese), and cardiovascular diseases (de Almeida et al. 2012; Gildengers et al. 2008; Hoblyn 2004).

Because of the pervasive medical problems in older adults with bipolar disorder, assessments of such individuals need to include not only thorough psychiatric examinations, but also careful medical evaluations. The latter include personal and family medical history, physical and neurological examinations, routine laboratory assessments (including metabolic, hepatic, and renal panels, and complete blood cell count), and more specialized testing as indicated. The individualized tests may include additional neurological assessments such as neuropsychological testing, neurological consultation, neuroimaging, electroencephalogram, and lumbar puncture. Important neurological disorders to consider in the differential diagnosis include delirium (which entails fluctuating level of consciousness, orientation, memory, and language), dementia (which entails sustained deterioration of orientation, memory, and language), and mild neurocognitive disorder (mild NCD, which is described in the following paragraphs). Agitation and disinhibition due to mania need to be distinguished from those due to dementia and delirium, whereas cognitive deficits due to depression need to be distinguished from those due to dementia or mild NCD. Finally, concurrent medical or neurological disorders and their treatments need to be characterized as comorbid/contributory in patients with primary mood disorders as opposed to causative in those with secondary mood disorders.

Arguably one of the most important recent psychiatric diagnostic developments with respect to older adults in general, and those with bipolar disorder in particular, is the status change for mild NCD in DSM-5 in 2013 (American Psychiatric Association 2013), which superseded DSM-IV-TR (American Psychiatric Association 2000). Specifically, mild NCD had its criteria modified and was moved from DSM-IV-TR Appendix B, "Criteria Sets and Axes Provided for Further Study," to the neurocognitive disorders section in the main body of DSM-5 (see Box 7–1). These changes were based on accumulating research that the largely congruent neurological disorder mild cognitive impairment (MCI) was common in the community (occurring in up to 10% of people over age 65 years) and associated with a fivefold greater risk of developing dementia (5%–10% per year vs. 1%–2% per year in those without MCI) (Petersen 2011). Mild NCD was added to DSM-5 to facilitate early detection (and hopefully in the future early treatment) of cognitive changes that may progress to major NCDs (or dementias). As with any effort to enhance sensitivity by including milder forms of illness that are on a continuum with health, mild NCD and MCI are controversial, with their inclusion being lauded by some and criticized by others (Blazer 2013; Ganguli et al. 2011; Morris 2012; Petersen 2011; Rabins and Lyketsos 2011).

Box 7–1. DSM-5 Criteria for Mild Neurocognitive Disorder

A. Evidence of modest cognitive decline from a previous level of performance in one or more cognitive domains (complex attention, executive function, learning and memory, language, perceptual-motor, or social cognition) based on:
  1. Concern of the individual, a knowledgeable informant, or the clinician that there has been a mild decline in cognitive function; and
  2. A modest impairment in cognitive performance, preferably documented by standardized neuropsychological testing or, in its absence, another quantified clinical assessment.
B. The cognitive deficits do not interfere with capacity for independence in everyday activities (i.e., complex instrumental activities of daily living such as paying bills or managing medications are preserved, but greater effort, compensatory strategies, or accommodation may be required).
C. The cognitive deficits do not occur exclusively in the context of a delirium.
D. The cognitive deficits are not better explained by another mental disorder (e.g., major depressive disorder, schizophrenia).

Specify whether due to:
   Alzheimer's disease
   Frontotemporal lobar degeneration
   Lewy body disease
   Vascular disease
   Traumatic brain injury
   Substance/medication use
   HIV infection
   Prion disease
   Parkinson's disease
   Huntington's disease
   Another medical condition
   Multiple etiologies
   Unspecified

Coding note: For mild neurocognitive disorder due to any of the medical etiologies listed above, code **331.83 (G31.84).** Do *not* use additional codes for the presumed etiological medical conditions. For substance/medication-induced mild neurocognitive disorder, code based on type of substance; see "Substance/Medication-Induced Major or Mild Neurocognitive Disorder" [in DSM-5]. For unspecified mild neurocognitive disorder, code **799.59 (R41.9).**

Specify:
   Without behavioral disturbance: If the cognitive disturbance is not accompanied by any clinically significant behavioral disturbance.
   With behavioral disturbance *(specify disturbance):* If the cognitive disturbance is accompanied by a clinically significant behavioral disturbance (e.g., psychotic symptoms, mood disturbance, agitation, apathy, or other behavioral symptoms).

Source. Reprinted from the *Diagnostic and Statistical Manual of Mental Disorders,* 5th Edition. Arlington, VA, American Psychiatric Association, 2013. Used with permission. Copyright © 2013 American Psychiatric Association.

Most (perhaps two-thirds of) individuals with MCI (which overlaps with DSM-5 mild NCD) have memory problems as the most prominent challenges and are therefore said to have *amnestic* MCI, although a substantive minority (perhaps one-third) of people with MCI have *nonamnestic* MCI, which is characterized more by prominent difficulties with attention, language, or visuospatial skills than with memory (Petersen 2011). Preliminary evidence suggests that amnestic and nonamnestic MCI might be harbingers of Alzheimer's and non-Alzheimer's (e.g., frontotemporal lobar deterioration or Lewy body disease) dementias, respectively (Petersen 2011). Assessment of older individuals with bipolar disorder and mild NCD includes the above-mentioned approach to assessment of older adults with bipolar disorder, but additionally entails particularly careful evaluation of potential adverse cognitive effects of medications, as well as neuropsychological testing (or, in its absence, other quantified clinical cognitive assessment), careful monitoring for deterioration of cognitive function over time, and more liberal use of neurological consultation and neuroimaging (e.g., magnetic resonance imaging to detect frontal or hippocampal atrophy). Neuropsychological testing is part of the standard evaluation of mild NCD, but if this is not available, simpler quantified clinical cognitive assessment metrics such as the Short Test of Mental Status (STMS; Tang-Wai et al. 2003) and the Montreal Cognitive Assessment (MoCA; Nasreddine et al. 2005) may be considered. In contrast, Folstein et al.'s (1975) Mini-Mental State Examination (which is sufficiently sensitive for dementia) is *not* appropriate for MCI assessment because it is commonly insensitive to the mild deficits seen in MCI.

Neurological consultation is often necessary to provide accurate specification of the medical etiology (or lack thereof) for mild NCD. Although biomarkers (including those in cerebrospinal fluid) are important research tools, these are not yet considered clinical tools (Petersen 2011). Treatments for MCI are in the very early stage of development, with no pharmacotherapies approved by the U.S. Food and Drug Administration (FDA) for MCI, and FDA-approved pharmacotherapies for dementia of the Alzheimer's type, such as donepezil, galantamine, and rivastigmine, lacking robust evidence of efficacy in MCI (Corey-Bloom 2012). Although disease-modifying treatments for MCI have not yet emerged, clinical research has suggested potential benefit for cognitive rehabilitation (e.g., use of mnemonics, association strategies, and computerized training) (Jean et al. 2010). Thus, clinical recommendations for patients with MCI commonly include conservative approaches, such as longitudinal quantified clinical cognitive assessments, and engaging in aerobic exercise, intellectually stimulating activities, and social activities (Petersen 2011).

■ Psychopharmacology Trends in Older Adults With Bipolar Disorder

Pharmacotherapy in older adults with bipolar disorder is evolving. For example, in the 1990s in North America and in German-speaking European countries, there was a shift away from lithium and toward divalproex for the management of older adults with bipolar disorder (Shulman et al. 2003), which was considered by some to lack a sufficient evidence base (Shulman 2010). Moreover, in mixed-age populations in the 2000s in at least some regions, lamotrigine appeared to move toward overtaking lithium and valproate (Bramness et al. 2009; Centorrino et al. 2010; Depp et al. 2008; Greil et al. 2012; Hooshmand et al. 2014; Reimers 2009; Walpoth-Niederwanger et al. 2012), and in a more widespread fashion, several second-generation antipsychotics (SGAs) overtook first-generation antipsychotics (Bowers et al. 2004; Depp et al. 2008; Greil et al. 2012; Hayes et al. 2011; Hooshmand et al. 2014; Pillarella et al. 2012; Walpoth-Niederwanger et al. 2012; Wilting et al. 2008; Wolfsperger et al. 2007; Yang et al. 2008). These pharmacotherapy trends in bipolar disorder may have been driven in part by perceived efficacy and tolerability advantages of new treatment options, although pharmaceutical company promotion of new proprietary medications likely also contributed.

Data from STEP-BD have been consistent with the above-mentioned prescribing trends. In one study, 193 older (ages ≥60 years) compared with 2,249 younger (ages 20–59 years) recovered STEP-BD patients were less often prescribed lithium (29.5% vs. 37.8%) but were statistically similarly prescribed valproate (39.4% vs. 34.0%), lamotrigine (21.2% vs. 25.6%), carbamazepine (6.7% vs. 5.1%), antidepressants (47.2% vs. 42.9%), SGAs (30.6% vs. 33.4%), and benzodiazepines (21.8% vs. 19.6%), with both age groups taking, on average, 2.1 psychotropic medications (Al Jurdi et al. 2008). Moreover, older compared with younger STEP-BD patients took significantly lower mean doses of lithium (31% lower, with use of lower doses evident in patients over age 50 years), valproate (22% lower, with use of lower doses evident in patients over 60 years), and risperidone (50% lower; age threshold for use of lower doses was not reported), but not other medications (Al Jurdi et al. 2008).

In the EMBLEM study, 475 older (age >60 years) compared with 2,286 younger (age <50 years) patients were more frequently taking psychotropic monotherapy and antidepressants, and less frequently taking SGAs, but had statistically similar rates of lithium, anticonvulsant, and first-generation antipsychotic use (Oostervink et al. 2009). The differential usage of medications across the age range could reflect a reluctance (among clinicians and/or patients) to alter a preexisting medication regimen that is associated with stability. Alternatively, the potential adverse metabolic profiles of older SGAs can make them less well-suited for older patients. Regardless, data regarding both adverse effects and potential efficacy of SGAs in older adults with bipolar disorder are severely lacking.

■ Treatment of Acute Manic and Mixed Episodes in Older Adults

Lithium

Although lithium remains an important option for relatively medically well older adults with acute mania (Abou-Saleh and Coppen 1983; Chen et al. 1999; Gildengers et al. 2005; Himmelhoch et al. 1980; Murray et al. 1983; Sajatovic 2002; Sajatovic et al. 2005b; Schaffer and Garvey 1984; Schneider and Wilcox 1998; Shulman et al. 1992; Snowdon 1991), older compared with younger manic adults have poorer responses to lithium (Van der Velde 1970). This may be due in part to lithium providing suboptimal efficacy in nonclassic presentations that are common in older adults with bipolar disorder, such as mixed episodes (Freeman et al. 1992; Keller et al. 1986; Secunda et al. 1985), dysphoric mania (i.e., DSM-5 manic episodes with mixed features) (Swann et al. 2002), secondary mania (Krauthammer and Klerman 1978), and rapid-cycling bipolar disorder (Kukopulos et al. 1980).

Lithium's utility in older adults may be additionally limited by tolerability challenges, such as neurological (e.g., tremor, ataxia, cognitive impairment) (Chacko et al. 1987; Dias et al. 2012; Gyulai 2013; Himmelhoch et al. 1980; Jacoby 2004; Juurlink et al. 2004; Murray et al. 1983; Smith and Helms 1982; Stone 1989), renal (e.g., renal impairment, polyuria/polydipsia) (Chacko et al. 1987; Hardy et al. 1987; Hewick et al. 1977; McKnight et al. 2012; Rej et al. 2012), endocrine/metabolic (e.g., hypothyroidism, weight gain) (Head and Dening 1998; McKnight et al. 2012; Roose et al. 1979; Stone 1989; van Melick et al. 2010), and other medical adverse effects (Eastham et al. 1998; Roose et al. 1979), which may necessitate using substantially lower lithium doses (e.g., with lithium serum concentrations of 0.4–0.8 mEq/L) or even discontinuing lithium. In addition, because of drug interactions, older adults with bipolar disorder who are taking nonsteroidal anti-inflammatory agents, thiazide diuretics, or angiotensin-converting enzyme inhibitors, as well as those with sodium-restricted diets or dehydration, may need to decrease lithium doses or even discontinue the medication (Roose et al. 1979; Schaffer and Garvey 1984; Sproule et al. 2000). Lithium's adverse effects must be considered in context with hypotheses that its mood stabilization and neuroprotective effects may attenuate the risk of dementia in patients with bipolar disorder (Kessing et al. 2008; Nunes et al. 2007).

Divalproex (Valproate)

Divalproex (valproate) is an important more recent (compared with lithium) treatment option for older adults with acute manic or mixed episodes (Chen et al. 1999; Gildengers et al. 2005; Kando et al. 1996; McFarland et al. 1990; Niedermier and Nasrallah 1998; Noaghiul et al. 1998; Puryear et al. 1995, Schneider and Wilcox 1998) and may be superior to lithium in treating secondary mania (Evans et al. 1995). Divalproex may be better tolerated than lithium in older adults (Conney and Kaston 1999; Puryear et al. 1995), although lithium and divalproex may yield comparable rates of delirium (Shulman et al. 2005). In older adults in skilled nursing facilities, divalproex compared with lithium therapy may yield better tolerability and mood outcomes and may also prove less expensive (Conney and Kaston 1999). However, the putative efficacy of divalproex in dementia-related agitation (Tariot et al. 2001) has been called into question in a meta-analysis (Lonergan and Luxenberg 2009). Moreover, divalproex can be associated with gastrointestinal (e.g., nausea, vomiting, dyspepsia, diarrhea), hepatic (e.g., transaminase elevations), central nervous system (e.g., tremor, sedation, dizziness, ataxia), and metabolic (e.g., weight gain, osteoporosis) side effects that may necessitate using substantially lower doses in older adults than in their younger counterparts (e.g., with valproate serum concentrations of 40–80 μg/mL) or even discontinuing or avoiding divalproex (Chen et al. 1999; Gyulai 2013; Hewick et al. 1977; Mezuk et al. 2010; Tariot et al. 2001).

In a recent 3-week, multicenter, randomized, double-blind trial in older adults ($\geq$ age 60 years) with bipolar I disorder and current acute manic, hypomanic, or mixed episodes, 112 patients taking lithium (0.8–1.0 mEq/L in ~60%, and 0.4–0.8 mEq/L in ~40%) compared with 112 taking valproate (80–100 μg/mL in ~60%, and 40–80 μg/mL in ~40%) had statistically similar improvements in mean Young Mania Rating Scale scores and complaints of weight gain and sedation, but more tremor and polydipsia (Gyulai 2013).

Very limited data suggest that divalproex combined with lithium may yield benefit in some older adults with bipolar disorder who are partial lithium responders (Goldberg et al. 2000; Schneider and Wilcox 1998) or who have a rapid-cycling course (Schneider and Wilcox 1998; Sharma et al. 1993).

Carbamazepine

Carbamazepine may have merit in treating secondary mania (Evans et al. 1995), although its use in older adults is limited by central nervous system (e.g., diplopia, blurred vision, fatigue, sedation, dizziness, and ataxia) and gastrointestinal (e.g., nausea, vomiting) problems, hyponatremia, drug interactions (Ketter et al. 1991a, 1991b), rash (Cates and Powers 1998), blood dyscrasias (Cates and Powers 1998; Saetre et al. 2007), and other medical (e.g., cardiac) problems. Carbamazepine tolerability limitations may necessitate having some older compared with younger adults taking lower doses (yielding carbamazepine serum concentrations as low as 6 μg/mL) or even discontinuing or avoiding carbamazepine (Battino et al. 2003). Carbamazepine decreases blood concentrations of multiple psychotropic and general medical medications through induction of multiple hepatic enzymes, including cytochrome P450 3A4, thus potentially compromising their efficacy (Ketter et al. 1991a, 1991b). Therefore, carbamazepine's challenging side-effect and drug interaction profiles, in addition to a lack of efficacy studies, make it a less desirable choice than lithium or divalproex for most older adults.

Second-Generation Antipsychotics

Emerging data suggest that SGAs may provide adequate efficacy and safety/tolerability in some older adults with acute manic or mixed episodes (Baruch et al. 2013; Frye et al. 1996; Madhusoodanan et al. 1995, 1999, 2000; Nicolato et al. 2006; Sajatovic et al. 2008a, 2008b; Shulman et al. 1997; Tariot et al. 2000, 2004). In spite of limited evidence of efficacy, these agents were used in almost one-third of older adult STEP-BD patients (Al Jurdi et al. 2008), and it may be that these agents are being used in most older adults with bipolar disorder living in nursing homes (Crystal et al. 2009). However, as a class these agents tend to have more adverse-effect challenges than mood stabilizers and antidepressants. Of particular concern in older adults are weight gain/metabolic problems, somnolence, cognitive impairment, extrapyramidal symptoms (although less than with first-generation antipsychotics), fall risk, and neuroleptic malignant syndrome (Gareri et al. 2006). Older adults may be at greater risk for SGA-induced metabolic syndrome, which in turn increases the risk of cardiovascular disease (Correll et al. 2006). Hence, there is a clear need to assess the benefits and harms of SGAs in older adults with bipolar disorder (Aziz et al. 2006). The need for systematic ascertainment of risks with SGAs for older adults with bipolar disorder is underscored by U.S. prescribing information, which includes boxed warnings indicating that each of these agents may increase mortality in older adults with dementia-related psychosis (primarily due to cardiac and infectious processes, already the most common causes of death in the older population). Moreover, most SGAs (with quetiapine and ziprasidone being important exceptions) have also been associated with increased risk of cerebrovascular accidents in older adults with dementia.

Electroconvulsive Therapy

Although electroconvulsive therapy (ECT) appears effective and safe in acute late-life depression (van der Wurff et al. 2003) and in mixed-age samples of adults with acute manic or mixed episodes (Mukherjee et al. 1994), its efficacy and safety/tolerability in older adults with acute manic or mixed episodes remain to be definitively established.

■ Treatment of Acute Bipolar Depression in Older Adults

Second-Generation Antipsychotics

All of the FDA-approved treatments for acute bipolar depression (olanzapine plus fluoxetine combination, quetiapine monotherapy, and lurasidone monotherapy and adjunctive therapy) include SGA agents. However, as noted in the previous section on acute manic and mixed episodes, this class of medications raises substantial but incompletely understood safety/tolerability challenges in older adults. Moreover, data are very limited regarding SGA efficacy in older adults with acute bipolar depression. For example, a post hoc analysis of data from 72 older adults (ages 55–65 years) extracted from data pooled from two 8-week multicenter, randomized, double-blind, mixed-age adult trials suggested that quetiapine (300 or 600 mg/day) compared with placebo might have adequate efficacy in older adults with acute bipolar depression (Sajatovic 2007). As might be expected, sedation, somnolence, and dizziness were the side effects most often leading to quetiapine discontinuation in depressed older adults with bipolar disorder, although the incidence of such side effects was not greater than in 906 depressed younger adults (ages 18–55 years) with bipolar disorder. Similarly, a post hoc analysis of data from 338 older adults (ages ≥66 years) with acute unipolar depression in a 9-week multicenter, randomized, double-blind, mixed-age adult trial suggested that extended-release quetiapine (50–300 mg/day) compared with placebo reduced Montgomery-Åsberg Depression Rating Scale (MADRS) scores in patients with both higher and lower anxiety, sleep disturbance, and pain (Montgomery et al. 2014). Very limited data are available regarding the treatment of acute psychotic depression in older adults with bipolar disorder. In older adults with acute psychotic unipolar depression, antipsychotics need to be combined with antidepressants, and possibly with ECT (Frank 2014).

Assessment of the olanzapine plus fluoxetine combination in older adults with acute bipolar depression appears to be a rather low priority, probably because of olanzapine's prominent metabolic side effects and sedation. Efficacy issues more than safety/tolerability limitations in mixed-age adult samples make assessment of the newer and somewhat better-tolerated SGAs aripiprazole and ziprasidone in older adults with acute bipolar depression a relatively low priority.

In contrast, in view of lurasidone's demonstrated efficacy and enhanced safety/tolerability (at least compared with the olanzapine plus fluoxetine combination and quetiapine monotherapy) in mixed-age adult samples, there appears to be a pressing need for systematic evaluation of lurasidone's efficacy as well as safety/tolerability in older adults with bipolar depression.

Lamotrigine

Lamotrigine, compared with valproate and carbamazepine, may have fewer side effects (including cognitive side effects) in older adults (Dias et al. 2012). In view of lamotrigine's generally adequate tolerability and utility in delaying depressive episodes in mixed-age adult populations, it is commonly prescribed for older adults with bipolar disorder, despite the lack of an FDA indication for acute bipolar depression. Indeed, in STEP-BD, 21.2% of older adults with bipolar disorder were taking lamotrigine (Al Jurdi et al. 2008). However, data are very limited regarding the efficacy and safety/tolerability of lamotrigine in older adults with acute bipolar depression. In a 12-week, uncontrolled, multicenter trial in 57 older adults (ages ≥60 years) with acute bipolar (type I>type II) depression, open adjunctive lamotrigine (mean dosage=151 mg/day) yielded response in 65%, with a rash discontinuation rate of 7% (Sajatovic et al. 2011). In this study, approximately 60% of patients had medical comorbidity, which was related to degree of depression, impaired cognition, and disability (Gildengers et al. 2013b).

Other Mood Stabilizers

Although lithium, divalproex, and carbamazepine appear better tolerated than most SGAs in older adults with bipolar disorder, safety/tolerability limitations compared with those of lamotrigine and antidepressants, along with lack of FDA indications or compelling evidence of efficacy in acute bipolar depression, limit the utility of these mood stabilizers for depressed older adults with bipolar disorder in clinical settings.

Antidepressants

Compared with most mood stabilizers and SGAs, most antidepressants have superior somatic safety/tolerability profiles, and this likely contributes at least in part to antidepressants being commonly administered to older adults with acute bipolar depression, despite the lack of FDA indications or evidence of efficacy. Indeed, 47.2% of older adults in STEP-BD were taking these agents (Al Jurdi et al. 2008). In geriatric unipolar depression, selective serotonin reuptake inhibitor (SSRI) antidepressants may yield limited (but adequate) acute efficacy (Nelson et al. 2008), with fair somatic tolerability in most patients (Wilson and Mottram 2004). Although the risks of inefficacy and treatment-emergent affective switch with antidepressants are of concern in mixed-age samples of patients with bipolar disorder, a small ($N=32$) retrospective study suggested that older adults with bipolar disorder treated with mood stabilizers and antidepressants may be at decreased risk of attempting suicide (Aizenberg et al. 2006), while a Canadian epidemiological study found that older adults with bipolar disorder taking antidepressants had a decreased rate of hospitalization for manic/mixed (but not depressive) episodes (Schaffer et al. 2006).

In view of the limited evidence base, clinicians may be faced with imputing information regarding the efficacy and safety/tolerability of antidepressants in older adults with acute bipolar depression from data in older patients with unipolar major depressive disorder. In a review of 51 randomized, double-blind, placebo-controlled acute antidepressant trials in older adults with unipolar major depressive disorder, the numbers needed to treat (NNTs) for response and remission compared with placebo for all antidepressants (tricyclic antidepressants, SSRIs, and other antidepressants) were 7 and 15, respectively (Kok et al. 2012). In older adults with psychotic unipolar depression, antidepressants need to be combined with antipsychotics, and possibly with ECT (Frank 2014).

Electroconvulsive Therapy

Although ECT appears to be effective and safe in acute late-life depression, its cost-effectiveness remains to be established (van der Wurff et al. 2003). Moreover, there is a dearth of randomized controlled ECT trial data to inform clinicians how to safely and effectively use this modality in older adults with acute bipolar depression. ECT's potential adverse effects of concern include cognitive/memory impairment, and, less often, cardio-vascular complications, prolonged seizures, prolonged apnea, headaches, muscle soreness, nausea, treatment-emergent mania, and posttreatment delirium (Kamat et al. 2003). Older adults with space-occupying lesions and brain tumors, cerebrovascular disease, cardiovascular disease, diabetes mellitus, seizure disorders, hyperthyroidism, and electrolyte disturbances, and those taking theophylline, benzodiazepines, anticonvulsants, lithium, diuretics, hypoglycemic agents, and levodopa/carbidopa may be at particular risk for problems with ECT (Kamat et al. 2003). Hence, in older adults, as in mixed-age populations, feasibility and acceptability concerns lead ECT to be held in reserve for patients with urgent, severe (e.g., psychotic), or refractory depression (Frank 2014).

Other Neuromodulation Therapies

Repetitive transcranial magnetic stimulation and other neuromodulation therapies (e.g., subconvulsive, focal, or subconvulsive and focal) are possible alternatives for treatment-resistant depression in the elderly, although to date these therapies have been used primarily in older adults with unipolar major depressive disorder (Riva-Posse et al. 2013).

Other Somatic Treatments

Limitations of somatic therapies in older adults have raised interest in complementary and alternative medicine interventions such as nutriceuticals (e.g., St. John's wort, fish oil, S-adenosylmethionine, folate), exercise, yoga, tai chi, massage therapy, music therapy, and religion and spirituality, although to date these therapies have been used primarily in older adults with unipolar major depressive disorder (Nyer et al. 2013) rather than with bipolar disorder.

Adjunctive Psychotherapy

As noted in the preceding chapters in this volume on the treatment of acute bipolar depression (Chapter 2) and bipolar preventive treatment (Chapter 4), there is growing appreciation of adjunctive psychosocial interventions in bipolar disorder (Geddes and Miklowitz 2013), with a substantial evidence base emerging to inform therapeutics in mixed-age populations, particularly for bipolar preventive treatment, and to a lesser extent for acute bipolar depression. Importantly, depressed older adults may prefer psychotherapy to pharmacotherapy (Gum et al. 2006).

However, very limited data are available regarding the efficacy of adjunctive psychotherapies in older adults with acute bipolar depression. For example, as of early 2015, the largest psychosocial intervention study to date in mixed-age adults with acute bipolar depression was the STEP-BD multicenter, randomized, controlled effectiveness trial, in which 163 patients receiving adjunctive intensive cognitive-behavioral therapy (CBT), family focused therapy, or interpersonal and social rhythm therapy were compared with 130 patients receiving a brief psychoeducation control intervention, yet there has not been a published report regarding efficacy and safety/tolerability in the subgroup of older adults who participated in this study. Thus, clinicians are faced with imputing information regarding the utility of psychosocial interventions from data in mixed-age adults with bipolar disorder or in older adults with unipolar major depressive disorder.

Data suggest that CBT has utility in depressed unipolar older adults, with meta-analyses of randomized controlled trials suggesting that CBT is more effective than treatment as usual or a wait-list control condition (Gould et al. 2012; Wilson et al. 2008). Also, in a recent meta-analysis, group CBT and computerized CBT compared with wait-list control appeared effective in older adults with acute unipolar subsyndromal depression (Krishna et al. 2013). Indeed, an expert consensus guideline included CBT among the preferred psychotherapy techniques for treating depression in older adults (Alexopoulos et al. 2001). Substantial evidence also supports roles in acute late-life unipolar depression for Problem Solving Therapy (which teaches problem solving to reduce psychological distress) (Arean et al. 1993, 2008, 2010) and Life Review (reminiscence) Therapy (Arean et al. 1993; Korte et al. 2012; Serrano et al. 2004). In contrast, evidence supporting Interpersonal Therapy in unipolar depressed older adults is more limited (Mossey; van Schaik et al. 2006).

■ Bipolar Preventive Treatment in Older Adults

Lithium

As described in Chapter 4, "Bipolar Disorder Preventive Treatment," lithium is the classic mood stabilizer for bipolar preventive treatment in mixed-age adult populations. Indeed, lithium continues to be an important preventive treatment option for relatively medically well older adults with classic bipolar disorder (i.e., with pure rather than mixed mania, and without rapid cycling). However, as described earlier in this chapter (see "Psychopharmacology Trends in Older Adults With Bipolar Disorder"), efficacy limitations in nonclassic bipolar disorder and safety/tolerability limitations in older adults have resulted in some migration from lithium to valproate in North America and German-speaking European countries.

Limited data are available regarding the efficacy and safety/tolerability of lithium bipolar preventive treatment in older adults (Hewick et al. 1977; Murray et al. 1983; Stone 1989), in spite of considerable clinical use. For example, in a retrospective study of 60 middle-aged and older adults (age >60 years) with unipolar depression and bipolar disorder, lithium preventive treatment yielded decreased depressive and manic relapses compared with prior to starting lithium, with only the expected tolerability challenges (Lepkifker et al. 2007).

As described in Chapter 4, multicenter, randomized, double-blind, placebo-controlled bipolar preventive treatment trials in mixed-age adult samples using divalproex, lamotrigine, and quetiapine monotherapy, as well as adjunctive (added to lithium or valproate) quetiapine, aripiprazole, risperidone, and ziprasidone, have had lithium (or lithium/valproate) monotherapy arms. However, in most instances such mixed-age adult bipolar preventive treatment trials had insufficient numbers of older patients to permit assessment of efficacy and safety/tolerability in older adults. An exception to this pattern was a secondary analysis of the pooled mixed-age adult lamotrigine monotherapy preventive treatment trials (with lithium as the active comparator) (Goodwin et al. 2004), in which the pattern of efficacy and tolerability findings among 98 older adults (age≥55 years) resembled that in the larger mixed-age adult analysis, with lithium (modal dosage=750 mg/day) and lamotrigine (modal dosage=240 mg/day) being more effective in delaying manic/hypomanic/mixed and depressive relapses, respectively, and lamotrigine being better tolerated than lithium (Sajatovic et al. 2005b). In this analysis, older adults taking lithium, relative to placebo, had unfavorable (single-digit) numbers needed to harm (NNHs) for adverse-event discontinuation (7), tremor (7), headache (8), and amnesia (9). There was no serious rash, although 2 of 34 older adults taking lithium, compared with none of 31 taking placebo, had benign rash.

Divalproex (Valproate)

Although it is clear that divalproex compared with lithium can provide superior acute efficacy and/or safety/tolerability in some older adults with bipolar disorder, there is a dearth of information regarding long-term use of divalproex in this population. In the absence of such information for divalproex (and for most other pharmacotherapies), providers commonly consider continuing divalproex for longer-term treatment in individuals with good acute affective responses and tolerability, based on the principle of the multiphase treatment strategy (i.e., continuing effective and adequately tolerated acute treatments to prevent relapse). Clearly, studies are needed to establish adequate evidence regarding the efficacy and safety/tolerability of longer-term divalproex in older adults with bipolar disorder.

Lamotrigine

In view of lamotrigine's generally good tolerability and ability to delay depressive episodes in mixed-age adult populations, it is commonly prescribed in older adults. In the older-adult secondary analysis of lamotrigine monotherapy preventive treatment trials described earlier (see subsection "Lithium"), lamotrigine and lithium appeared more effective in delaying bipolar depressive and manic/hypomanic/mixed relapses, respectively, with lamotrigine appearing better tolerated than lithium (Sajatovic et al. 2005b). In this analysis, older adults taking lamotrigine compared with placebo had unfavorable (single-digit) NNHs for back pain (7) and headache (9). There was no serious rash, although 1 of 33 older adults taking lamotrigine, compared with none of 31 taking placebo, had benign rash.

Second-Generation Antipsychotics

As described in Chapter 4, several SGAs have FDA indications for bipolar preventive treatment in mixed-age adult populations, but the efficacy and safety/tolerability of these agents for bipolar preventive treatment in older adults remain to be established. Given the tolerability challenges of these agents in older adults (described earlier in this chapter, in the sections on SGAs in the treatment of acute manic and mixed episodes and of acute bipolar depression), careful assessment of the potential benefits versus harms is indicated when contemplating their longer-term use in older adults with bipolar disorder. Indeed, some experts suggest that if sustained remission is achieved, antipsychotics and antidepressants ought to be gradually tapered and discontinued (Young et al. 2004).

The three large longer-term comparative effectiveness trials that assessed lithium, valproate, and quetiapine in mixed-age adult bipolar disorder populations—Bipolar Affective Disorder Lithium/Anticonvulsant

Evaluation (BALANCE; Geddes et al. 2010), Lithium Treatment Moderate-Dose Use Study (LiTMUS; Nierenberg et al. 2013), and Bipolar Clinical and Health Outcomes Initiative in Comparative Effectiveness (Bipolar CHOICE; Nierenberg et al. 2014), which were described in Chapter 4 on bipolar preventive treatment—did not have sufficient numbers of older adults with bipolar disorder to assess efficacy and safety/tolerability differences in older compared with younger patients with bipolar disorder.

Antidepressants

As noted in Chapters 2 and 4, on the treatment of acute bipolar depression and bipolar preventive treatment, respectively, a limited evidence base and highly variable opinions exist regarding the role of antidepressants in mixed-age adults with bipolar disorder, with particular controversy regarding their use in preventive treatment (Pacchiarotti et al. 2013). Some clinicians may emphasize the somatic safety/tolerability profiles of antidepressants, compared with mood stabilizers and SGAs, and invoke the multiphase treatment strategy (i.e., continuing effective and adequately tolerated acute treatments in efforts to prevent relapse) to advocate using adjunctive antidepressants as preventive agents in older adults with bipolar disorder. In contrast, other clinicians may emphasize the risk of mood destabilization with longer-term antidepressants and advocate limiting exposure to these agents in older adults with bipolar disorder. In view of the limited evidence base, clinicians are faced with imputing information regarding the efficacy and safety/tolerability of longer-term antidepressants in older adults with bipolar disorder from data in mixed-age patients with bipolar disorder or in older adults with unipolar major depressive disorder.

In a review of eight randomized, double-blind, placebo-controlled, longer-term (i.e., with durations ranging from 24 weeks to 3 years) antidepressant trials in 925 older adults with unipolar major depressive disorder, the NNT to prevent recurrence compared with placebo was an encouraging 4 for all antidepressants, 3 for tricyclic antidepressants, and 5 for SSRIs (Kok et al. 2011). Indeed, it is recommended that treatment of unipolar geriatric depression be for a minimum of 12 months (and up to 2 years) from the time of remission, with indefinite treatment considered for patients with severe or recurrent depression, those requiring ECT, or those having only partial resolution of symptoms; moreover, if antidepressants are discontinued, it is recommended that the dose be tapered down over several months, with careful monitoring for evidence of relapse (Frank 2014).

Electroconvulsive Therapy

Although ECT appears to be effective and safe in acute late-life depression, its efficacy and safety/tolerability in bipolar preventive treatment in older adults remain to be definitively established (van der Wurff et al. 2003).

Adjunctive Psychotherapy

There is growing appreciation for the utility of adjunctive psychosocial interventions in bipolar disorders (Geddes and Miklowitz 2013), with evidence of their utility in mixed-age samples of adults with bipolar disorder being more robust for bipolar preventive treatment than for acute bipolar depression. However, there are limited data regarding the efficacy of such interventions as preventive treatments in older adults with bipolar disorder. Thus, clinicians are faced with imputing information regarding the utility of adjunctive psychosocial bipolar preventive interventions from data in mixed-age patients with bipolar disorder or in older patients with unipolar major depressive disorder.

A review of earlier controlled trials in older adults indicated that problem-solving therapy (Ciechanowski et al. 2004; Williams et al. 2000), life review therapy (Pot et al. 2010), Internet/group CBT (Spek et al. 2008), and CBT/problem-solving therapy (van't Veer-Tazelaar et al. 2009) were safe and cost-effective methods to reduce the public health burden of depression among older adults with subthreshold depression (Lee et al. 2012). However, more recent data have been less encouraging. For example, in late-life unipolar subsyndromal depression, although individual CBT may prevent relapse (Lee et al. 2012), group CBT may not (Krishna et al. 2013). Also, in a recent meta-analysis, group CBT compared with wait-list control did *not* appear effective in preventing unipolar subsyndromal depression in older adults (Krishna et al. 2013).

Although integrated psychosocial interventions may help mixed-age adult samples of patients with bipolar disorder, there are few data regarding such interventions in older adults. In 441 mixed-age adult patients with bipolar disorder, systematic care management (including structured group psychoeducation, monthly telephone monitoring, and feedback to and coordination with a mental health treatment team) provided by nurse care managers yielded lower mean mania ratings over 24 months (Simon et al. 2006). In another randomized controlled trial in 306 mixed-age adult veterans with bipolar disorder, a collaborative model for chronic care (including group psychoeducation, nurse care coordinators to improve information flow and access to and continuity of care, and clinician decision support with simplified practice guidelines) was found to reduce weeks in (primarily manic) mood episodes and to improve social role function, mental quality of life, and treatment satisfaction over 36 months (Bauer et al. 2006). Moreover, there is evidence supporting integrated psychosocial interventions for geriatric depression. For example, an expert consensus guideline regarding the management of depression in older adults strongly supported including appropriate psychosocial interventions (e.g., psychoeducation, family counseling, and visiting nurse services) in treatment programs (Alexopoulos et al. 2001).

■ Conclusion

Age-specific complex psychiatric and medical presentations and differential treatment responses make the diagnosis and treatment of bipolar disorder in older adults challenging. Systematic data demonstrating therapeutic efficacy in older adults with bipolar disorder are very limited. Moreover, certain medications entail distinctive safety/tolerability concerns when administered to older adults in general and to those with bipolar disorder in particular (Table 7–1). Lithium administration in older adults may be limited by risks of neurotoxicity (e.g., tremor, ataxia, cognitive impairment) (Gyulai 2013), as well as thyroid and renal problems (McKnight et al. 2012). Divalproex may be somewhat better tolerated than lithium in older adults but can cause somnolence (Tariot et al. 2001) and weight gain (Gyulai 2013). Carbamazepine is a potent enzyme inducer that can affect efficacy of multiple psychotropic and nonpsychotropic medications (Ketter et al. 1991a, 1991b), as well as cause rash and blood dyscrasias (Cates and Powers 1998). In contrast, lamotrigine may have fewer adverse-effect limitations in older adults than do lithium, divalproex, and carbamazepine (Sajatovic et al. 2011). SGA-related sedation and weight gain/metabolic problems are of substantive concern in older adults (Gareri et al. 2006). In geriatric unipolar depression, SSRI antidepressants may yield limited efficacy (Nelson et al. 2008) but fair somatic tolerability in most patients (although nausea, vomiting, dizziness, and drowsiness occur in some patients) (Wilson and Mottram 2004), whereas the risk of mood destabilization in older patients with bipolar disorder may be limited (Schaffer et al. 2006). Although anxiolytics/hypnotics have abuse potential, they can be effective, well-tolerated adjuncts in some younger adults with bipolar disorder. However, in older adults with bipolar disorder, the ability of these agents to yield neurotoxicity (e.g., sedation, ataxia), cognitive impairment, and delir-

TABLE 7–1. Medication safety/tolerability challenges in older adults with bipolar disorder

Lithium	Neurotoxicity (e.g., tremor, ataxia, cognitive impairment) (Gyulai 2013), thyroid problems (McKnight et al. 2012), renal problems (McKnight et al. 2012)
Divalproex	Somnolence (Tariot et al. 2001), weight gain (Gyulai 2013)
Carbamazepine	Drug interactions (Ketter et al. 1991a, 1991b), rash (Cates and Powers 1998), blood dyscrasias (Cates and Powers 1998)
Lamotrigine	Relatively well tolerated (Sajatovic et al. 2011)
Second-generation antipsychotics	Sedation, weight gain/metabolic problems (Gareri et al. 2006)
Antidepressants	Limited efficacy (?) (Nelson et al. 2008), relatively good somatic tolerability (Wilson and Mottram 2004), limited mood destabilization risk (Schaffer et al. 2006)
Anxiolytics/hypnotics	Neurotoxicity (e.g., sedation, ataxia) (Lechin et al. 1996), cognitive impairment (Lechin et al. 1996), delirium (Lechin et al. 1996), falls (Softic et al. 2013)

ium (Lechin et al. 1996), as well as falls (Softic et al. 2013), is of particular concern.

In view of the limitations of somatic therapies and the dearth of controlled trials of adjunctive psychosocial therapies in older adults with bipolar disorder, it appears particularly necessary for future research to provide systematic assessment of adjunctive psychosocial therapies for older adults with bipolar disorder.

■ References

Abou-Saleh MT, Coppen A: The prognosis of depression in old age: the case for lithium therapy. Br J Psychiatry 143:527–528, 1983 6416345

Aizenberg D, Olmer A, Barak Y: Suicide attempts amongst elderly bipolar patients. J Affect Disord 91(1):91–94, 2006 16434107

Al Jurdi RK, Marangell LB, Petersen NJ, et al: Prescription patterns of psychotropic medications in elderly compared with younger participants who achieved a "recovered" status in the Systematic Treatment Enhancement Program for Bipolar Disorder. Am J Geriatr Psychiatry 16(11):922–933, 2008 18978253

Alexopoulos GS, Katz IR, Reynolds CF 3rd, et al: The expert consensus guideline series. Pharmacotherapy of depressive disorders in older patients. Postgrad Med Spec No Pharmacotherapy:1–86, 2001

American Psychiatric Association: Diagnostic and Statistical Manual of Mental Disorders, 4th Edition, Text Revision. Washington, DC, American Psychiatric Association, 2000

American Psychiatric Association: Diagnostic and Statistical Manual of Mental Disorders, 5th Edition. Washington, DC, American Psychiatric Association, 2013

Aprahamian I, Ladeira RB, Diniz BS, et al: Cognitive impairment in euthymic older adults with bipolar disorder: a controlled study using cognitive screening tests. Am J Geriatr Psychiatry 22(4):389–397, 2014 23567429

Arean PA, Perri MG, Nezu AM, et al: Comparative effectiveness of social problem-solving therapy and reminiscence therapy as treatments for depression in older adults. J Consult Clin Psychol 61(6):1003–1010, 1993 8113478

Arean P, Hegel M, Vannoy S, et al: Effectiveness of problem-solving therapy for older, primary care patients with depression: results from the IMPACT project. Gerontologist 48(3):311–323, 2008 18591356

Areán PA, Raue P, Mackin RS, et al: Problem-solving therapy and supportive therapy in older adults with major depression and executive dysfunction. Am J Psychiatry 167(11):1391–1398, 2010 20516155

Aziz R, Lorberg B, Tampi RR: Treatments for late-life bipolar disorder. Am J Geriatr Pharmacother 4(4):347–364, 2006 17296540

Bartels SJ, Forester B, Miles KM, Joyce T: Mental health service use by elderly patients with bipolar disorder and unipolar major depression. Am J Geriatr Psychiatry 8(2):160–166, 2000 10804077

Baruch Y, Tadger S, Plopski I, Barak Y: Asenapine for elderly bipolar manic patients. J Affect Disord 145(1):130–132, 2013 22877962

Battino D, Croci D, Rossini A, et al: Serum carbamazepine concentrations in elderly patients: a case-matched pharmacokinetic evaluation based on therapeutic drug monitoring data. Epilepsia 44(7):923–929, 2003 12823575

Bauer MS, McBride L, Williford WO, et al; Cooperative Studies Program 430 Study Team: Collaborative care for bipolar disorder, Part II: impact on clinical outcome, function, and costs. Psychiatr Serv 57(7):937–945, 2006 16816277

Beyer JL, Kuchibhatla M, Cassidy F, Krishnan KR: Stressful life events in older bipolar patients. Int J Geriatr Psychiatry 23(12):1271–1275, 2008 18613269

Blazer D: Neurocognitive disorders in DSM-5. Am J Psychiatry 170(6):585–587, 2013 23732964

Bowers L, Callaghan P, Clark N, et al: Comparisons of psychotropic drug prescribing patterns in acute psychiatric wards across Europe. Eur J Clin Pharmacol 60(1):29–35, 2004 14747883

Bramness JG, Grøholt B, Engeland A, et al: The use of lithium, valproate or lamotrigine for psychiatric conditions in children and adolescents in Norway 2004–2007—a prescription database study. J Affect Disord 117(3):208–211, 2009 19189871

Brooks JO 3rd, Hoblyn JC, Kraemer HC, et al: Factors associated with psychiatric hospitalization of individuals diagnosed with dementia and comorbid bipolar disorder. J Geriatr Psychiatry Neurol 19(2):72–77, 2006 16690991

Brown SL: Variations in utilization and cost of inpatient psychiatric services among adults in Maryland. Psychiatr Serv 52(6):841–843, 2001 11376239

Cacilhas AA, Magalhães PV, Ceresér KM, et al: Bipolar disorder and age-related functional impairment. Rev Bras Psiquiatr 31(4):354–357, 2009 20098826

Cates M, Powers R: Concomitant rash and blood dyscrasias in geriatric psychiatry patients treated with carbamazepine. Ann Pharmacother 32(9):884–887, 1998 9762374

Centorrino F, Ventriglio A, Vincenti A, et al: Changes in medication practices for hospitalized psychiatric patients: 2009 versus 2004. Hum Psychopharmacol 25(2):179–186, 2010 20196186

Chacko RC, Marsh BJ, Marmion J, et al: Lithium side effects in elderly bipolar outpatients. Hillside J Clin Psychiatry 9(1):79–88, 1987 3653845

Chen ST, Altshuler LL, Melnyk KA, et al: Efficacy of lithium vs. valproate in the treatment of mania in the elderly: a retrospective study. J Clin Psychiatry 60(3):181–186, 1999 10192594

Ciechanowski P, Wagner E, Schmaling K, et al: Community-integrated home-based depression treatment in older adults: a randomized controlled trial. JAMA 291(13):1569–1577, 2004 15069044

Conney J, Kaston B: Pharmacoeconomic and health outcome comparison of lithium and divalproex in a VA geriatric nursing home population: influence of drug-related morbidity on total cost of treatment. Am J Manag Care 5(2):197–204, 1999 10346515

Corey-Bloom J: Treatment trials in aging and mild cognitive impairment. Curr Top Behav Neurosci 10:347–356, 2012 21786037

Correll CU, Frederickson AM, Kane JM, et al: Metabolic syndrome and the risk of coronary heart disease in 367 patients treated with second-generation antipsychotic drugs. J Clin Psychiatry 67(4):575–583, 2006 16669722

Crystal S, Olfson M, Huang C, et al: Broadened use of atypical antipsychotics: safety, effectiveness, and policy challenges. Health Aff (Millwood) 28(5):w770–w781, 2009 19622537

de Almeida KM, Moreira CL, Lafer B: Metabolic syndrome and bipolar disorder: what should psychiatrists know? CNS Neurosci Ther 18(2):160–166, 2012 22070636

Depp CA, Lindamer LA, Folsom DP, et al: Differences in clinical features and mental health service use in bipolar disorder across the lifespan. Am J Geriatr Psychiatry 13(4):290–298, 2005 15845754

Depp C, Ojeda VD, Mastin W, et al: Trends in use of antipsychotics and mood stabilizers among Medicaid beneficiaries with bipolar disorder, 2001–2004. Psychiatr Serv 59(10):1169–1174, 2008 18832503

Dhingra U, Rabins PV: Mania in the elderly: a 5–7 year follow-up. J Am Geriatr Soc 39(6):581–583, 1991 2037748

Dias VV, Balanzá-Martinez V, Soeiro-de-Souza MG, et al: Pharmacological approaches in bipolar disorders and the impact on cognition: a critical overview. Acta Psychiatr Scand 126(5):315–331, 2012 22881296

Dols A, Rhebergen D, Beekman A, et al: Psychiatric and medical comorbidities: results from a bipolar elderly cohort study. Am J Geriatr Psychiatry Jan 4, 2014 [Epub ahead of print] 24495405

Eastham JH, Jeste DV, Young RC: Assessment and treatment of bipolar disorder in the elderly. Drugs Aging 12(3):205–224, 1998 9534021

Elshahawi HH, Essawi H, Rabie MA, et al: Cognitive functions among euthymic bipolar I patients after a single manic episode versus recurrent episodes. J Affect Disord 130(1–2):180–191, 2011 21074274

Evans DL, Byerly MJ, Greer RA: Secondary mania: diagnosis and treatment. J Clin Psychiatry 56(Suppl 3):31–37, 1995 7883741

Folstein MF, Folstein SE, McHugh PR: "Mini-mental state": a practical method for grading the cognitive state of patients for the clinician. J Psychiatr Res 12(3):189–198, 1975 1202204

Frank C: Pharmacologic treatment of depression in the elderly. Can Fam Physician 60(2):121–126, 2014 24522673

Freeman TW, Clothier JL, Pazzaglia P, et al: A double-blind comparison of valproate and lithium in the treatment of acute mania. Am J Psychiatry 149(1):108–111, 1992 1728157

Frye MA, Altshuler LL, Bitran JA: Clozapine in rapid cycling bipolar disorder. J Clin Psychopharmacol 16(1):87–90, 1996 8834431

Ganguli M, Blacker D, Blazer DG, et al: Classification of neurocognitive disorders in DSM-5: a work in progress. Am J Geriatr Psychiatry 19(3):205–210, 2011 21425518

Gareri P, De Fazio P, De Fazio S, et al: Adverse effects of atypical antipsychotics in the elderly: a review. Drugs Aging 23(12):937–956, 2006 17154659

Geddes JR, Miklowitz DJ: Treatment of bipolar disorder. Lancet 381(9878):1672–1682, 2013 23663953

Geddes JR, Goodwin GM, Rendell J, et al; BALANCE investigators and collaborators: Lithium plus valproate combination therapy versus monotherapy for relapse prevention in bipolar I disorder (BALANCE): a randomised open-label trial. Lancet 375(9712):385–395, 2010 20092882

Gildengers AG, Butters MA, Seligman K, et al: Cognitive functioning in late-life bipolar disorder. Am J Psychiatry 161(4):736–738, 2004 15056521

Gildengers AG, Mulsant BH, Begley AE, et al: A pilot study of standardized treatment in geriatric bipolar disorder. Am J Geriatr Psychiatry 13(4):319–323, 2005 15845758

Gildengers AG, Whyte EM, Drayer RA, et al: Medical burden in late-life bipolar and major depressive disorders. Am J Geriatr Psychiatry 16(3):194–200, 2008 18310550

Gildengers AG, Mulsant BH, Al Jurdi RK, et al; GERI-BD Study Group: The relationship of bipolar disorder lifetime duration and vascular burden to cognition in older adults. Bipolar Disord 12(8):851–858, 2010 21176032

Gildengers AG, Chisholm D, Butters MA, et al: Two-year course of cognitive function and instrumental activities of daily living in older adults with bipolar disorder: evidence for neuroprogression? Psychol Med 43(4):801–811, 2013a 22846332

Gildengers A, Tatsuoka C, Bialko C, et al: Correlates of disability in depressed older adults with bipolar disorder. Cut Edge Psychiatry Pract 2013(1):332–338, 2013b

Goldberg JF, Sacks MH, Kocsis JH: Low-dose lithium augmentation of divalproex in geriatric mania. J Clin Psychiatry 61(4):304, 2000 10830157

Goldstein BI, Fagiolini A, Houck P, et al: Cardiovascular disease and hypertension among adults with bipolar I disorder in the United States. Bipolar Disord 11(6):657–662, 2009 19689508

Goodwin GM, Bowden CL, Calabrese JR, et al: A pooled analysis of 2 placebo-controlled 18-month trials of lamotrigine and lithium maintenance in bipolar I disorder. J Clin Psychiatry 65(3):432–441, 2004 15096085

Gould RL, Coulson MC, Howard RJ: Cognitive behavioral therapy for depression in older people: a meta-analysis and meta-regression of randomized controlled trials. J Am Geriatr Soc 60(10):1817–1830, 2012 23003115

Greil W, Häberle A, Hauels P, et al: Pharmacotherapeutic trends in 2231 psychiatric inpatients with bipolar depression from the International AMSP Project between 1994 and 2009. J Affect Disord 136(3):534–542, 2012 22134044

Gum AM, Areán PA, Hunkeler E, et al: Depression treatment preferences in older primary care patients. Gerontologist 46(1):14–22, 2006 16452280

Gyulai L: GERI-BD: first randomized, double blind controlled trial comparing lithium and valproate in late-life mania. Paper presented at the 10th International Conference on Bipolar Disorder, Miami Beach, FL, June 13–16, 2013

Hardy BG, Shulman KI, Mackenzie SE, et al: Pharmacokinetics of lithium in the elderly. J Clin Psychopharmacol 7(3):153–158, 1987 3110219

Hayes J, Prah P, Nazareth I, et al: Prescribing trends in bipolar disorder: cohort study in the United Kingdom THIN primary care database 1995–2009. PLoS ONE 6(12):e28725, 2011 22163329

Head L, Dening T: Lithium in the over-65s: who is taking it and who is monitoring it? A survey of older adults on lithium in the Cambridge Mental Health Services catchment area. Int J Geriatr Psychiatry 13(3):164–171, 1998 9565838

Hewick DS, Newbury P, Hopwood S, et al: Age as a factor affecting lithium therapy. Br J Clin Pharmacol 4(2):201–205, 1977 861133

Himmelhoch JM, Neil JF, May SJ, et al: Age, dementia, dyskinesias, and lithium response. Am J Psychiatry 137(8):941–945, 1980 7416295

Hirschfeld RM, Calabrese JR, Weissman MM, et al: Screening for bipolar disorder in the community. J Clin Psychiatry 64(1):53–59, 2003 12590624

Hoblyn J: Bipolar disorder in later life. Older adults presenting with new onset manic symptoms usually have underlying medical or neurologic disorder. Geriatrics 59(6):41–44, 2004 15224795

Hooshmand F, Miller S, Dore J, et al: Trends in pharmacotherapy in patients referred to a bipolar specialty clinic, 2000–2011. J Affect Disord 155:283–287, 2014 24314912

Jacoby R: Concomitant loop diuretics and ACE inhibitors increase risk of lithium toxicity in elderly people. Evid Based Ment Health 7(4):120, 2004 15504808

Jean L, Bergeron ME, Thivierge S, et al: Cognitive intervention programs for individuals with mild cognitive impairment: systematic review of the literature. Am J Geriatr Psychiatry 18(4):281–296, 2010 20220584

Juurlink DN, Mamdani MM, Kopp A, et al: Drug-induced lithium toxicity in the elderly: a population-based study. J Am Geriatr Soc 52(5):794–798, 2004 15086664

Kamat SM, Lefevre PJ, Grossberg GT: Electroconvulsive therapy in the elderly. Clin Geriatr Med 19(4):825–839, 2003 15024814

Kando JC, Tohen M, Castillo J, et al: The use of valproate in an elderly population with affective symptoms. J Clin Psychiatry 57(6):238–240, 1996 8666559

Keller MB, Lavori PW, Coryell W, et al: Differential outcome of pure manic, mixed/cycling, and pure depressive episodes in patients with bipolar illness. JAMA 255(22):3138–3142, 1986 3702024

Kessing LV: Diagnostic subtypes of bipolar disorder in older versus younger adults. Bipolar Disord 8(1):56–64, 2006 16411981

Kessing LV, Andersen PK: Does the risk of developing dementia increase with the number of episodes in patients with depressive disorder and in patients with bipolar disorder? J Neurol Neurosurg Psychiatry 75(12):1662–1666, 2004 15548477

Kessing LV, Nilsson FM: Increased risk of developing dementia in patients with major affective disorders compared to patients with other medical illnesses. J Affect Disord 73(3):261–269, 2003 12547295

Kessing LV, Olsen EW, Mortensen PB, et al: Dementia in affective disorder: a case-register study. Acta Psychiatr Scand 100(3):176–185, 1999 10493083

Kessing LV, Søndergård L, Forman JL, et al: Lithium treatment and risk of dementia. Arch Gen Psychiatry 65(11):1331–1335, 2008 18981345

Kessler RC, Berglund P, Demler O, et al: Lifetime prevalence and age-of-onset distributions of DSM-IV disorders in the National Comorbidity Survey Replication. Arch Gen Psychiatry 62(6):593–602, 2005 15939837

Ketter TA, Post RM, Worthington K: Principles of clinically important drug interactions with carbamazepine. Part I. J Clin Psychopharmacol 11(3):198–203, 1991a 2066459

Ketter TA, Post RM, Worthington K: Principles of clinically important drug interactions with carbamazepine. Part II. J Clin Psychopharmacol 11(5):306–313, 1991b 1765573

Kok RM, Heeren TJ, Nolen WA: Continuing treatment of depression in the elderly: a systematic review and meta-analysis of double-blinded randomized controlled trials with antidepressants. Am J Geriatr Psychiatry 19(3):249–255, 2011 21425505

Kok RM, Nolen WA, Heeren TJ: Efficacy of treatment in older depressed patients: a systematic review and meta-analysis of double-blind randomized controlled trials with antidepressants. J Affect Disord 141(2–3):103–115, 2012 22480823

Korte J, Bohlmeijer ET, Cappeliez P, et al: Life review therapy for older adults with moderate depressive symptomatology: a pragmatic randomized controlled trial. Psychol Med 42(6):1163–1173, 2012 21995889

Krauthammer C, Klerman GL: Secondary mania: manic syndromes associated with antecedent physical illness or drugs. Arch Gen Psychiatry 35(11):1333–1339, 1978 757997

Krishna M, Honagodu A, Rajendra R, et al: A systematic review and meta-analysis of group psychotherapy for sub-clinical depression in older adults. Int J Geriatr Psychiatry 28(9):881–888, 2013 23147496

Kukopulos A, Reginaldi D, Laddomada P, et al: Course of the manic-depressive cycle and changes caused by treatment. Pharmakopsychiatr Neuropsychopharmakol 13(4):156–167, 1980 6108577

Lala SV, Sajatovic M: Medical and psychiatric comorbidities among elderly individuals with bipolar disorder: a literature review. J Geriatr Psychiatry Neurol 25(1):20–25, 2012 22467842

Lechin F, van der Dijs B, Benaim M: Benzodiazepines: tolerability in elderly patients. Psychother Psychosom 65(4):171–182, 1996 8843497

Lee SY, Franchetti MK, Imanbayev A, et al: Non-pharmacological prevention of major depression among community-dwelling older adults: a systematic review of the efficacy of psychotherapy interventions. Arch Gerontol Geriatr 55(3):522–529, 2012 22483200

Lepkifker E, Iancu I, Horesh N, et al: Lithium therapy for unipolar and bipolar depression among the middle-aged and older adult patient subpopulation. Depress Anxiety 24(8):571–576, 2007 17133442

Lewandowski KE, Sperry SH, Malloy MC, et al: Age as a predictor of cognitive decline in bipolar disorder. Am J Geriatr Psychiatry Oct 6, 2013 [Epub ahead of print] 24262287

Lonergan E, Luxenberg J: Valproate preparations for agitation in dementia. Cochrane Database Syst Rev (3):CD003945, 2009 19588348

Madhusoodanan S, Brenner R, Araujo L, et al: Efficacy of risperidone treatment for psychoses associated with schizophrenia, schizoaffective disorder, bipolar disorder, or senile dementia in 11 geriatric patients: a case series. J Clin Psychiatry 56(11):514–518, 1995 7592504

Madhusoodanan S, Suresh P, Brenner R, et al: Experience with the atypical antipsychotics—risperidone and olanzapine in the elderly. Ann Clin Psychiatry 11(3):113–118, 1999 10482120

Madhusoodanan S, Brenner R, Alcantra A: Clinical experience with quetiapine in elderly patients with psychotic disorders. J Geriatr Psychiatry Neurol 13(1):28–32, 2000 10753004

McFarland BH, Miller MR, Straumfjord AA: Valproate use in the older manic patient. J Clin Psychiatry 51(11):479–481, 1990 1977740

McKnight RF, Adida M, Budge K, et al: Lithium toxicity profile: a systematic review and meta-analysis. Lancet 379(9817):721–728, 2012 22265699

Mezuk B, Morden NE, Ganoczy D, et al: Anticonvulsant use, bipolar disorder, and risk of fracture among older adults in the Veterans Health Administration. Am J Geriatr Psychiatry 18(3):245–255, 2010 20224520

Montgomery SA, Altamura AC, Katila H, et al: Efficacy of extended release quetiapine fumarate monotherapy in elderly patients with major depressive disorder: secondary analyses in subgroups of patients according to baseline anxiety, sleep disturbance, and pain levels. Int Clin Psychopharmacol 29(2):93–105, 2014 24162081

Morris JC: Revised criteria for mild cognitive impairment may compromise the diagnosis of Alzheimer disease dementia. Arch Neurol 69(6):700–708, 2012 22312163

Mossey, JM, Knott KA, Higgins M, et al: Effectiveness of a psychosocial intervention, interpersonal counseling, for subdysthymic depression in medically ill elderly. J Gerontol A Biol Sci Med Sci 51(4):M172–M178, 1996 8681000

Mukherjee S, Sackeim HA, Schnur DB: Electroconvulsive therapy of acute manic episodes: a review of 50 years' experience. Am J Psychiatry 151(2):169–176, 1994 8296883

Murray N, Hopwood S, Balfour DJ, et al: The influence of age on lithium efficacy and side-effects in out-patients. Psychol Med 13(1):53–60, 1983 6405416

Nasreddine ZS, Phillips NA, Bédirian V, et al: The Montreal Cognitive Assessment, MoCA: a brief screening tool for mild cognitive impairment. J Am Geriatr Soc 53(4):695–699, 2005 15817019

Nelson JC, Delucchi K, Schneider LS: Efficacy of second generation antidepressants in late-life depression: a meta-analysis of the evidence. Am J Geriatr Psychiatry 16(7):558–567, 2008 18591576

Nicolato R, Romano-Silva MA, Correa H, et al: Stuporous catatonia in an elderly bipolar patient: response to olanzapine. Aust NZ J Psychiatry 40(5):498, 2006 16683979

Niedermier JA, Nasrallah HA: Clinical correlates of response to valproate in geriatric inpatients. Ann Clin Psychiatry 10(4):165–168, 1998 9988057

Nierenberg AA, Friedman ES, Bowden CL, et al: Lithium treatment moderate-dose use study (LiTMUS) for bipolar disorder: a randomized comparative effectiveness trial of optimized personalized treatment with and without lithium. Am J Psychiatry 170(1):102–110, 2013 23288387

Nierenberg AA, Sylvia LG, Leon AC, et al; Bipolar CHOICE Study Group: Clinical and Health Outcomes Initiative in Comparative Effectiveness for Bipolar Disorder (Bipolar CHOICE): a pragmatic trial of complex treatment for a complex disorder. Clin Trials 11(1):114–127, 2014 24346608

Noaghiul S, Narayan M, Nelson JC: Divalproex treatment of mania in elderly patients. Am J Geriatr Psychiatry 6(3):257–262, 1998 9659958

Nunes PV, Forlenza OV, Gattaz WF: Lithium and risk for Alzheimer's disease in elderly patients with bipolar disorder. Br J Psychiatry 190:359–360, 2007 17401045

Nyer M, Doorley J, Durham K, et al: What is the role of alternative treatments in late-life depression? Psychiatr Clin North Am 36(4):577–596, 2013 24229658

Oostervink F, Boomsma MM, Nolen WA, et al; EMBLEM Advisory Board: Bipolar disorder in the elderly; different effects of age and of age of onset. J Affect Disord 116(3):176–183, 2009 19087895

Pacchiarotti I, Bond DJ, Baldessarini RJ, et al: The International Society for Bipolar Disorders (ISBD) task force report on antidepressant use in bipolar disorders. Am J Psychiatry 170(11):1249–1262, 2013 24030475

Petersen RC: Clinical practice. Mild cognitive impairment. N Engl J Med 364(23):2227–2234, 2011 21651394

Pillarella J, Higashi A, Alexander GC, et al: Trends in use of second-generation antipsychotics for treatment of bipolar disorder in the United States, 1998–2009. Psychiatr Serv 63(1):83–86, 2012 22227765

Post RM: Transduction of psychosocial stress into the neurobiology of recurrent affective disorder. Am J Psychiatry 149(8):999–1010, 1992 1353322

Pot AM, Bohlmeijer ET, Onrust S, et al: The impact of life review on depression in older adults: a randomized controlled trial. Int Psychogeriatr 22(4):572–581, 2010 20128949

Puryear LJ, Kunik ME, Workman R Jr: Tolerability of divalproex sodium in elderly psychiatric patients with mixed diagnoses. J Geriatr Psychiatry Neurol 8(4):234–237, 1995 8561838

Rabins PV, Lyketsos CG: A commentary on the proposed DSM revision regarding the classification of cognitive disorders. Am J Geriatr Psychiatry 19(3):201–204, 2011 21425503

Reimers A: Trends and changes in the clinical use of lamotrigine. Pharmaco-epidemiol Drug Saf 18(2):132–139, 2009 19089845

Rej S, Herrmann N, Shulman K: The effects of lithium on renal function in older adults—a systematic review. J Geriatr Psychiatry Neurol 25(1):51–61, 2012 22467847

Riva-Posse P, Hermida AP, McDonald WM: The role of electroconvulsive and neuromodulation therapies in the treatment of geriatric depression. Psychiatr Clin North Am 36(4):607–630, 2013 24229660

Roose SP, Bone S, Haidorfer C, et al: Lithium treatment in older patients. Am J Psychiatry 136(6):843–844, 1979 443475

Saetre E, Perucca E, Isojärvi J, Gjerstad L; LAM 40089 Study Group: An international multicenter randomized double-blind controlled trial of lamotrigine and sustained-release carbamazepine in the treatment of newly diagnosed epilepsy in the elderly. Epilepsia 48(7):1292–1302, 2007 17561956

Sajatovic M: Treatment of bipolar disorder in older adults. Int J Geriatr Psychiatry 17(9):865–873, 2002 12221662

Sajatovic M: Quetiapine for the treatment of depressive episodes in adults aged 55 to 65 years with bipolar disorder. Paper presented at the 44th Annual Meeting of the American Association of Geriatric Psychiatry, New Orleans, LA, March 2007

Sajatovic M, Kales HC: Diagnosis and management of bipolar disorder with comorbid anxiety in the elderly. J Clin Psychiatry 67(Suppl 1):21–27, 2006 16426113

Sajatovic M, Popli A, Semple W: Health resource utilization over a ten-year period by geriatric veterans with schizophrenia and bipolar disorder. J Geriatr Psychiatry Neurol 15:128–133, 1996 12230082

Sajatovic M, Blow FC, Ignacio RV, et al: New-onset bipolar disorder in later life. Am J Geriatr Psychiatry 13(4):282–289, 2005a 15845753

Sajatovic M, Gyulai L, Calabrese JR, et al: Maintenance treatment outcomes in older patients with bipolar I disorder. Am J Geriatr Psychiatry 13(4):305–311, 2005b 15845756

Sajatovic M, Calabrese JR, Mullen J: Quetiapine for the treatment of bipolar mania in older adults. Bipolar Disord 10(6):662–671, 2008a 18837860

Sajatovic M, Coconcea N, Ignacio RV, et al: Aripiprazole therapy in 20 older adults with bipolar disorder: a 12-week, open-label trial. J Clin Psychiatry 69(1):41–46, 2008b 18312036

Sajatovic M, Gildengers A, Al Jurdi RK, et al: Multisite, open-label, prospective trial of lamotrigine for geriatric bipolar depression: a preliminary report. Bipolar Disord 13(3):294–302, 2011 21676132

Samuels S, Fang M: Olanzapine may cause delirium in geriatric patients. J Clin Psychiatry 65(4):582–583, 2004 15119927

Schaffer A, Mamdani M, Levitt A, et al: Effect of antidepressant use on admissions to hospital among elderly bipolar patients. Int J Geriatr Psychiatry 21(3):275–280, 2006 16477586

Schaffer CB, Garvey MJ: Use of lithium in acutely manic elderly patients. Clin Gerontol 3:58–60, 1984

Schneider AL, Wilcox CS: Divalproate augmentation in lithium-resistant rapid cycling mania in four geriatric patients. J Affect Disord 47(1–3):201–205, 1998 9476762

Schouws SN, Comijs HC, Stek ML, et al: Cognitive impairment in early and late bipolar disorder. Am J Geriatr Psychiatry 17(6):508–515, 2009 19461259

Schouws SN, Stek ML, Comijs HC, et al: Risk factors for cognitive impairment in elderly bipolar patients. J Affect Disord 125(1–3):330–335, 2010 20079932

Secunda SK, Katz MM, Swann A, et al: Mania. Diagnosis, state measurement and prediction of treatment response. J Affect Disord 8(2):113–121, 1985 3157719

Serrano JP, Latorre JM, Gatz M, Montanes J: Life review therapy using autobiographical retrieval practice for older adults with depressive symptomatology. Psychol Aging 19(2):270–277, 2004 15222820

Sharma V, Persad E, Mazmanian D, et al: Treatment of rapid cycling bipolar disorder with combination therapy of valproate and lithium. Can J Psychiatry 38(2):137–139, 1993 8467440

Shulman KI: Lithium for older adults with bipolar disorder: Should it still be considered a first-line agent? Drugs Aging 27(8):607–615, 2010 20658789

Shulman KI, Tohen M, Satlin A, et al: Mania compared with unipolar depression in old age. Am J Psychiatry 149(3):341–345, 1992 1536272

Shulman KI, Rochon P, Sykora K, et al: Changing prescription patterns for lithium and valproic acid in old age: shifting practice without evidence. BMJ 326(7396):960–961, 2003 12727769

Shulman KI, Sykora K, Gill S, et al: Incidence of delirium in older adults newly prescribed lithium or valproate: a population-based cohort study. J Clin Psychiatry 66(4):424–427, 2005 15816783

Shulman RW, Singh A, Shulman KI: Treatment of elderly institutionalized bipolar patients with clozapine. Psychopharmacol Bull 33(1):113–118, 1997 9133761

Simon GE, Ludman EJ, Bauer MS, et al: Long-term effectiveness and cost of a systematic care program for bipolar disorder. Arch Gen Psychiatry 63(5):500–508, 2006 16651507

Smith RE, Helms PM: Adverse effects of lithium therapy in the acutely ill elderly patient. J Clin Psychiatry 43(3):94–99, 1982 7061409

Snowdon J: A retrospective case-note study of bipolar disorder in old age. Br J Psychiatry 158:485–490, 1991 2054563

Softic A, Beganlic A, Pranjic N, et al: The influence of the use of benzodiazepines in the frequency falls in the elderly. Med Arh 67(4):256–259, 2013 24520747

Spek V, Cuijpers P, Nyklícek I, et al: One-year follow-up results of a randomized controlled clinical trial on Internet-based cognitive behavioural therapy for subthreshold depression in people over 50 years. Psychol Med 38(5):635–639, 2008 18205965

Sproule BA, Hardy BG, Shulman KI: Differential pharmacokinetics of lithium in elderly patients. Drugs Aging 16(3):165–177, 2000 10803857

Stone K: Mania in the elderly. Br J Psychiatry 155:220–224, 1989 2597918

Swann AC, Bowden CL, Calabrese JR, et al: Pattern of response to divalproex, lithium, or placebo in four naturalistic subtypes of mania. Neuropsychopharmacology 26(4):530–536, 2002 11927177

Tang-Wai DF, Knopman DS, Geda YE, et al: Comparison of the Short Test of Mental Status and the Mini-Mental State Examination in mild cognitive impairment. Arch Neurol 60(12):1777–1781, 2003 14676056

Tariot PN, Salzman C, Yeung PP, et al: Long-term use of quetiapine in elderly patients with psychotic disorders. Clin Ther 22(9):1068–1084, 2000 11048905

Tariot PN, Schneider LS, Mintzer JE, et al: Depakote Elderly Mania Study Group. Safety and tolerability of divalproex sodium in the treatment of signs and symptoms of mania in elderly patients with dementia: results of a double-blind, placebo-controlled trial. Curr Ther Res Clin Exp 62(1):51–67, 2001

Tariot PN, Profenno LA, Ismail MS: Efficacy of atypical antipsychotics in elderly patients with dementia. J Clin Psychiatry 65 (suppl 11):11–15, 2004 15264966

Tohen M, Shulman KI, Satlin A: First-episode mania in late life. Am J Psychiatry 151(1):130–132, 1994 8267112

Van der Velde CD: Effectiveness of lithium carbonate in the treatment of manic-depressive illness. Am J Psychiatry 127(3):345–351, 1970 5458599

van der Wurff FB, Stek ML, Hoogendijk WJ, et al: The efficacy and safety of ECT in depressed older adults: a literature review. Int J Geriatr Psychiatry 18(10):894–904, 2003 14533122

van Melick EJ, Wilting I, Meinders AE, et al: Prevalence and determinants of thyroid disorders in elderly patients with affective disorders: lithium and nonlithium patients. Am J Geriatr Psychiatry 18(5):395–403, 2010 20429083

van Schaik A, van Marwijk H, Adèr H, et al: Interpersonal psychotherapy for elderly patients in primary care. Am J Geriatr Psychiatry 14(9):777–786, 2006 16943174

van't Veer-Tazelaar PJ, van Marwijk HW, van Oppen P, et al: Stepped-care prevention of anxiety and depression in late life: a randomized controlled trial. Arch Gen Psychiatry 66(3):297–304, 2009 19255379

Walpoth-Niederwanger M, Kemmler G, Grunze H, et al: Treatment patterns in inpatients with bipolar disorder at a psychiatric university hospital over a 9-year period: focus on mood stabilizers. Int Clin Psychopharmacol 27(5):256–266, 2012 22842799

Williams JW Jr, Barrett J, Oxman T, et al: Treatment of dysthymia and minor depression in primary care: A randomized controlled trial in older adults. JAMA 284(12):1519–1526, 2000 11000645

Wilson K, Mottram P: A comparison of side effects of selective serotonin reuptake inhibitors and tricyclic antidepressants in older depressed patients: a meta-analysis. Int J Geriatr Psychiatry 19(8):754–762, 2004 15290699

Wilson KC, Mottram PG, Vassilas CA: Psychotherapeutic treatments for older depressed people. Cochrane Database Syst Rev (1):CD004853, 2008 18254062

Wilting I, Souverein PC, Nolen WA, et al: Changes in outpatient lithium treatment in the Netherlands during 1996–2005. J Affect Disord 111(1):94–99, 2008 18342951

Wolfsperger M, Greil W, Rössler W, Grohmann R: Pharmacological treatment of acute mania in psychiatric in-patients between 1994 and 2004. J Affect Disord 99(1–3):9–17, 2007 16989907

Yang M, Barner JC, Lawson KA, et al: Antipsychotic medication utilization trends among Texas veterans: 1997–2002. Ann Pharmacother 42(9):1229–1238, 2008 18682544

Yassa R, Nair V, Nastase C, et al: Prevalence of bipolar disorder in a psychogeriatric population. J Affect Disord 14(3):197–201, 1988 2968383

Young RC, Gyulai L, Mulsant BH, et al: Pharmacotherapy of bipolar disorder in old age: review and recommendations. Am J Geriatr Psychiatry 12(4):342–357, 2004 15249272

8

Mood Stabilizers and Second-Generation Antipsychotics

Pharmacology, Drug Interactions, Adverse Effects, and Dosing

Terence A. Ketter, M.D.

Although the mood stabilizers lithium, carbamazepine, valproate, and lamotrigine may be argued to be the foundational pharmacotherapies for bipolar disorder, the second-generation antipsychotics (SGAs) olanzapine, risperidone, quetiapine, ziprasidone, aripiprazole, asenapine, and lurasidone have been increasingly used, so that some in the field opine that mood stabilizers and SGAs are the two most crucial medication classes in the management of bipolar disorder. In addition, antidepressants, anxiolytics/hypnotics, other anticonvulsants, and other medications are very commonly combined with mood stabilizers and SGAs in clinical settings, highlighting the importance of avoiding and managing side effects and drug interactions.

Mood stabilizers and SGAs have varying pharmacodynamics, pharmacokinetics, drug-drug interactions, and adverse effects. Thus, clinicians are challenged with integrating the complex data regarding efficacy spectra with the pharmacological properties described for mood stabilizers and SGAs in this chapter, in efforts to provide safe, effective, state-of-the-art pharmacotherapy. Readers interested in similar information organized by drug classes for antidepressants, anxiolytics, other anticonvulsants, and other medications used in the treatment of bipolar disorder are referred to the chapter "Antidepressants, Anxiolytics/Hypnotics, and Other Medication: Pharmacokinetics, Drug Interactions, Adverse Effects, and Administration" (Ketter and Wang 2010) in *Handbook of Diagnosis and Treatment of Bipolar Disorders* (Ketter 2010). To enhance brevity and readability in the current chapter, I have noted in this chapter only clinically significant drug interactions and adverse effects, and have limited literature citations. Readers interested in a more detailed (albeit older) review of the material in this chapter are referred to the chapter "Mood Stabilizers and Antipsychotics: Pharmacokinetics, Drug Interactions, Adverse Effects, and Administration" (Ketter and Wang 2010) in the aforementioned *Handbook of Diagnosis and Treatment of Bipolar Disorders.*

■ Mood Stabilizers

The term *mood stabilizer* is commonly used to refer to medications that are approved for the treatment of bipolar disorder that are not dopamine receptor antagonists or partial agonists. The mood stabilizers include lithium and the anticonvulsants valproate, carbamazepine, and lamotrigine. Unfortunately, as of early 2015, there was no consensus definition of the term *mood stabilizer,* leading the U.S. Food and Drug Administration (FDA) to avoid using the term and some experts to even suggest abandoning it. In this chapter, *mood stabilizer* is used as defined above, reflecting the common clinical usage of the term.

All four mood stabilizers are available in immediate-release and extended-release oral formulations. In addition, lithium, valproate, and carbamazepine are available in suspension formulations; valproate is available in an intravenous formulation; and lamotrigine is available in chewable dispersible tablet and orally disintegrating tablet formulations. Unfortunately, mood stabilizer rapid-acting injectable intramuscular and long-acting injectable formulations are not available.

Adverse effects with mood stabilizers are generally somewhat more frequent and more severe than with antidepressants but are somewhat less frequent and less severe than with antipsychotics, as depicted in Figure 2–1 in Chapter 2, "Treatment of Acute Bipolar Depression." However, the newer mood stabilizer lamotrigine has tolerability superior to that of the older mood stabilizers (lithium, valproate, and carbamazepine) and comparable to that of antidepressants. Administering mood stabilizers (e.g., due to differential efficacy spectra across illness phases and to differential side effects and drug interactions) is arguably as complex and challenging as administering antipsychotics.

In view of the relative complexity of mood stabilizer therapy, patient education regarding common and serious adverse events is crucial. Information sheets or booklets describing clinical monitoring for problems, such as neurotoxicity with lithium, hepatic and pancreatic reactions and teratogenicity with valproate, hematological reactions and drug interactions with carbamazepine, and dermatological reactions with lamotrigine, can aid in prevention and early detection of adverse events to enhance tolerability and safety.

Lithium

Lithium is a cation with multiple biochemical effects. Although intracellular signaling (Quiroz et al. 2004) is a crucial area of exploration of lithium mechanisms, this ion also has effects on γ-aminobutyric acid (GABA), glutamate, calcium, and monoamines. Lithium received FDA approval for acute mania monotherapy in 1970 and as a bipolar preventive treatment in 1974.

Lithium is well absorbed, with a bioavailability close to 100%; is not bound to plasma proteins; and has a half-life of approximately 24 hours (Marcus 1994). Sustained-release formulations can decrease peak serum concentrations and hence adverse effects related to peak concentrations (Castrogiovanni 2002). Lithium is almost exclusively (>95%) renally excreted unchanged, with a clearance about one-fourth that of creatinine (generally ranging from 10 to 40 mL/min), so that the dosage may need to be decreased in patients with decreased renal function. This, considered with evidence suggesting adverse renal effects of lithium, suggests that patients with decreased renal function may not be good candidates for lithium therapy. Lower lithium doses may be necessary in older adults, due to decreased clearance and/or increased sensitivity to side effects (Physicians' Desk Reference 2014).

Because of its near-exclusive renal excretion unchanged, lithium has renally mediated rather than hepatically mediated pharmacokinetic drug-drug interactions (Finley et al. 1995). Therefore, lithium does not usually have clinically significant pharmacokinetic interactions with most psychotropic medications (which most often have hepatic metabolism), including other mood stabilizers and SGAs (Table 8–1), or with most anticonvulsants, although a single-case report suggests that topiramate could occasionally yield clinically significant increases in serum lithium concentrations in some individuals (Abraham and Owen 2004).

However, other case reports suggest that occasional individuals may experience pharmacodynamic drug interactions when combining lithium with carbamazepine (neurotoxicity) (Shukla et al. 1984), SGAs (neuroleptic malignant syndrome [NMS]) (Ali et al. 2006), first-generation antipsychotics (encephalopathic syndrome with weakness, lethargy, fever, tremulousness, confusion, extrapyramidal symptoms [EPS], leukocytosis, elevated serum enzymes, blood urea nitrogen, and fasting blood sugar that may overlap NMS) (Murphy et al. 1989), antidepressants (serotonin syndrome) (Adan-Manes et al. 2006), and benzodiaze-

TABLE 8–1. Clinically significant pharmacokinetic interactions of mood stabilizers with one another and with second-generation antipsychotics

Class/Medication	Lithium	Valproate	Carbamazepine	Lamotrigine
Mood stabilizers				
Lithium	—			
Valproate	—	—		
Carbamazepine	—	↑Carbamazepine-E ↓Valproate	↓Carbamazepine	
Lamotrigine	—	↑Lamotrigine	↓Lamotrigine	—
Second-generation antipsychotics				
Clozapine	—	—	↓Clozapine	—
Olanzapine	—	↓(?) Olanzapine	↓Olanzapine	—
Risperidone	—	—	↓Risperidone	—
Quetiapine	—	↑(?) Quetiapine	↓Quetiapine ↑(?) Carbamazepine-E	↓(?) Quetiapine
Ziprasidone	—	—	↓(?) Ziprasidone	—(?)
Aripiprazole	—	—	↓Aripiprazole	—
Asenapine	—	—	—	—(?)
Lurasidone	—	—	↓(?) Lurasidone	—(?)

Note. Carbamazepine-E=carbamazepine-10,11-epoxide; ↑=increased; ↓=decreased; (?)=limited data; —=no reported pharmacokinetic interaction.

pines (neurotoxicity) (Koczerginski et al. 1989). Nevertheless, for most patients, lithium lacks clinically significant drug interactions with most psychotropic and anticonvulsant medications encountered in the management of patients with bipolar disorder.

In contrast, several agents with prominent renal effects that are commonly used in general medical practice have been clearly implicated in routinely altering lithium pharmacokinetics (Finley et al. 1995) (Table 8–2). For example, thiazide diuretics, certain nonsteroidal anti-inflammatory drugs (NSAIDs), angiotensin I converting enzyme inhibitors (ACEIs), and angiotensin II receptor type 1 (AT_1) antagonists can increase lithium reabsorption in the proximal tubule, yielding increased serum lithium concentrations and lithium toxicity. In contrast, methylxanthines such as aminophylline, theophylline, and possibly caffeine can increase lithium clearance, potentially yielding inefficacy.

Physiological and disease states can have varying effects on lithium clearance. Increasing age is associated with decreased renal clearance and increased sensitivity to adverse effects, yielding the need for lower (on average approximately 40%–50% lower) lithium doses and serum concentrations in older adults (Shulman et al. 1987). Dehydration, renal disease, and sodium depletion also decrease renal lithium clearance, increasing the risk of toxicity (Atherton et al. 1987). In contrast, lithium clearance increases during pregnancy (Schou and Weinstein 1980) and may also increase during strenuous exercise (Jefferson et al. 1982). Patients who become manic or hypomanic often have dramatic increases in physical activity, which in some individuals may yield increased cardiac output and increased renal lithium filtration and excretion, as well as decreased serum lithium concentrations at the very time when this medication is needed most (Kukopoulos et al. 1985). However, there do not appear to be statistically significant changes in mean lithium clearance in groups of patients with mania (Swann et al. 1990).

Common, dose-related adverse effects with lithium include central nervous system (CNS) (sedation, tremor, ataxia, lethargy, decreased coordination, and cognitive problems), gastrointestinal (nausea, vomiting, diarrhea), renal (polyuria, polydipsia), endocrine/metabolic (hypothyroidism, weight gain), and dermatological (hair loss, acne) problems, as well as edema (Gelenberg 1988) (Table 8–3).

The U.S. prescribing information (USPI) for lithium includes a boxed warning regarding the risk of lithium toxicity that can occur at doses close to therapeutic levels (Physicians' Desk Reference 2014). Lithium intoxication can present with CNS, gastrointestinal, cardiovascular, and renal symptoms (Livingstone and Rampes 2006). In severe cases, lithium intoxication can yield irreversible CNS (Verdoux and Bourgeois

TABLE 8–2. Factors affecting lithium clearance

Decreased by:	Not changed by:	Increased by:
Diuretics	**Diuretics**	**Diuretics**
Thiazides	Amiloride	Acetazolamide
Older NSAIDs	Furosemide	Mannitol
Diclofenac	**Analgesics**	**Methylxanthines**
±Ibuprofen	±ASA	Aminophylline
Indomethacin	Acetaminophen	±Caffeine
Ketoprofen		Theophylline
Mefenamic acid		
Meloxicam		
Naproxen (smaller effect with OTC dose)		
Piroxicam		
±Sulindac		
COX-2 inhibitors		
Celecoxib		
Rofecoxib		
ACEIs		
Captopril		
Enalapril		
Fosinopril		
Lisinopril		
Perindopril		
AT$_1$ antagonists		
Candesartan		
Losartan		
Valsartan		
Physiological/disease states		
Advanced age	Pregnancy	
Dehydration	±Mania	
Renal disease		
Sodium depletion		

Note. ±=conflicting data; ACEI=angiotensin I converting enzyme inhibitor; ASA = acetylsalicylic acid; AT$_1$=angiotensin II receptor type 1; COX-2 = cyclooxygenase-2; NSAID=nonsteroidal anti-inflammatory drug; OTC=over-the-counter.

TABLE 8–3.   Treatment of mood stabilizer adverse effects

Adverse effect	Management options
General	Decrease/divide dose. Change mood stabilizer.
Gastrointestinal upset	Give with food or in divided doses. Change to extended release if nausea or vomiting. Change to suspension or immediate release if diarrhea. Provide symptomatic relief with gastrointestinal agents.
Weight gain	Give prior warning. Recommend diet and exercise. Aggressively treat hyperphagic, anergic depression (e.g., add bupropion, thyroid medication). Add topiramate, zonisamide, atomoxetine, or metformin. Caution with prescription weight-loss agents and stimulants.
Neurotoxicity	Dose at bedtime. Initiate gradually to improve tolerability (especially with lithium and carbamazepine).
Tremor	Add propranolol, atenolol, or pindolol.
Hair loss	Add selenium 25–100 µg/day or zinc 10–50 mg/day.
Polyuria	Prescribe single daily dose. Add amiloride, thiazide, or indomethacin.
Hypothyroidism	Prescribe thyroid hormone replacement.
Hepatotoxicity	Discontinue carbamazepine or valproate if hepatic indices are >3×upper limit of normal.
Rash	Initiate gradually. Limit other new antigens during initiation (?). Refer for dermatology consultation regarding desensitization. Discontinue carbamazepine or lamotrigine if rash is not clearly unrelated to drug.
Leukopenia	Add lithium. Discontinue carbamazepine if white blood cell count is <3,000 or neutrophils are <1,000.
Hyponatremia	Add lithium, demeclocycline, or doxycycline (?).

Note.   (?)=limited data.

1990), cardiac (Terao et al. 1996), or renal problems (Hetmar 1988), and even death (Amdisen et al. 1974). The risk of lithium toxicity is high in patients with significant renal or cardiovascular disease, severe debilitation, dehydration, or sodium depletion, or in those patients taking diuretics or ACEIs. However, in medically healthy individuals, at dosages of 900 mg/day or less, lithium is commonly adequately tolerated, and even with low serum levels may yield benefit in milder forms of bipolar disorders or when used as an adjunct to other mood stabilizers or anti-depressants.

Other lithium USPI warnings include risks of renal problems (e.g., nephrogenic diabetes insipidus, and morphological changes with glo-merular and interstitial fibrosis and nephron atrophy with chronic ther-apy, as described later in this section), as well as drug interactions (as described later in this section), such as encephalopathic syndrome when taken with neuroleptics. Patients need to maintain adequate fluid and so-dium intake, and caution is indicated in the setting of protracted sweating, diarrhea, infection, and fever. Lithium can also yield thyroid problems, as described later in this section.

Lithium can cause digestive tract disturbances. The lithium citrate so-lution has more proximal absorption and thus exacerbates upper (nausea and vomiting) or attenuates lower (diarrhea) gastrointestinal adverse effects; the reverse holds for sustained-release preparations. Administra-tion of divided doses and with food can help attenuate gastrointesti-nal adverse effects.

Although lithium is commonly given in divided doses to decrease peak serum levels and thus minimize adverse effects, doses can also be weighted toward bedtime, and patients receiving low to moderate doses may tolerate a single daily dose at bedtime. The latter regimen may aid sleep, attenuate daytime neurotoxicity, and possibly even decrease poly-uria. β-Blocking agents can attenuate lithium-induced tremor.

Lithium has endocrine adverse effects and can yield hypothyroidism in up to one-third of patients, with women and patients with rapid cy-cling possibly being at particular risk (Livingstone and Rampes 2006). Moreover, lower serum levothyroxine concentrations appear to be asso-ciated with more frequent affective episodes and more depression in pa-tients with mood disorders (Frye et al. 1999). Patients with hypothyroid-ism (increased thyroid-stimulating hormone [TSH] and decreased free thyroxine) need levothyroxine replacement therapy. However, there is controversy regarding the management of subclinical hypothyroidism (increased TSH and normal free thyroxine). One proposed approach en-tails 1) administering levothyroxine if TSH exceeds 10 mU/L, even in the absence of clinical symptoms, in view of the risk of progression of thyroid disease, and 2) increasing laboratory monitoring and considering levo-thyroxine if TSH is between 5 and 10 mU/L (Kleiner et al. 1999). Hyperthy-roidism, although far less common, can also occur with lithium therapy (Barclay et al. 1994). Hypercalcemia and hyperparathyroidism can also be seen with lithium (Livingstone and Rampes 2006); if hypercalcemia is detected on electrolyte screening, serum parathyroid hormone needs to be assessed.

As noted earlier in this section, lithium has significant interactions with renal function. Lithium can cause common benign as well as rare serious renal adverse effects (Livingstone and Rampes 2006). Nephrogenic diabetes insipidus may occur in up to 10% of patients with chronic lithium therapy (Bendz and Aurell 1999). Polyuria and polydipsia can be attenuated by lithium dose reduction or single daily dose, and by administration of diuretics, although care must be taken because such agents can influence lithium clearance. For example, hydrochlorothiazide 50 mg/day may attenuate polyuria, but using this agent requires decreasing lithium dose and replacing potassium. Indomethacin has also been considered, but this agent also decreases lithium clearance and could yield renal problems. Amiloride 5–10 mg twice a day has been suggested to be a preferable option for lithium-induced nephrogenic diabetes insipidus. Chronic lithium less commonly yields more long-standing and serious renal complications that are apparently more prevalent in cases with repeated lithium toxicity, advanced age, and concurrent NSAID therapy or chronic medical illness (Timmer and Sands 1999). Clinical and laboratory monitoring may help detect problems early, thus allowing interventions to attenuate adverse effects.

Many of the agents used in treating patients with bipolar disorder can yield weight gain. Weight gain can occur with lithium therapy (Bowden et al. 2000, 2006a) and can be a significant contributor to adherence problems. Weight gain appears to be more of a challenge with lithium than with lamotrigine (Sachs et al. 2006a), particularly in patients who are already obese (Bowden et al. 2006a), but less of a problem than with valproate (Bowden et al. 2000) or olanzapine (Tohen et al. 2005).

Counseling regarding weight gain early in the preventive phase of treatment may allow early attention to diet and exercise to attenuate this effect. In some cases, early detection of a rising high-normal or modestly elevated TSH can allow crossing over to another mood stabilizer, thus avoiding the need for chronic thyroid hormone replacement, which can be necessary in more advanced cases of lithium-induced hypothyroidism. Even in some euthyroid patients, addition of thyroid hormones may offer adjunctive antidepressant effects, increasing energy and activity, and thus attenuating weight gain. Another important approach is to minimize the number of concurrent medications that also yield weight gain, thus avoiding potential synergistic weight increases. Classical prescription weight-loss agents and stimulants need to be considered with caution, because they can destabilize mood and result in abuse or dependence. Adjunctive anticonvulsants such as topiramate (Bray et al. 2003) and zonisamide (Gadde et al. 2003), the norepinephrine reuptake inhibitor atomoxetine (McElroy et al. 2007), and the antidiabetic agent metformin (Correll et al. 2013) may allow patients to lose weight without routinely destabilizing mood, provided there is adequate concurrent antimanic therapy.

Acneiform and maculopapular eruptions, psoriasis, and folliculitis can occur with lithium (Yeung and Chan 2004). In occasional patients, switching to or adding another mood stabilizer to allow lithium dosage decrease or discontinuation is necessary.

Lithium can have adverse cardiac effects, which include benign eletrocardiographic T-wave morphological changes, clinically significant sinus node dysfunction or sinoatrial block, and onset or aggravation of ventricular irritability (Terao et al. 1996).

Lithium is a teratogen (FDA pregnancy category D[1]), yielding cardiac malformations at a rate of 0.1%–1.0% (Cohen et al. 1994). Thus, pregnant women taking lithium during organogenesis should undergo fetal echocardiography and level 2 ultrasound (Diav-Citrin et al. 2014). In patients with mild enough illness, a medication-free interval during pregnancy may be feasible. Because rapid discontinuation of lithium may yield rebound episodes (Baldessarini et al. 1996), gradual tapering off of lithium is a preferable strategy when feasible. Some patients have sufficiently severe illness to merit continuing lithium during pregnancy. Frank counseling and discussion of the risks and benefits of this approach is crucial in the management of such cases. Lithium and other mood stabilizers generally should be restarted immediately postpartum, in view of the risk of relapse, which may be as high as 60% (Cohen et al. 1995). Because lithium and other mood stabilizers are excreted to varying degrees in breast milk, the most conservative approach is to not breastfeed while taking mood stabilizers. However, because data suggest that lithium concentrations fall 50% from maternal serum to milk, and another 50% from milk to infant serum, yielding adequate tolerability in infants, recommendations against lithium during breastfeeding may need to be reassessed (Viguera et al. 2007).

In acute settings, such as the inpatient treatment of mania, lithium therapy is commonly initiated at 600–1,200 mg/day in two or three di-

---

[1]In late 2014, the FDA decided to do away with letter-based pregnancy categories in favor of a text-based descriptive approach. Although this change was planned to take effect in June of 2015, in this chapter we present the FDA's still current (as of early 2015) letter-based pregnancy categories.

vided doses, and increased as necessary and tolerated every 1–4 days by 300 mg/day, with final dosages commonly not exceeding 1,800 mg/ day (Table 8–4). Some patients may better tolerate weighting the dose toward bedtime or even taking the entire daily dose at bedtime. Euthymic or depressed patients tend to tolerate aggressive initiation less well than manic patients. Thus, in less acute situations, such as the initiation of prophylaxis or adjunctive use, lithium can be started at 300–600 mg/day, and increased as necessary and tolerated by 300 mg/day every 4–7 days. Target dosages are commonly between 900 and 1,800 mg/day, yielding serum levels from 0.6 to 1.2 mEq/L, with the higher dosages used acutely and the lower dosages used in adjunctive therapy or prophylaxis (Sproule 2002). In acute mania studies of adjunctive SGAs (added to lithium or valproate), target serum lithium concentrations ranged from 0.6 to 1.4 mEq/L, yet actual mean serum lithium concentrations ranged between only 0.70 and 0.76 mEq/L (Sachs et al. 2002; Tohen et al. 2002; Yatham et al. 2004).

Older data suggest that during maintenance treatment, serum lithium concentrations maintained at 0.4–0.6 (median average 0.54) mEq/L compared with 0.8–1.0 (median average 0.83) mEq/L were better tolerated but less effective (Gelenberg et al. 1989). However, in a European lithium versus carbamazepine maintenance study, serum trough lithium concentrations were targeted at 0.6–0.8 mEq/L, with an actual mean of only 0.63 mEq/L (Greil et al. 1997). In an American lithium versus carbamazepine maintenance study, serum trough lithium concentrations were targeted at 0.5–1.2 mEq/L, with an actual mean of 0.84 mEq/L (Denicoff et al. 1997). In a lithium versus divalproex versus placebo maintenance study, trough serum lithium concentrations were targeted at 0.8–1.2 mEq/L, with an actual mean of 1.0 mEq/L (Bowden et al. 2000). In a lithium versus lamotrigine versus placebo maintenance study, trough serum lithium concentrations were targeted at 0.8–1.1 mEq/L, with an actual steady state mean of only 0.8 mEq/L (Calabrese et al. 2003). In a lithium versus olanzapine maintenance study, trough serum lithium concentrations were targeted at 0.6–1.2 mEq/L, with an actual mean of 0.76 mEq/L (Tohen et al. 2005). In two recent American comparative effectiveness studies, lithium combined with other treatments was administered at either low dosages (median dosage=600 mg/day, mean serum lithium concentration = 0.47 mEq/L) (Nierenberg et al. 2013) or more conventional dosages (median dosage=900 mg/day, mean serum lithium concentration = 0.6 mEq/L) (Nierenberg et al. 2014).

Patients need to be advised of lithium adverse effects, drug interactions, and the importance of adequate hydration. Clinical assessments with lithium therapy include a baseline physical examination and rou-

TABLE 8–4. Dosing of mood stabilizers and second-generation antipsychotics

Class/Medication	Start (mg/day or mg/kg/day)	Target range (mg/day)	Blood levels/comments
Mood stabilizers			
Lithium	600–1,200 acute	900–1,800 acute	0.9–1.2 mEq/L acute
	300–600 less acute	600–1,200 less acute	0.6–0.9 mEq/L less acute
			div/qhs
Valproate	25 mg/kg/day acute	2,000–3,000 acute	85–125 µg/mL acute
	250–500 less acute	1,000–2,000 less acute	50–85 µg/mL less acute
			DR div, ER qhs
Carbamazepine	400–800 acute	800–1,600 acute	9–12 µg/mL acute (?)
	200–400 less acute (?)	600–1,200 less acute (?)	4–9 µg/mL less acute (?)
			div
Lamotrigine	25×2 wks, 50×2 wks, 100×1 wk, then 200	200–400 (occasionally 500)	3–15 µg/mL (?)
			qam

TABLE 8–4. Dosing of mood stabilizers and second-generation antipsychotics *(continued)*

Class/Medication	Start (mg/day or mg/kg/day)	Target range (mg/day)	Blood levels/comments
Second-generation antipsychotics			
Aripiprazole	15–30 acute	15–30 acute	qam (qhs if sedating)
	2–5 less acute (?)	5–10 less acute (?)	
Aripiprazole IM	9.75	15–30	q2h
Clozapine	25, ↑25 qd acute (?)	50–400 acute (?)	qhs>div
	12.5, ↑25 q4d less acute (?)	25–200 less acute (?)	
Olanzapine	10–15 acute	10–20 acute	qhs
	5 less acute	5–10 less acute	
Olanzapine IM	5–10	10–30	q2h–q4h
Quetiapine IR	100, ↑100 qd acute	400–800 acute	qhs>div
	50, ↑50–100 qd less acute	300–600 less acute	
Quetiapine XR	300, ↑600 day 2, 800 day 3 acute	400–800 acute	q evening
	50, ↑100 day 2, 200 day 3, 300 day 4 less acute	300 less acute	
Risperidone	2–3 acute	1–6 acute	qhs
	0.25–0.5 less acute (?)	1–3 less acute (?)	

TABLE 8–4. Dosing of mood stabilizers and second-generation antipsychotics (*continued*)

Class/Medication	Start (mg/day or mg/kg/day)	Target range (mg/day)	Blood levels/comments
Second-generation antipsychotics (continued)			
Risperidone LAI	25 q2wks	25–50 q2wks	q2wks
Ziprasidone	80 acute	120–160 acute	div/qd, with food
	80 less acute (?)	120–160 less acute (?)	240–320 in occasional patients (?)
Ziprasidone IM	10	40	q2h—schizophrenia[a]
Asenapine	10 acute	20 acute	qhs>div
	5 less acute	10 acute	
Lurasidone	20	20–120 (average 60)	qd, with food

Note. Acute=manic or mixed inpatients; less acute=depressed, euthymic, or hypomanic outpatients. DR=direct release; ER=extended release; IM=intramuscular (rapid-acting injectable); IR=immediate release; LAI=long-acting injectable; XR=extended release. div=divided doses recommended, but dose commonly weighted toward bedtime; qam=each morning; qd=once daily; qhs=daily at bedtime; q2h=every 2 hours; q2wks=every 2 weeks; q4d=every 4 days; (?)=limited data.
[a]As of early 2015, approved for schizophrenia but not bipolar disorder.

tine querying of patients regarding CNS (sedation, tremor, ataxia), gastrointestinal (nausea, vomiting, diarrhea), metabolic (weight gain), and renal (polyuria, polydipsia) disorders and adverse effects at baseline and during treatment. Laboratory monitoring includes baseline pregnancy test, electrocardiogram (ECG) in patients over age 40 years, and renal (blood urea nitrogen, serum creatinine and electrolytes) and thyroid (TSH) indices, with reevaluation of renal and thyroid indices at 3 and 6 months, and then every 6–12 months thereafter, and as clinically indicated (American Psychiatric Association 2002). Serum lithium concentrations are commonly assessed at steady state, which occurs at about 5 days after a dosage change, and then as clinically indicated by inefficacy or adverse effects. More frequent laboratory monitoring is prudent in the medically ill and in patients with abnormal baseline or after-treatment indices.

Divalproex (Valproate)

Divalproex (or valproate) is a fatty acid with a variety of biochemical actions, including effects on sodium channels, GABA, glutamate, dopamine, and intracellular signaling (Li et al. 2002).

Valproate is well absorbed, with bioavailability close to 100%, and is 80%–90% bound to plasma proteins (DeVane 2003). Binding is saturable, so that at higher doses a greater percentage of the drug may be in the free form. Valproate is quite hydrophilic, with a low volume of distribution of only about 0.1 L/kg. Thus, at higher doses, the increased free fraction may remain in the blood compartment (rather than escaping into the tissues) and thus be cleared by the liver. This may yield "sublinear" kinetics, so that with higher serum concentrations, greater increases in dose may be required to yield the desired increase in serum level (Graves 1995).

In monotherapy valproate has a half-life of approximately 12 hours, although when combined with enzyme inducers such as carbamazepine, valproate's half-life falls 50% to approximately 6 hours. Valproate is available as valproic acid (commonly referred to as valproate); as divalproex delayed-release (DR) formulation (commonly referred to as divalproex), which has better gastrointestinal tolerability than valproic acid (Zarate et al. 1999); and as divalproex extended-release (ER) formulation (commonly referred to as divalproex-ER), which has potentially even better tolerability than the divalproex-DR formulation (Smith et al. 2004).

Valproate is extensively metabolized, with three principal routes of elimination: 1) conjugation to inactive glucuronides and other inactive metabolites (approximately 50% of disposition), 2) β-oxidation in the mitochondria (approximately 40% of disposition), and 3) cytochrome P450 (CYP) oxidation (approximately 10% of disposition) (Potter and Ketter 1993). Valproate has a somewhat more favorable therapeutic index than lithium or carbamazepine, with a lower incidence of neurotoxicity being an important advantage. This relatively favorable therapeutic index, along with the existence of three principal metabolic pathways, may contribute to the fact that clinical drug-drug interactions yielding clinical toxicity with valproate may be less prominent than with lithium or carbamazepine.

Valproate should not be taken by 1) patients with hepatic disease or significant hepatic dysfunction, 2) patients with mitochondrial disorders caused by mutations in mitochondrial DNA polymerase γ (POLG; e.g., Alpers-Huttenlocher syndrome) and children under age 2 years who are suspected of having a POLG-related disorder, and 3) patients with urea cycle disorders (Physicians' Desk Reference 2014). Limited data indicate that lower valproate doses may commonly be necessary in older adults. In contrast, lower valproate doses do not appear to be routinely necessary in patients with renal impairment.

Valproate inhibits hepatic metabolism (including epoxide hydrolase, some glycosyltransferase[s], and some CYP isoforms) and therefore has metabolic interactions with some drugs (Bourgeois 1988). Thus, valproate can yield increased serum concentrations of carbamazepine-10,11-epoxide (carbamazepine-E) (Pisani et al. 1990) (Tables 8–1 and 8–5). In contrast, carbamazepine induces valproate metabolism, yielding decreased serum valproate concentrations (Levy et al. 1982; Jann et al. 1988) (Tables 8–1, 8–5, and 8–6). Valproate doubles serum lamotrigine concentrations (Anderson et al. 1996; Rambeck and Wolf 1993; Rowland et al. 2006) (Tables 8–1 and 8–5) and thus increases the risk of rash with lamotrigine, so that it is particularly important to take care to introduce lamotrigine even more conservatively (halving lamotrigine doses) in patients who are taking valproate (Faught et al. 1999).

In contrast, for most patients, combining valproate with SGAs (Table 8–1), antidepressants, or benzodiazepines is well tolerated and does not entail clinically significant pharmacokinetic drug interactions. However, valproate decreased dose-corrected olanzapine concentrations in four patients (Bergemann et al. 2006), and valproate may (Aichhorn et al. 2006) or may not (Physicians' Desk Reference 2014) increase quetiapine serum concentrations (Table 8–1). Also, valproate can increase serum amitriptyline/nortriptyline concentrations (Table 8–5) (Wong et al. 1996). Moreover, limited data suggest that in at least some patients, combining valproate with lorazepam might yield serious CNS depression (Lee et al. 2002), combining valproate with clonazepam may in-

TABLE 8–5. Selected valproate metabolic drug interactions

VPA →↑Drug	Drug →↑VPA	Drug →↓VPA
Amitriptyline	Aspirin	Carbamazepine
Carbamazepine-E	Felbamate	Meropenem
Ethosuximide		Phenobarbital
Felbamate		Phenytoin
Lamotrigine		Rifampin
Nortriptyline		
Phenobarbital		
Phenytoin		
Zidovudine		

Note. Carbamazepine-E = carbamazepine-10,11-epoxide; VPA = valproate.

duce absence status in patients with a history of absence status (Watson 1979), and combining valproate with zolpidem might yield somnambulism (Sattar et al. 2003).

Valproate can yield increased serum concentrations of ethosuximide, felbamate, phenobarbital, and phenytoin; felbamate can yield increased valproate concentrations, whereas phenobarbital and phenytoin can yield decreased serum valproate concentrations (Table 8–5) (Physicians' Desk Reference 2014).

Aspirin can yield decreased valproate clearance (Table 8–5), as well as decreased valproate protein binding. The antimicrobials rifampin and meropenem can yield decreased serum valproate concentrations, whereas valproate can yield increased serum concentrations of zidovudine. In contrast to carbamazepine, valproate does *not* yield clinically significant decreases in serum concentrations of hormonal contraceptives.

Plasma protein binding interactions can also occur, so that valproate can increase free fractions of diazepam, carbamazepine, phenytoin, tiagabine, tolbutamide, and warfarin, whereas the NSAIDs aspirin, diflunisal, tolmetin, mefenamic acid, fenoprofen, ibuprofen, and naproxen can increase free valproate.

Common dose-related adverse effects with valproate include CNS (tremor, sedation, dizziness), gastrointestinal (nausea, vomiting, dyspepsia, diarrhea), hepatic (transaminase elevations), and metabolic (weight gain, osteoporosis) problems, and hair loss (Dreifuss and Langer 1988). CNS adverse effects may be attenuated by weighting valproate dosage toward bedtime or dosage reduction, and β-blockers may attenuate valproate-induced tremor. Valproate can cause weight gain, which appears to be more of a problem than with lithium (Bowden et al. 2000) but less of a challenge than with olanzapine (Tohen et al. 2003a). Valproate-related weight gain can be approached in a fashion similar to that described earlier in this chapter for lithium. Limited data suggest that valproate-induced hair loss may be avoided or attenuated by the addition of selenium 25–100 µg/day and/or zinc 10–50 mg/day.

The USPI for valproate includes boxed warnings regarding the risks of hepatotoxicity, teratogenicity, and pancreatitis (Physicians' Desk Reference 2014). Hepatic fatalities are of concern in infants receiving valproate along with enzyme-inducing agents, although rates for patients over age 10 years are only approximately 1 per 609,000 with valproate monotherapy and approximately 1 per 28,000 when valproate is given with enzyme inducers (Bryant and Dreifuss 1996). Valproate, like carbamazepine, is generally discontinued if hepatic indices rise above three times the upper limit of normal. Rates of major congenital malformations (spina bifida, heart defects, urogenital defects, and multiple anomalies) with valproate appear higher compared with rates with carbamazepine or lamotrigine or with no anticonvulsant (Cunnington et al. 2005; Morrow et al. 2006; Vajda et al. 2007; Wyszynski et al. 2005). Valproate also appears to increase the risks of neurodevelopmental or neurocognitive defects (Adab et al. 2001; Gaily et al. 2004). Valproate-induced pancreatitis may occur in as many as 1 in 1,000 patient-years of exposure and is detectable by assessing serum amylase in patients with persistent or severe gastrointestinal problems. Other valproate USPI warnings include the risks of hyperammonemic encephalopathy in patients with urea cycle disorders, somnolence in older adults, thrombocytopenia, and suicidality (an anticonvulsant class warning).

For over two decades, there have been reports regarding an association between valproate therapy and polycystic ovarian syndrome in women with epilepsy (Isojärvi et al. 1993; Rasgon 2004). Studies in patients with bipolar disorder consistent with the possibility of a 6%–10% risk of polycystic ovarian syndrome with valproate in women with bipolar disorder have indicated the need for prospective trials to systematically assess this issue (Joffe et al. 2006; Rasgon et al. 2005).

Valproate is a teratogen (FDA pregnancy category D), with risks from valproate therapy in pregnancy appearing to be more problematic than those from other mood stabilizers. Folate supplementation may attenuate the risk of spina bifida, and ultrasound may allow early detection. Although valproate concentrations in breast milk and infant serum are low (<10% of maternal serum levels), the FDA recommends that "consideration should be given to discontinuing nursing when [valproate] is administered to a nursing woman."

In acute settings, such as the inpatient treatment of mania, valproate therapy in the past was commonly initiated at 750 mg/day and increased as necessary and tolerated by 250 mg/day every 1–2 days. More recent studies have described more aggressive valproate initiation in acute mania utilizing divalproex formulations. Thus, with the divalproex delayed-release formulation, initiating at 20 mg/kg or even loading with 30 mg/kg/day for 1 or 2 days, followed by 20 mg/kg/day, appeared generally well tolerated in patients with acute mania (Lima et al. 1999; McElroy et al. 1996) (Table 8–4). Because of lower bioavailability, doses with the divalproex ER formulation may need to be 6%–20% higher than with the divalproex direct-release formulation. In the acute mania registration study, the divalproex ER formulation was started at 25 mg/kg/day (rounded up to the nearest 500 mg), increased by 500 mg on day 3, and intermittently adjusted based on clinical effects targeting serum levels from 85 to 125 µg/mL (600–850 µM/L) (Bowden et al. 2006b). However, euthymic or depressed patients tend to tolerate aggressive initiation less well than manic patients. Thus, in less acute situations, such as the initiation of prophylaxis or adjunctive use, valproate is often started at 250–500 mg/day and increased, as necessary and tolerated, by 250 mg/day every 4–7 days. Target doses in the past have commonly been between 750 and 2,500 mg/day, yielding serum levels from 50 to 125 µg/mL (350–850 µM/L) (Bowden et al. 1996), with the higher portion of the range used acutely and lower doses used in adjunctive therapy or prophylaxis. All or the majority of the divalproex delayed-release formulation dose can commonly be given in a single dose at bedtime. In a meta-analysis of controlled acute mania studies, therapeutic effect size increased linearly with serum valproate concentrations (Allen et al. 2006). In acute mania studies of adjunctive SGAs, target serum valproate concentrations ranged from 50 to 125 µg/mL, while actual mean serum valproate concentrations ranged between only 64 and 70 µg/mL (Sachs et al. 2002; Tohen et al. 2002; Yatham et al. 2004). In a maintenance study of divalproex delayed-release formulation versus lithium versus placebo, serum trough valproate concentrations were targeted at 71–125 µg/mL, with an actual mean of 85 µg/mL (Bowden et al. 2000).

Patients need to be advised of valproate adverse effects and drug interactions. Clinical assessments with valproate therapy include a baseline physical examination and routinely querying patients regarding hepatic and hematological disorders and adverse effects at baseline and during treatment. Laboratory monitoring during valproate therapy commonly includes baseline complete blood count, differential, platelets, and hepatic indices, and reevaluation every 6–12 months and as clinically indicated (American Psychiatric Association 2002). Most of the concerning hematological reactions occur in the first 3 months of therapy (Tohen et al. 1995). Serum valproate concentrations are typically assessed at steady state and then as clinically indicated by inefficacy or adverse effects.

Carbamazepine

Carbamazepine has a tricyclic structure and a wide array of biochemical effects, including effects on sodium channels, GABA, glutamate, somatostatin, adenosine, and intracellular signaling (Li et al. 2002).

Carbamazepine's pharmacokinetic properties are atypical among medications prescribed by psychiatrists and necessitate special care when treating patients concurrently with other medications (Ketter et al. 1991a, 1991b). Carbamazepine has erratic absorption and a bioavailability of approximately 80% and is about 75% bound to plasma proteins, with the most important metabolic pathway being via CYP3A4, and accounting for approximately 40% of disposition (although throughput triples with enzyme induction) (Kerr et al. 1994). Aromatic hydroxylation via CYP1A2 accounts for another approximately 40% of disposition, whereas glucuronidation by uridine diphosphate glycosyltransferase (UGT) accounts for approximately 15% of disposition (Staines et al. 2004). Carbamazepine's half-life is about 24 hours before autoinduction but falls to about 8 hours after autoinduction (2–4 weeks into therapy). This variation may require dose adjustment to maintain adequate blood levels and therapeutic effects.

Lower carbamazepine doses may be necessary in older adults, because of decreased clearance and/or increased sensitivity to side effects (Physicians' Desk Reference 2014). Although lower carbamazepine doses may be necessary in patients with hepatic impairment, data are insufficient to determine whether or not lower carbamazepine doses are necessary in patients with renal impairment.

Carbamazepine induces conjugation, CYP3A4, and presumably other CYP isoforms. Therefore, carbamazepine decreases the serum levels not only of carbamazepine itself (autoinduction) but also of many other medications (heteroinduction) (Tables 8–1 and 8–6). Carbamazepine-induced decreases in serum levels of certain concurrent medications can render them ineffective, whereas if carbamazepine is discontinued, serum levels of such other medications can rise, leading to toxic effects from these agents. Finally, carbamazepine metabolism can be inhibited by CYP3A4 inhibitors, yielding increased serum carbamazepine levels and intoxication (Table 8–7).

TABLE 8–6. Selected drugs with increased clearance with carbamazepine

Alprazolam (?)	Itraconazole
Amitriptyline	Lamotrigine
Aripiprazole	Levetiracetam (?)
Bupropion	Levothyroxine
Carbamazepine	Lurasidone (?)
Chlorpromazine (?)	Methadone
Citalopram	Midazolam
Clobazam	Mirtazapine
Clonazepam	Nortriptyline
Clozapine	Olanzapine
Cyclosporine (?)	Oxcarbazepine
Delavirdine	Oxiracetam (?)
Desipramine	Pancuronium
Dexamethasone	Perampanel
Diazepam	Phenytoin
Dicumarol (?)	Praziquantel
Doxacurium	Prednisolone
Doxepin	Primidone
Doxycycline	Quetiapine
Escitalopram	Risperidone
Eslicarbazepine (?)	Sertraline
Ethosuximide	Theophylline (?)
Felbamate	Thiothixene (?)
Felodipine	Tiagabine
Fentanyl (?)	Topiramate
Fluphenazine (?)	Valproate
Glucocorticoids	Vecuronium
Haloperidol	Warfarin
Hormonal contraceptives	Ziprasidone (?)
Imipramine	Zonisamide
Indinavir	

Note. (?)=limited data.

TABLE 8–7. Selected drugs that decrease clearance of carbamazepine

Acetazolamide	Nefazodone
Cimetidine	Nelfinavir
Clarithromycin	Nicotinamide
Danazol	Ponsinomycin
Diltiazem	Propoxyphene
Erythromycin	D-Propoxyphene
Fluoxetine	Quetiapine ($\uparrow$carbamazepine-E) (?)
Flurithromycin	Quinine
Fluvoxamine	Ritonavir
Grapefruit juice	Troleandomycin
Isoniazid	Valproate ($\uparrow$carbamazepine-E)
Itraconazole	Verapamil
Josamycin	Viloxazine
Ketoconazole	

Note. Carbamazepine-E = carbamazepine-10,11-epoxide; $\uparrow$ = increased; (?) = limited data.

Carbamazepine has a wide variety of (primarily pharmacokinetic) drug-drug interactions (Tables 8–1, 8–6, and 8–7), in excess of those seen with other mood stabilizers. Knowledge of carbamazepine drug-drug interactions is crucial for effective management. Advances in molecular pharmacology have characterized specific CYP isoforms responsible for metabolism of various medications (Ketter et al. 1991a, 1991b). This information may allow clinicians to anticipate and avoid pharmacokinetic drug-drug interactions and thus provide more effective combination pharmacotherapies. The reader interested in detailed reviews of carbamazepine drug-drug interactions may find these elsewhere (Ketter et al. 1991a, 1991b).

Although carbamazepine and lithium do not usually have significant pharmacokinetic interactions (Table 8–1), a few case reports suggest that some individuals may experience neurotoxicity with the carbamazepine plus lithium combination—despite having serum concentrations of both drugs within the therapeutic range—presumably related to a pharmacodynamic interaction (Shukla et al. 1984).

Carbamazepine induces valproate metabolism, yielding decreased serum valproate concentrations (Jann et al. 1988) (Tables 8–1, 8–5, and 8–6).

This interaction can potentially confound clinicians because patients can have neurotoxicity due to elevated carbamazepine-E or free carbamazepine concentrations in spite of therapeutic total carbamazepine levels. Thus, in view of increased carbamazepine-E levels, carbamazepine levels as low as about one-half of those seen without valproate may be required. Carbamazepine decreases serum valproate levels, and its discontinuation can yield increased serum valproate levels and toxicity. As a general rule, clinicians should carefully monitor patients taking the carbamazepine plus valproate combination for side effects and consider decreasing the carbamazepine dose in advance (because of the expected displacement of carbamazepine from plasma proteins and increase in carbamazepine-E) and ultimately increasing the valproate dose (because of expected carbamazepine-induced decrements in valproate).

Carbamazepine induces lamotrigine metabolism (May et al. 1996) (Tables 8–1 and 8–6) so that, as described in the following subsection, lamotrigine therapy in the presence of carbamazepine requires higher doses of lamotrigine. Although lamotrigine does not usually yield clinically significant changes in serum carbamazepine concentrations, lamotrigine may enhance carbamazepine neurotoxicity, probably by a pharmacodynamic interaction (Besag et al. 1998).

Carbamazepine has pharmacokinetic drug interactions with multiple SGAs (Tables 8–1 and 8–6). Carbamazepine induces clozapine metabolism, and this combination is not recommended in view of possible (but not proven) synergistic bone marrow suppression (Junghan et al. 1993). Carbamazepine also increases metabolism of olanzapine, risperidone, quetiapine, aripiprazole, and potentially ziprasidone and lurasidone. Although the clinical significance of carbamazepine-induced decreases in ziprasidone serum concentrations remains to be determined, carbamazepine interactions with risperidone and olanzapine have been confirmed to be clinically significant. Finally, carbamazepine is expected to decrease lurasidone serum concentrations (Physicians' Desk Reference 2014).

Carbamazepine increases metabolism of haloperidol (Yasui-Furukori et al. 2003) and possibly other first-generation antipsychotics. Some patients may have improvement or no deterioration in psychiatric status or fewer neuroleptic side effects during combination treatment, whereas others may have deterioration in psychiatric status (Kahn et al. 1990).

Carbamazepine appears to induce metabolism of tricyclic antidepressants, bupropion, citalopram, sertraline, mirtazapine, mianserin, and to some extent trazodone (Table 8–6). Carbamazepine may increase rather than decrease serum levels of transdermal selegiline and its metabolites (Physicians' Desk Reference 2014). Although theoretical grounds have been stated for concern about combining carbamazepine with monoamine oxidase inhibitors, preliminary data suggest that the addition of phenelzine or tranylcypromine to carbamazepine may be well tolerated, does not affect carbamazepine levels, and may provide relief of refractory depressive symptoms in some patients (Ketter et al. 1995). The CYP3A4 inhibitors fluoxetine, fluvoxamine, and nefazodone can inhibit carbamazepine metabolism, yielding increased carbamazepine levels and toxicity (Table 8–7). Viloxazine and perhaps trazodone can also increase carbamazepine levels.

Carbamazepine may decrease serum levels of clonazepam, alprazolam, clobazam, and midazolam (Table 8–6), and the hypnotics eszopiclone and zolpidem, potentially decreasing the efficacy of these agents.

Carbamazepine induction of hepatic metabolism yields clinically significant decreases in serum concentrations of multiple anticonvulsants, including felbamate, topiramate, tiagabine, oxcarbazepine, zonisamide, perampanel, and possibly levetiracetam and eslicarbazepine (Table 8–6). There is controversy regarding pharmacokinetic drug interactions between carbamazepine and vigabatrin. The older anticonvulsants phenytoin, phenobarbital, primidone, methsuximide, and possibly felbamate can yield clinically significant decreases in serum carbamazepine levels. In addition, carbamazepine may have a pharmacodynamic interaction with levetiracetam.

The commonly used calcium channel blockers verapamil and diltiazem can increase carbamazepine levels and cause clinical toxicity (Table 8–7), whereas enzyme-inducing anticonvulsants such as carbamazepine can decrease nimodipine and felodipine levels (Table 8–6).

Carbamazepine decreases levothyroxine (T_4), free T_4 index, and, less consistently, liothyronine (T_3) concentrations.

Drug-drug interactions between carbamazepine and other (nonpsychotropic) drugs are also of substantial clinical importance. Carbamazepine induces metabolism of diverse medications, raising the possibility of undermining the efficacy of steroids such as hormonal contraceptives (Table 8–6) (Doose et al. 2003). In women taking carbamazepine, oral contraceptive preparations need to contain at least 50 μg of ethinyl estradiol, levonorgestrel implants are contraindicated because of cases of contraceptive failure, and medroxyprogesterone injections need to be given every 10 rather than 12 weeks.

Carbamazepine also induces metabolism of prednisolone and methylprednisolone; the methylxanthines theophylline and aminophylline; the antibiotic doxycycline; the neuromuscular blockers pancuronium, vecuronium, and doxacurium; and the anticoagulant warfarin, and possibly dicumarol (Table 8–6). Coadministration of carbamazepine and delavirdine may lead to delavirdine inefficacy.

In contrast, a variety of medications can increase serum carbamaze-pine levels and potentially yield clinical toxicity. Such agents include nicotinamide, the antibiotics erythromycin, troleandomycin (triacety-loleandomycin), clarithromycin, and isoniazid; the protease inhibitors ritonavir and nelfinavir; and the carbonic anhydrase inhibitor acetazol-amide (Table 8–7). In addition, other medications such as cisplatin and doxorubicin may decrease serum carbamazepine levels, potentially yield-ing inefficacy.

Carbamazepine therapy is associated with adverse events that are common and benign as well as ones that are rare and serious. The most common dose-related adverse effects with carbamazepine involve the CNS (diplopia, blurred vision, fatigue, sedation, dizziness, ataxia) or gas-trointestinal system (nausea, vomiting). Carbamazepine CNS adverse effects tend to occur early in therapy before autoinduction and the de-velopment of some tolerance to carbamazepine's central adverse ef-fects. Gradual initial dosing and careful attention to potential drug-drug interactions can help attenuate this problem. Carbamazepine-induced gastrointestinal disturbance can be approached in a fashion similar to that described for lithium (see earlier subsection "Lithium").

The carbamazepine USPI includes boxed warnings regarding the risks of serious dermatological reactions and the human leukocyte an-tigen (HLA) allele HLA-B*1502, as well as aplastic anemia (16 per mil-lion patient-years) and agranulocytosis (48 per million patient-years) (Physicians' Desk Reference 2014). Other carbamazepine USPI warn-ings include the risks of teratogenicity, and increased intraocular pres-sure due to mild anticholinergic activity. Carbamazepine can also yield hematological (benign leukopenia, benign thrombocytopenia), derma-tological (benign rash), electrolyte (asymptomatic hyponatremia), and hepatic (benign transaminase elevations) problems.

Much less commonly, carbamazepine can yield analogous serious problems. For example, mild leukopenia and benign rash occur in as many as 1 in 10 patients, with the slight possibility that these usually be-nign phenomena are heralding malignant aplastic anemia, occurring in approximately 1 per 100,000 patients, or Stevens-Johnson syndrome or toxic epidermal necrolysis, occurring in approximately 1–6 per 10,000 patients (Tohen et al. 1995). The risk of serious rash with carbamazepine may be 10 times as high in some Asian countries and is strongly linked to HLA-B*1502 (Hung et al. 2006). Thus, the carbamazepine USPI states that Asians ought to be genetically tested and, if HLA-B*1502 positive, should not be treated with carbamazepine unless the benefit clearly outweighs the risk. Hematological monitoring needs to be intensified in patients with low or marginal leukocyte counts, and carbamazepine is generally discontinued if the leukocyte count falls below 3,000/μL or the granulocyte count is below 1,000/μL. Rash presenting with systemic illness, or involvement of the eyes, mouth, or bladder (dysuria) constitutes a medical emergency, and carbamazepine ought to be immediately discontinued and the patient assessed emergently. For more benign presentations, immediate dermatological consultation is required to assess the risks of continuing therapy. In carefully selected cases, with the collaboration of dermatology, it may be worth attempting desensitization by decreasing the dose and adding antihistamine or prednisone, although these agents entail additional risks of sedation and mood destabilization, respectively. Carbamazepine can rarely cause clinically significant hepatic problems, and it generally needs to be discontinued if hepatic indices rise above three times the upper limit of normal. The carbamazepine USPI also includes an anticonvulsant class warning regarding the risk of suicidality.

Although carbamazepine can cause modest increases TSH levels, frank hypothyroidism is very uncommon. Carbamazepine may affect cardiac conduction and should be used with caution in patients with cardiac disorders. A baseline ECG is worth consideration if there is any indication of cardiac problems.

Carbamazepine appears less likely than lithium or valproate to yield weight gain. For this reason, carbamazepine may provide an important alternative to lithium or valproate for patients who struggle with this problem. Carbamazepine-induced hyponatremia is commonly adequately tolerated in young physically well individuals, although it can yield serious sequelae in medically frail older adults.

Carbamazepine is a teratogen (FDA pregnancy category D). Thus, carbamazepine can yield minor anomalies (craniofacial malformations and digital hypoplasia) in up to 20% of patients and spina bifida in approximately 1%. For the latter, folate supplementation may attenuate the risk, and ultrasound may allow early detection. Overall rates of major congenital malformations with carbamazepine could be comparable to rates with lamotrigine or no anticonvulsant and lower compared to rates with valproate. The issue of carbamazepine therapy in pregnancy can be approached in a fashion similar to that described above for lithium. Although carbamazepine concentrations in breast milk are variable, and there is very little evidence of adverse effects in newborns exposed to carbamazepine via breast milk, the USPI recommends that "a decision should be made whether to discontinue nursing or to discontinue the drug, taking into account the importance of the drug to the mother."

In acute settings, such as the inpatient treatment of mania, carbamazepine therapy is commonly initiated at 200–400 mg/day and then increased as necessary and tolerated by 200 mg/day every 2–4 days (Table 8–4). In controlled acute mania studies, a beaded extended-release capsule formulation was started at 200 mg twice daily and titrated by daily increments of 200 mg to final dosages as high as 1,600 mg/day (Weisler et al. 2004, 2005). In a report of open extension therapy after these controlled acute mania studies, beaded extended-release capsule carbamazepine was started at 200 mg twice daily and titrated by increments of 200 mg every 3 days (vs. daily in the acute studies) to final dosages as high as 1,600 mg/day (Ketter et al. 2004). This approach decreased the incidence of CNS (dizziness, somnolence, ataxia), digestive (nausea, vomiting), and dermatological (pruritus) adverse effects by approximately 50%. Euthymic or depressed patients tend to tolerate aggressive initiation less well than manic patients. Thus, in less acute situations, such as the initiation of prophylaxis or adjunctive use, carbamazepine is commonly started at 100–200 mg/day and increased as necessary and tolerated by 200 mg/day every 4–7 days. Even this gradual initiation may cause adverse effects. Thus, starting with 50 mg (half of a chewable 100-mg tablet) at bedtime and increasing by 50 mg every 4–7 days may yield a better-tolerated initiation. Because of autoinduction, doses after 2–4 weeks of therapy may need to be twice as high as in the first week to yield comparable serum levels. Target doses are commonly between 600 and 1,200 mg/day, yielding serum levels from 6 to 12 μg/mL (20 to 60 μM/L), with the higher portion of the range used acutely and the lower doses used in prophylaxis or adjunctive therapy. In a European carbamazepine versus lithium maintenance study, serum trough carbamazepine concentrations targeted a range of 4–12 μg/mL, with an actual mean of 6.4 μg/mL (Greil et al. 1997). In an American carbamazepine versus lithium maintenance study, serum trough carbamazepine concentrations targeted a range of 4–12 μg/mL, with an actual mean of 7.7 μg/mL (Denicoff et al. 1997).

Patients need to be advised of carbamazepine adverse effects and drug interactions. Clinical assessments with carbamazepine therapy include a baseline physical examination and routinely querying patients regarding hepatic and hematological disorders and adverse effects at baseline and during treatment. In the past, recommended laboratory monitoring during carbamazepine therapy included baseline complete blood count, differential, platelets, hepatic indices, and serum sodium, with reevaluation at 2, 4, 6, and 8 weeks, and then every 3 months, and as clinically indicated (American Psychiatric Association 2002). As with valproate, most of the dangerous hematological reactions occur in the first 3 months of therapy (Tohen et al. 1995). In contemporary clinical practice, somewhat less focus is placed on scheduled monitoring, and clinically indicated monitoring (e.g., when a patient becomes ill with a fever) is emphasized. Patients who have abnormal or marginal indices at any point merit carefully scheduled and clinically indicated monitoring. The USPI for the beaded extended-release capsule carbamazepine formulation approved for the treatment of acute mania recommends monitoring baseline complete blood count, including platelets possibly with reticulocytes and serum iron, and hepatic function; closely monitoring patients with low or decreased white blood cell count or platelets; and considering discontinuation of carbamazepine if there is evidence of bone marrow depression (Physicians' Desk Reference 2014). Serum carbamazepine concentrations are typically assessed at steady state and then as indicated by inefficacy or adverse effects.

Lamotrigine

Lamotrigine has a phenyltriazine structure, is a sodium channel and weak serotonin 5-HT$_3$ receptor blocker, and decreases glutamate release (Ketter et al. 2003). Although lamotrigine appears to modestly inhibit reuptake of serotonin, this effect may not be clinically significant because sexual dysfunction is not a major concern.

Lamotrigine has bioavailability of approximately 98%, is 55% bound to plasma proteins, and has a linear dose–plasma concentration relationship (Mikati et al. 1989). In monotherapy, lamotrigine's half-life is approximately 28 hours. Lamotrigine is extensively metabolized, mostly by glucuronidation, with only approximately 10% excreted unchanged in the urine. Lamotrigine does not yield clinically significant induction or inhibition of CYP isoforms and therefore is more a target of than an instigator of drug interactions. Combined with the enzyme inducer carbamazepine, lamotrigine's half-life falls 50% to approximately 14 hours (Tables 8–1 and 8–6). Combined with the enzyme inhibitor valproate, lamotrigine's half-life doubles to approximately 56 hours (Tables 8–1 and 8–5).

Lower lamotrigine doses may be necessary in older adults, because of decreased clearance and/or increased sensitivity to side effects. In view of the limited data regarding lamotrigine in patients with hepatic or renal impairment, cautious lamotrigine dosing is recommended (Physicians' Desk Reference 2014).

The enzyme-inducing mood-stabilizing anticonvulsant carbamazepine decreases serum lamotrigine concentrations (May et al. 1996) (Tables 8–1 and 8–6), whereas the enzyme-inhibiting mood-stabilizing anticonvulsant valproate increases lamotrigine levels (Anderson et al. 1996) (Tables 8–1 and 8–5). In addition, lamotrigine can enhance carbamazepine neurotoxicity, probably by a pharmacodynamic interaction.

Lamotrigine appears to lack clinically significant pharmacokinetic drug interactions with most other psychotropics (Table 8–1). However, therapeutic drug monitoring database information suggests that lamotrigine could substantively decrease serum quetiapine concentrations (Andersson et al. 2011) (Table 8–1), and single cases of increased clozapine (Kossen et al. 2001) and risperidone levels (Bienentreu and Kronmüller 2005) with lamotrigine have been reported. Case reports also suggest that sertraline may increase serum lamotrigine levels in some patients (Kaufman and Gerner 1998), that lamotrigine combined with escitalopram could yield myoclonus (Rosenhagen et al. 2006), and that lamotrigine combined with venlafaxine in overdose could yield seizures, ventricular tachycardia, and rhabdomyolysis (Peano et al. 1997).

Oxcarbazepine may decrease serum lamotrigine concentrations (May et al. 1999), and a possible pharmacodynamic interaction has been reported with this combination (Sabers and Gram 2000).

Lamotrigine has clinically significant pharmacokinetic interactions with a few other medications. Hormonal contraceptives cause clinically significant decreases in serum lamotrigine concentrations (Christensen et al. 2007), and serum lamotrigine concentrations may be decreased with lopinavir/ritonavir and with atazanavir/ritonavir. Also, rifampin increases lamotrigine clearance.

Lamotrigine is generally well tolerated, particularly in comparison to other treatment options for patients with bipolar disorder. The most common adverse events in bipolar disorder patients in clinical trials were headache, benign rash, dizziness, diarrhea, dream abnormality, and pruritus.

The lamotrigine USPI includes a boxed warning regarding the risk of serious rashes requiring hospitalization, which have included Stevens-Johnson syndrome, in 0.8% and 0.3% of pediatric and adult epilepsy patients receiving adjunctive therapy, respectively, and in 0.08% and 0.13% of adult mood disorder patients taking monotherapy and adjunctive therapy, respectively (Physicians' Desk Reference 2014). The risk of rash is higher in patients under age 16 years, and may be higher when coadministered with valproate, when the recommended initial lamotrigine dose is exceeded, and when the recommended lamotrigine dose escalation is exceeded. Benign rash may be seen in 10% of patients; however, because any rash is potentially serious, rashes require discontinuation of lamotrigine, unless they are clearly not drug related. Nearly all cases of life-threatening rashes have occurred within 2–8 weeks of starting lamotrigine. Other lamotrigine USPI warnings include the risks of hypersensitivity reactions (with fever and lymphadenopathy, but not necessarily rash), acute multiorgan failure (fatalities observed in about

1 in 400 pediatric and 1 in 1,800 adult epilepsy patients, but not in bipolar disorder patients), blood dyscrasia, and possibly withdrawal seizures in patients with bipolar disorder, so that unless safety concerns demand abrupt discontinuation, lamotrigine should be tapered over 2 weeks. The lamotrigine USPI also includes an anticonvulsant class warning regarding the risk of suicidality.

Lamotrigine can cause CNS (headache, somnolence, insomnia, dizziness, tremor) and gastrointestinal (nausea, diarrhea) adverse effects. These problems most often attenuate or resolve with time or lamotrigine dose adjustment but in occasional patients may require discontinuation of the lamotrigine. Unlike other mood stabilizers, lamotrigine has not been associated with weight gain. Also of clinical importance, lamotrigine may be less likely than selective serotonin reuptake inhibitors or other anticonvulsants to cause sexual dysfunction.

Lamotrigine is a teratogen (FDA pregnancy category C). Overall rates of major congenital malformations with lamotrigine could be comparable to rates with carbamazepine or no anticonvulsant, and lower compared with rates with valproate (Cunnington et al. 2005; Morrow et al. 2006; Vajda et al. 2007; Wyszynski et al. 2005). Nevertheless, lamotrigine may increase the risk of certain malformations, namely cleft lip and cleft palate. Lamotrigine concentrations in breast milk are variable but in some instances may approach "therapeutic ranges." Despite the lack of evidence of adverse effects in newborns exposed to lamotrigine via breast milk, the FDA has taken a conservative stance, considering lamotrigine administration "not recommended" during lactation.

Lamotrigine dosage is initially titrated *very slowly* to decrease the risk of rash. When lamotrigine is given without valproate, the USPI recommends starting lamotrigine at 25 mg/day for 2 weeks, increasing to 50 mg/day for 2 weeks, then 100 mg/day for 1 week, and then 200 mg/day in a single daily dose (Table 8–4), with doses exceeding 200 mg/day not recommended unless concurrent hormonal contraceptives (which decrease serum lamotrigine concentrations) are administered (Physicians' Desk Reference 2014). Nevertheless, even in the absence of hormonal contraceptive, selected patients may benefit from further gradual lamotrigine titration to final doses as high as 400–500 mg/day. Even more gradual lamotrigine initial titration—starting with 25 mg/day for 2 weeks, then increasing to 50 mg/day for the next 2 weeks, and then increasing weekly by 25 mg/day—may further decrease the risk of rash (Ketter et al. 2005).

When lamotrigine is added to valproate, recommended lamotrigine doses are halved, so lamotrigine is started at 25 mg every other day (although 12.5 mg/day may be worth considering) for 2 weeks, then increased to 25 mg/day for 2 weeks, then 50 mg/day for 1 week, and then 100 mg/day in a single daily dose, with doses exceeding 100 mg/day not recommended unless concurrent hormonal contraceptives (which decrease serum lamotrigine concentrations) are administered (Physicians' Desk Reference 2014). Nevertheless, even in the absence of hormonal contraceptive, selected patients concurrently taking valproate may benefit from further gradual lamotrigine titration to final dosages as high as 250 mg/day.

When lamotrigine is given with carbamazepine, recommended lamotrigine doses are doubled, so that lamotrigine may be started at 50 mg/day for 2 weeks, increased to 100 mg/day for 2 weeks, then 300 mg/day for 1 week, and then 400 mg/day in divided doses, with dosages exceeding 400 mg/day not recommended unless concurrent hormonal contraceptives (which decrease serum lamotrigine concentrations) are administered (Physicians' Desk Reference 2014). Nevertheless, even in the absence of hormonal contraceptive, selected patients concurrently taking carbamazepine may benefit from further gradual lamotrigine titration to final dosages as high as 800 mg/day.

Patients should be advised that if they fail to take lamotrigine for 5 half-lives (e.g., approximately 5 days in the absence of carbamazepine, or 3 days in the presence of carbamazepine), gradual reintroduction as described above is necessary, because rashes have been reported with rapid reintroduction.

Patients need to be advised of lamotrigine's adverse effects and drug interactions. Clinical assessments with lamotrigine therapy include a baseline physical examination and routinely querying patients regarding rash at baseline and during treatment. Lamotrigine is generally well tolerated and serum concentrations have not been related to therapeutic effects in patients with bipolar disorder, and therefore therapeutic drug monitoring with lamotrigine is not generally performed. Nevertheless, in patients taking lamotrigine at higher dosages (e.g., 400 mg/day without valproate, 200 mg/day with valproate, or 800 mg/day with carbamazepine) with inadequate therapeutic response and good tolerability, assessing serum lamotrigine concentration may be worthwhile in order to provide an assessment of adherence and/or metabolic abnormalities. In epilepsy patients, serum lamotrigine concentrations range from approximately 3 to 15 µg/mL (10 to 60 µM/L). Therefore, in a patient with bipolar disorder taking lamotrigine at higher dosages with inadequate therapeutic response, serum lamotrigine concentrations of less than 3 µg/mL or in excess of 15 µg/mL may suggest adherence/pharmacokinetic or nonresponse problems, respectively.

■ Second-Generation Antipsychotics

Psychotic symptoms may occur in up to 50% of patients with acute mania and also may arise (albeit less often) in patients with acute bipolar depression. Mood stabilizers may fail to provide adequate efficacy in such circumstances. Also, acutely manic patients with profound agitation may require parenteral medication, whereas less acutely ill patients with poor adherence for bipolar disorder preventive treatment may benefit from depot formulations. Unfortunately, as of early 2015, mood stabilizers were not available in parenteral or depot formulations. However, such formulations of SGAs, also referred to as *atypical antipsychotics*, were available. Thus, because of both efficacy and formulation availability limitations of mood stabilizers, SGAs have been commonly used (largely replacing older antipsychotics due to superior tolerability) in the treatment of bipolar disorder.

Clozapine, the prototypical SGA, has potent antipsychotic effects but lacks the risks of acute EPS and tardive dyskinesia. Nevertheless, clozapine still has a very challenging safety/tolerability profile (that includes risk of agranulocytosis); therefore, other SGAs were developed in hopes of finding agents with antipsychotic effects that entailed less risk of EPS than older antipsychotics and better overall safety/tolerability than clozapine. Hypotheses regarding the mechanisms contributing to SGAs having fewer problems with EPS than older antipsychotics include that SGAs tend to be more robust antagonists of serotonin 5-HT$_{2A}$ receptors than of dopamine D$_2$ receptors (Meltzer and Massey 2011), as well as that SGAs bind more loosely to dopamine D$_2$ receptors than does dopamine itself (whereas older antipsychotics bind to dopamine D$_2$ receptors more tightly than does dopamine itself) (Seeman 2002). SGAs block (or have partial agonist effects at) not only dopamine D$_2$ receptors (as do the antimanic first-generation antipsychotics) but also serotonin 5-HT$_2$ receptors (as does the antidepressant nefazodone) and, therefore, perhaps depending on the relative size of these as well as other receptor actions, could have antimanic, antidepressant, or even mood-stabilizing properties.

Compared with mood stabilizers, SGAs tend to entail more frequent and severe safety/tolerability challenges (e.g., weight gain/metabolic problems with olanzapine, acute EPS/hyperprolactinemia with risperidone, somnolence/sedation with quetiapine, and akathisia with newer SGAs), which can limit their utility (Table 8–8). SGAs may be broadly subdivided into two subgroups based on side-effect profiles: 1) older

TABLE 8–8. Differential adverse effects of second-generation antipsychotics

Medication	Somnolence/ sedation	Weight/ metabolic effects	Akathisia	EPS	Hyperprolactinemia	Orthostasis	Anticholinergic effects
Older							
Clozapine	+++	+++	+/–	+/–	+/–	+++	+++
Olanzapine	+++	+++	+	+	+	+	++
Risperidone	++	++	+	++	+++	+	+
Quetiapine	+++	++	+/–	+/–	+	++	+
Newer							
Aripiprazole	+	+	++	+	+/–	+/–	+/–
Ziprasidone	+	+/–	++	+	+	+/–	+/–
Asenapine	++	++	+	+/–	+	+	+/–
Lurasidone	+	+	+	+/–	+	+	+/–

Note. EPS=extrapyramidal symptoms.
Risk: +/–=minimal/none; +=low; ++=intermediate; +++=high.
Source. Adapted from American Diabetes Association et al. 2004; Lehman et al. 2004.

SGAs (clozapine, olanzapine, risperidone, and quetiapine) with generally more somnolence/sedation and weight gain but less akathisia than newer SGAs and 2) newer SGAs (aripiprazole, ziprasidone, asenapine, and lurasidone) with generally less somnolence/sedation and weight gain but more akathisia than older SGAs.

SGA side effects (more than therapeutic effects) have been associated with actions at specific receptors to varying extents, so that EPS/hyperprolactinemia (and antipsychotic benefits) have been most associated with dopamine D_2 receptor antagonism, somnolence/sedation and weight gain with histamine H_1 receptor antagonism, orthostasis with α_1 adrenergic receptor antagonism, and dry mouth, constipation, and blurred vision with muscarinic cholinergic receptor antagonism. In contrast, there is far less evidence for consistent biochemical actions underlying SGA-related akathisia and antidepressant effects.

The USPI for SGAs includes multiple warnings/precautions (Physicians' Desk Reference 2014). Indeed, as of early 2015, the seven SGAs with FDA bipolar disorder indications (olanzapine, risperidone, quetiapine, ziprasidone, aripiprazole, asenapine, and lurasidone) had in common 12 such USPI warnings/precautions, including the risks of 1) increased mortality in elderly patients with dementia-related psychosis (a boxed warning, with a reminder that SGAs are not approved for dementia-related psychosis); 2) NMS (discontinue and monitor closely); 3) tardive dyskinesia (discontinue if clinically appropriate); 4) hyperglycemia and diabetes mellitus (monitor hyperglycemia symptoms such as polydipsia, polyuria, polyphagia, and weakness, and monitor glucose if diabetes risk); 5) orthostatic hypotension with or without syncope (caution if cardiovascular/cerebrovascular disease); 6) leukopenia, neutropenia, and agranulocytosis (monitor if prior/baseline leukopenia, and discontinue if the white blood cell count decreases in the absence of other causative factors); 7) seizures (caution if seizure disorder or seizure risk); 8) potential for cognitive and motor impairment (caution operating machinery); 9) body temperature dysregulation (pyrexia, feeling hot; caution if strenuous exercise, extreme heat exposure, anticholinergic medication, dehydration); 10) suicide (risk related to bipolar disorder/schizophrenia; closely supervise high-risk patients); 11) dysphagia (caution if aspiration pneumonia risk); and 12) use in patients with concomitant illness (caution if cardiovascular or other systemic disease).

Regarding the hyperglycemia and diabetes mellitus SGA class warning (item 4 in list above), the report of a consensus development conference suggested that the risks of obesity, diabetes, and hyperlipidemia were higher with the older SGAs clozapine and olanzapine, intermediate with the older SGAs risperidone and quetiapine, and lower with the newer SGAs ziprasidone and aripiprazole, and recommended clinical and (as indicated) laboratory monitoring for obesity, diabetes, and hyperlipidemia for patients taking SGAs (American Diabetes Association et al. 2004). As of early 2015, evidence is consistent with the risks of weight gain and metabolic complications with additional newer SGAs being lower (e.g., with lurasidone) or similar (e.g., with asenapine) compared with older SGAs (De Hert et al. 2012).

The presence or absence of additional USPI warnings/precautions indicates within-class safety/tolerability differences across individual SGAs. For example, as of early 2015, USPIs included four additional warnings/precautions for all of the above-mentioned SGAs, with the following exceptions: 1) weight gain (monitor weight)—ziprasidone excepted; 2) hyperprolactinemia (galactorrhea, amenorrhea, gynecomastia, and impotence risk)—aripiprazole excepted; 3) hyperlipidemia/dyslipidemia (monitor lipids)—ziprasidone and asenapine excepted; and 4) cerebrovascular accidents, including stroke, in elderly patients with dementia-related psychosis (SGAs not approved for dementia-related psychosis)—quetiapine and ziprasidone excepted.

In addition, the USPIs for SGAs with indications for bipolar depression (i.e., olanzapine plus fluoxetine combination, quetiapine, and lurasidone) or unipolar depression (i.e., adjunctive aripiprazole, adjunctive quetiapine, and olanzapine plus fluoxetine combination) included (antidepressant class) boxed warnings of increased risk of suicidal thinking and behavior in children, adolescents, and young adults taking antidepressants, and the need to monitor for worsening and emergence of suicidal thoughts and behaviors.

Clozapine

Clozapine is a dibenzodiazepine derivative, which is distinctive in that it is the prototypical SGA, with high affinities for serotonin 5-HT_{2A}, 5-HT_{2C}, 5-HT_6, and 5-HT_7, histamine H_1, and muscarinic acetylcholine receptors, but only moderate to low dopamine receptor affinity (Bymaster et al. 1996). Clozapine was considered an important advance in psychopharmacology because it provided marked efficacy in psychosis combined with absence of risks of acute EPS and tardive dyskinesia.

Unfortunately, blood dyscrasias and other side effects limit clozapine's utility. Indeed, after its introduction in clinical studies in the United States in the early 1970s, clozapine was withdrawn in 1974 due to the risk of agranulocytosis, and was not approved for schizophrenia until 1989. Although as of early 2015 clozapine lacked any FDA indication for bipolar disorder, clozapine remained of interest because it was the first SGA, and the only agent approved for treatment-resistant schizophrenia and for decreasing suicidal behavior in patients with schizophrenia (Meltzer et al. 2003). Uncontrolled reports (for a review, see Frye et al. 1998) and a controlled trial (Suppes et al. 1999) suggested that clozapine may be effective in patients with treatment-refractory bipolar disorder.

Clozapine is well absorbed, with 70% bioavailability, 97% protein binding, a linear dose–serum concentration relationship, and a half-life of 12 hours (Byerly and DeVane 1996). Clozapine is extensively metabolized by CYP1A2 and to a lesser extent by CYP3A4 and does not appear to robustly induce or inhibit CYP isozymes, so that other medications influencing clozapine pharmacokinetics account for most clozapine pharmacokinetic drug interactions. Caution is advised when administering clozapine to older adults or patients with hepatic or renal impairment (Physicians' Desk Reference 2014).

Case report data suggest that sporadic individuals taking clozapine with lithium could develop NMS (Pope et al. 1986). Limited data suggest that valproate could decrease clozapine levels in some patients (Longo and Salzman 1995). Clozapine metabolism is consistently increased with carbamazepine (Tiihonen et al. 1995) (Tables 8–1 and 8–6), and the combination of clozapine with carbamazepine is not recommended in view of possible (but not proven) synergistic bone marrow suppression (Junghan et al. 1993). A single case of increased clozapine with lamotrigine has been reported (Kossen et al. 2001).

The CYP1A2 inhibitor fluvoxamine can yield clinically significant increases in serum clozapine concentrations (Wang et al. 2004). Nefazodone may increase serum clozapine concentrations, but the clinical significance of this interaction has been questioned. Clozapine may modestly inhibit CYP2C9 and CYP2D6, and thus could increase serum nortriptyline concentrations (Smith and Riskin 1994).

Caution needs to be exercised when combining clozapine with benzodiazepines because some patients may develop respiratory depression or even arrest (Klimke and Klieser 1994).

Tobacco smoking induces CYP1A2 (Zevin and Benowitz 1999), decreasing serum clozapine concentrations (Meyer 2001). In contrast, caffeine in excess of 400 mg/day only modestly increases serum clozapine concentrations (Raaska et al. 2004). Phenytoin and rifampin may decrease clozapine plasma levels, whereas cimetidine, ciprofloxacin, and erythromycin may increase clozapine plasma levels. Clozapine may potentiate the hypotensive effects of antihypertensive drugs and side effects of anticholinergic drugs.

Clozapine generally has a challenging adverse-effect profile compared with other treatment options, and thus tends to be held in reserve for patients with treatment-resistant bipolar disorder (Suppes et al. 1999). The most common adverse effects associated with clozapine discontinuation include fever and CNS (sedation, seizures, dizziness), cardiovascular (tachycardia, hypotension, syncope, ECG changes), gastrointestinal (nausea, vomiting), and hematological (leukopenia, granulocytopenia, agranulocytosis) problems (Iqbal et al. 2003). Thus, the clozapine USPI includes boxed warnings regarding the risks of 1) agranulocytosis, 2) seizures, 3) myocarditis, 4) other adverse cardiovascular and respiratory effects, and 5) increased mortality (primarily cardiovascular or infectious) in older adults with dementia-related psychosis (an antipsychotic class warning) (Physicians' Desk Reference 2014). Other adverse cardiovascular and respiratory effects include orthostatic hypotension, syncope, respiratory/cardiac arrest (1 per 3,000 patients), tachycardia, and ECG repolarization changes. Clozapine adverse effects include cardiomyopathy (8.9 per 100,000 patient-years), fever, pulmonary embolism (fatal in 1 per 3,500 patient-years), increased transaminases, hepatitis, anticholinergic symptoms (constipation, urinary retention), hypersalivation, and headache. As of early 2015, clozapine had not been associated with congenital malformations in humans (FDA pregnancy category B).

Clozapine is commonly initiated at 25 mg/day and increased by 25–50 mg/day every 4–7 days, with 900 mg/day the maximum final dosage in schizophrenia (Table 8–4). In patients with treatment-refractory bipolar disorder, final dosages of clozapine often range between 50 and 250 mg/day, given all or mostly at bedtime, and commonly in combination with other medications. Indeed, in a controlled trial, mean dosages of adjunctive clozapine in bipolar disorder and schizoaffective disorder patients were 234 and 623 mg/day, respectively (Suppes et al. 1999).

Risperidone

Risperidone is a benzisoxazole derivative (structurally different from the benzepines clozapine, olanzapine, and quetiapine), which is distinctive in that although it yields substantial dopamine D_2 receptor antagonism (and thus is a potent antipsychotic that yields hyperprolactinemia), it has even greater serotonin 5-HT_{2A} antagonism, and perhaps for this reason at low dosages (i.e., <6 mg/day) is associated with only limited EPS. Risperidone blocks serotonin 5-HT_{2A} and 5-HT_{1A}, dopamine D_1 and D_2, α_1- and α_2-adrenergic, and histamine H_1 receptors (Bymaster et al. 1996).

Risperidone is well absorbed, with 70% bioavailability, 90% protein binding, a linear dose-to-serum concentration relationship, and a half-life of 6 hours in extensive CYP2D6 metabolizers and of 24 hours in poor CYP2D6 metabolizers (Byerly and DeVane 1996). Risperidone is substantially metabolized, with less than 30% excreted unchanged in the urine, whereas its main active metabolite, 9-hydroxy-risperidone (paliperidone), is removed primarily by renal excretion. The 9-hydroxy-risperidone metabolite has activity similar to that of risperidone, and risperidone with 9-hydroxy-risperidone are together referred to as the *active moiety*, which has a half-life of 20 hours and protein binding of 90% for risperidone and 70% for 9-hydroxy-risperidone. Based on pharmacokinetics related to the prominent renal excretion of the active moiety, risperidone dose reduction and cautious dose titration may be necessary in older adults and in patients with renal disease (Snoeck et al. 1995). Risperidone does not appear to induce or inhibit CYP isozymes (Shin et al. 1999), although lower risperidone doses may also be necessary in patients with hepatic impairment (Physicians' Desk Reference 2014).

Carbamazepine consistently yields clinically significant induction of risperidone metabolism (Yatham et al. 2003) (Tables 8–1 and 8–6). Case reports suggest that sporadic individuals could develop serious adverse effects such as NMS when risperidone is combined with lithium (Bourgeois and Kahn 2003). Also, a single case of increased risperidone with lamotrigine has been reported (Bienentreu and Kronmüller 2005).

Case studies suggest that some individuals taking risperidone with clozapine may experience increased serum clozapine (Koreen et al. 1995) or risperidone (Physicians' Desk Reference 2014) concentrations, and even a neurotoxic syndrome (mild NMS) (Kontaxakis et al. 2002). The CYP2D6 inhibitor thioridazine increases risperidone serum concentrations.

Paroxetine, fluoxetine, and fluvoxamine can also increase serum risperidone concentrations. Occasional patients may experience substantive increases in serum risperidone concentrations with sertraline.

A single case report suggested that risperidone could yield clinically significant decreases in serum zonisamide concentrations (Okumura 1999).

Rifampin induces and ketoconazole inhibits risperidone metabolism, whereas cimetidine and ranitidine can increase risperidone bioavailability. Risperidone may enhance hypotensive effects of other medications and antagonize the effects of levodopa and dopamine agonists.

The most common adverse events associated with risperidone discontinuation in acute mania trials were somnolence, dizziness, and EPS. Dose-related EPS are particularly evident above 6 mg/day.

In addition to the USPI SGA class warnings mentioned above (see introduction to "Second-Generation Antipsychotics"), the risperidone USPI includes warnings of the risk of thrombotic thrombocytopenic pur-

pura and antiemetic effects (Physicians' Desk Reference 2014). Other adverse effects include orthostatic hypotension, tachycardia, QTc prolongation, seizures (in 0.3% of patients), hyperprolactinemia, amenorrhea, galactorrhea, decreased libido and sexual function, rhinitis, constipation, and dysphagia. Concerns have been raised regarding an increased risk of prolactinoma with risperidone. As of early 2015, risperidone had not been associated with congenital malformations in humans (FDA pregnancy category C).

Risperidone in acute mania is commonly initiated at 2–3 mg/day and increased by 1 mg/day on a daily basis as necessary and tolerated, with final dosages ranging between 1 and 6 mg/day (Table 8–4), and averaging approximately 4–6 mg/day in controlled trials (Hirschfeld et al. 2004; Khanna et al. 2003; Sachs et al. 2002; Yatham et al. 2003). So that adverse effects can be limited in patients with less acute bipolar disorder, risperidone may be started at 0.25–0.5 mg/day and increased as necessary and tolerated every 4–7 days by 0.25–0.5 mg/day, with an initial target dose of 1–2 mg/day. In patients with bipolar disorder, risperidone is often administered all or mostly at bedtime, and commonly in combination with other medications. Risperidone long-acting injectable formulation (LAI) is initiated at 25 mg every 2 weeks, overlapping with oral risperidone or other oral antipsychotic, and increased monthly as necessary and tolerated to as high as 50 mg intramuscularly every 2 weeks. In a controlled trial in a type of rapid cycling called *frequently relapsing bipolar disorder* (patients with four or more mood episodes requiring treatment in the prior year), the mean dose of risperidone LAI added to treatment as usual was 29.7 mg every 2 weeks (Macfadden et al. 2009).

Olanzapine

Olanzapine is a thienobenzodiazepine derivative that is distinctive in that it was the first successful structural analog of clozapine, with a receptor binding profile overlapping that of clozapine, and thus blocking serotonin 5-HT_{2A}, 5-HT_{2C}, and 5-HT_3, dopamine D_1, D_2, and D_4, α_1-adrenergic, histamine H_1, and muscarinic cholinergic receptors (Bymaster et al. 1996).

Olanzapine is well absorbed, with greater than 80% bioavailability, 93% protein binding, a half-life of 30 hours, and linear pharmacokinetics at doses up to 20 mg (Callaghan et al. 1999). Olanzapine is extensively (>80%) metabolized, primarily via UGT1A4 glucuronidation and CYP1A2 oxidation, but does not induce or inhibit CYP isozymes. Lower olanzapine doses may be necessary in older adults but not routinely in patients with hepatic or renal impairment (Physicians' Desk Reference 2014).

Case reports suggest that sporadic individuals could develop serious adverse effects such as NMS when olanzapine is combined with lithium. Valproate may occasionally lower serum olanzapine concentrations. Carbamazepine substantially decreases olanzapine concentrations (Tables 8–1 and 8–6).

The CYP1A2 inhibitor fluvoxamine yields clinically significant increases in serum olanzapine concentrations, whereas CYP1A2 inducers such as omeprazole might decrease serum olanzapine concentrations. Ciprofloxacin may increase serum olanzapine concentrations. Tobacco smoking can decrease serum olanzapine concentrations, and women compared with men may have slightly (approximately 25%) decreased olanzapine clearance.

Olanzapine may enhance hypotensive effects of other medications, whereas diazepam and alcohol may enhance olanzapine's hypotensive effects. Olanzapine may antagonize the effects of levodopa and dopamine agonists.

The most common adverse effects with oral olanzapine are somnolence, dry mouth, dizziness, asthenia, constipation, dyspepsia, increased appetite, and tremor. Weight gain is more of a problem with olanzapine than with lithium or valproate. Olanzapine-related weight gain can be approached in a fashion similar to that described earlier in this chapter for lithium, but can be particularly challenging to manage. Somnolence is the most common adverse effect with intramuscular olanzapine. Maximal dosing of intramuscular olanzapine may yield substantial orthostatic hypotension, so that administration of additional doses to patients with clinically significant postural changes in systolic blood pressure is not recommended.

In addition to the USPI SGA class warnings mentioned above (see introduction to "Second-Generation Antipsychotics"), the olanzapine USPI includes a warning of the risk of priapism (Physicians' Desk Reference 2014). Other noteworthy adverse effects include orthostatic hypotension, syncope (in 0.6% of patients), seizures (in 0.9% of patients), hyperprolactinemia, and benign transaminase elevations (in 0.2% of patients). As of early 2015, olanzapine had not been associated with congenital malformations in humans (FDA pregnancy category C).

In acute mania monotherapy, olanzapine is commonly initiated at 10–15 mg/day and increased by 5 mg daily as necessary and tolerated, with final dosages ranging between 5 and 20 mg/day (Table 8–4), and averaging 15–16 mg/day in controlled trials (Tohen et al. 1999, 2000). In acute mania adjunctive therapy, olanzapine is commonly initiated at 10–15 mg/day and increased by 5 mg daily as necessary and tolerated, with final dosages ranging between 5 and 20 mg/day, and averaging

10.4 mg/day in a controlled trial (Tohen et al. 2002). In acute bipolar I depression, olanzapine was dosed more conservatively, with a mean final dosage of 7.4 mg/day (combined with a mean final dosage of fluoxetine of 39.3 mg/day) (Tohen et al. 2003b). In monotherapy maintenance treatment for bipolar I disorder, the mean final olanzapine dosage was 12.5 mg/day (Tohen et al. 2006). In patients with bipolar disorder, olanzapine is often administered all or mostly at bedtime, and commonly in combination with other medications. In acute agitation, intramuscular olanzapine is started with 10 mg, with repeat doses of 10 mg as necessary and tolerated after 2 hours and 6 hours, with a maximum dose of 30 mg in a 24-hour period. Lower doses are recommended in older adults (5 mg intramuscular once) or debilitated patients (2.5 mg intramuscular once).

Quetiapine

Quetiapine is a dibenzothiazepine derivative (structural analog of clozapine) that is distinctive in that, like clozapine, it has very low dopamine D_2 receptor affinity and, hence, very low risk of EPS (Bymaster et al. 1996; Nemeroff et al. 2002). However, unlike clozapine, quetiapine also has low serotonin $5-HT_{2A}$ receptor affinity (albeit greater than that for D_2 receptors). Quetiapine has high histamine H_1 receptor affinity (likely contributing to somnolence/sedation) and α_1-adrenergic receptor affinity (likely contributing to orthostasis), but it has low muscarinic cholinergic receptor affinity. Quetiapine has an active norquetiapine metabolite that blocks norepinephrine reuptake, potentially contributing to antidepressant effects (López-Muñoz and Alamo 2013).

Quetiapine is 100% bioavailable, with 83% protein binding, and has linear pharmacokinetics at dosages between 200 and 750 mg/day, and a short half-life of 6 hours (DeVane and Nemeroff 2001). Quetiapine is extensively metabolized, primarily by CYP3A4, and does not have clinically significant effects on CYP isozymes. Lower quetiapine doses may be necessary in older adults and in patients with hepatic (but not routinely with renal) impairment (Physicians' Desk Reference 2014).

Quetiapine metabolism is increased with carbamazepine, whereas valproate may or may not yield clinically significant increases in quetiapine serum concentrations (Tables 8–1 and 8–6). Therapeutic drug monitoring database information suggested that lamotrigine might substantively decrease serum quetiapine concentrations (Table 8–1).

Quetiapine metabolism is increased with phenytoin. The CYP3A4 inhibitors ketoconazole and erythromycin increase in serum quetiapine concentrations.

Quetiapine combined with medications with sedative effects may yield additive sedative effects. Quetiapine may enhance hypotensive effects of other medications, and may antagonize the effects of levodopa and dopamine agonists. False-positive urine drug screens using immunoassays for methadone or tricyclic antidepressants have been reported in patients taking quetiapine.

Caution is indicated when combining quetiapine with drugs known to cause electrolyte imbalance or to increase the QTc interval. Concerns regarding QTc prolongation have included the possibility of exacerbation of this problem if quetiapine is combined with other agents with this adverse effect, such as ziprasidone, asenapine, chlorpromazine, thioridazine, pimozide, and paliperidone. Systematic studies are lacking to assess the clinical significance of such putative pharmacodynamic interactions.

The most common adverse events with quetiapine are somnolence, dizziness (postural hypotension), dry mouth, constipation, increased serum glutamate pyruvate transaminase, weight gain, and dyspepsia (Adler et al. 2007).

In addition to the USPI SGA class warnings mentioned above (see introduction to "Second-Generation Antipsychotics"), the quetiapine USPI includes warnings of the risks of QTc prolongation, priapism, increased blood pressure in youth, cataracts, hypothyroidism, increased transaminases, and withdrawal symptoms. Concern regarding the development of cataracts in dogs has led to a recommendation of ophthalmological examinations, but the risk in humans appears to be low. Quetiapine therapy entails risks of syncope (in 1% of patients) and seizures (in 0.5% of patients). As of early 2015, quetiapine had not been associated with congenital malformations in humans (FDA pregnancy category C).

In acute mania, quetiapine is commonly initiated at 100 mg/day in two divided doses, and increased daily by 100 mg as necessary and tolerated, with final dosages ranging between 400 and 800 mg/day (Table 8–4), and averaging approximately 500–600 mg/day in responders in controlled trials (Bowden et al. 2005; McIntyre et al. 2005; Sachs et al. 2004; Yatham et al. 2004). In acute bipolar I or II depression, quetiapine is commonly initiated at 50 mg/day at bedtime, and increased daily by 100 mg as necessary and tolerated, with final dosages ranging between 300 and 600 mg/day in controlled trials (Calabrese et al. 2005; Thase et al. 2006). The USPI for the longer-term adjunctive use of quetiapine notes that dosages of 400–800 mg/day in divided doses were used in the registration studies and that generally patients in the maintenance phase ought to be continued on the same dose on which they were stabilized in the stabilization phase. However, the quetiapine USPI also states that patients should be treated with the lowest quetiapine dose needed to maintain remission. Given the risk of adverse effects, it is prudent to start quetiapine in euthymic patients in a gradual fashion similar to initiation in depressed patients, rather than in the rapid fashion used in manic patients.

The quetiapine extended-release (XR) formulation in adults with acute illness (e.g., acute mania) may be started at 300 mg in the evening and increased, as necessary and tolerated, to 600 mg in the evening on day 2 and to 800 mg in the evening on day 3, with the maximum dose being 800 mg in the evening. In adults with less acute illness (e.g., bipolar depression), quetiapine XR may be started at 50 mg in the evening, and increased, as necessary and tolerated, to 100 mg in the evening on day 2, to 200 mg in the evening on day 3, and to 300 mg in the evening on day 4, with the recommended and maximum dose being 300 mg in the evening.

Ziprasidone

Ziprasidone is a benzisothiazole derivative, which is distinctive in that it is a particularly robust serotonin 5-HT_{2A} compared with dopamine D_2 receptor antagonist. Ziprasidone blocks serotonin 5-HT_{2C} and 5-HT_{1D} receptors, is a partial agonist at serotonin 5-HT_{1A} receptors, and is a serotonin and norepinephrine reuptake inhibitor, but has low affinities for α_1-adrenergic, histamine H_1, and muscarinic cholinergic M_1 receptors (Stahl and Shayegan 2003).

Concurrent ingestion of food doubles ziprasidone absorption from approximately 30% to 60%. Ziprasidone is 99% bound to plasma proteins, has a half-life of 6.6 hours, and is extensively metabolized, two-thirds by aldehyde oxidase reduction and one-third by CYP3A4 oxidation; however, it does not have clinically significant effects on CYP isozymes. Ziprasidone dose adjustment is not routinely necessary in older adults or in patients with hepatic or renal impairment (Physicians' Desk Reference 2014).

Carbamazepine decreases serum ziprasidone concentrations, but the clinical significance of this interaction remains to be determined (Tables 8–1 and 8–6). Case reports suggest that sporadic individuals could develop serious adverse effects, such as NMS when ziprasidone is combined with lithium, blood dyscrasia with ziprasidone and quetiapine, and a possible serotonin syndrome with citalopram following cross-titration from clozapine to ziprasidone.

Ketoconazole increases serum ziprasidone concentrations, but the clinical significance of this interaction remains to be determined.

In addition to the USPI SGA class warnings mentioned above (see introduction to "Second-Generation Antipsychotics"), the ziprasidone USPI includes warnings of the risks of QTc prolongation and rash (Physicians' Desk Reference 2014). Concerns regarding QTc prolongation have included the possibility of exacerbation of this problem if ziprasidone is combined with other agents having this adverse effect, such as quetiapine, asenapine, chlorpromazine, thioridazine, pimozide, and paliperidone. Systematic studies are lacking to assess the clinical significance of such putative pharmacodynamic interactions.

The most common adverse events associated with discontinuation of ziprasidone in acute mania were akathisia, anxiety, depression, dizziness, dystonia, rash, and vomiting. The most common adverse events with intramuscular ziprasidone for agitation in schizophrenia patients were headache, nausea, and somnolence.

Ziprasidone and aripiprazole, compared with risperidone, olanzapine, and quetiapine, can yield less sedation but more akathisia. In patients with acute mania, akathisia is commonly accompanied by and at times difficult to distinguish from agitation and anxiety. These overlapping symptoms may attenuate with adjunctive benzodiazepine therapy. Indeed, meta-analysis suggests that benzodiazepines (e.g., clonazepam 0.5–2.5 mg/day) can reduce symptoms of akathisia in the short term (Lima et al. 2002). There are more limited data regarding the utility of other agents for antipsychotic-related akathisia. Meta-analyses suggest that there are insufficient data to recommend β-blockers and that there is no reliable evidence to support or refute the utility of anticholinergics. In other controlled studies, mirtazapine 15 mg/day and propranolol 80 mg/day were superior to placebo in a 90-patient, 1-week trial (Poyurovsky et al. 2006); vitamin B_6 1,200 mg/day tended to be superior to placebo in a 20-patient, 5-day trial; and the $5-HT_2$ antagonist mianserin 15 mg/day was superior to placebo in a 30-patient, 5-day trial. In some patients it may even be necessary to switch to clozapine to avoid akathisia (Bratti et al. 2007).

Other adverse effects include benign rash (in 5% of patients), orthostatic hypotension, syncope (in 0.6% of patients), and seizures (in 0.4% of patients). As of early 2015, ziprasidone had not been associated with congenital malformations in humans (FDA pregnancy category C).

In acute mania, ziprasidone is commonly initiated at 80 mg/day administered with food in two divided doses, and increased as necessary and tolerated on day 2 to 120–160 mg/day administered with food in two divided doses, with final doses ranging between 80 and 160 mg/day (Table 8–4) and averaging approximately 125–130 mg/day in controlled trials (Keck et al. 2003b; Potkin et al. 2005). In clinical practice, lower (e.g.,

<80 mg/day) compared with higher (e.g., ≥80 mg/day) ziprasidone dosages may increase the risk of akathisia (Oral et al. 2006), so that optimal titration of this agent may involve avoiding lower doses to prevent akathisia or abruptly increasing to higher doses if akathisia develops at lower doses. Also, for convenience, and in view of the risk of sedation, dosing may be weighted toward dinner time or bedtime with a snack. Although not recommended in the USPI, occasional patients may tolerate and benefit from dosages as high as 240–320 mg/day. For agitation in schizophrenia, intramuscular ziprasidone 10 mg is administered and repeated as often as every 2 hours as necessary and tolerated, with a maximum of 40 mg/day for 3 days.

Aripiprazole

Aripiprazole is a quinolinone derivative, which is distinctive in that it is a partial agonist at dopamine D_2 and serotonin 5-HT$_{1A}$ receptors (Burris et al. 2002). As a dopamine D_2 partial agonist, aripiprazole may "stabilize" dopaminergic neurotransmission, by decreasing dopamine neurotransmission in high dopamine states such as mania and by increasing dopamine neurotransmission in low dopamine states such as bipolar depression. Aripiprazole is also an antagonist at serotonin 5-HT$_{2A}$ receptors, with limited affinity for histamine H_1 receptors and low affinity for muscarinic cholinergic receptors (Lawler et al. 1999; Swainston Harrison and Perry 2004).

Aripiprazole has a bioavailability of 87%, is 99% bound to plasma proteins, has a long 72-hour half-life (Mallikaarjun et al. 2004), and is metabolized to an active dehydroaripiprazole metabolite that has an even longer half-life of 94 hours. Aripiprazole is extensively metabolized, primarily through oxidation by CYP2D6 and CYP3A4, although it does not have clinically significant effects on CYP isozymes (Swainston Harrison and Perry 2004). Although concerns have been raised regarding the possibility of inhibitors of CYP2D6 and CYP3A4 and inducers of CYP3A4 affecting aripiprazole pharmacokinetics, systematic data regarding such putative interactions are limited. Aripiprazole dose adjustment is not routinely necessary in older adults or in patients with hepatic or renal impairment (Physicians' Desk Reference 2014).

Carbamazepine induces aripiprazole metabolism (Nakamura et al. 2009) (Tables 8–1 and 8–6). Sporadic individuals could develop serious adverse effects such as NMS when aripiprazole is combined with lithium.

The USPI for aripiprazole notes that the CYP2D6 inhibitors fluoxetine and paroxetine could increase serum aripiprazole concentrations (Physicians' Desk Reference 2014), and case reports suggest that sporadic problems with aripiprazole combined with antidepressants may include possible NMS when aripiprazole is combined with fluoxetine (Duggal and Kithas 2005) and urinary obstruction when aripiprazole is combined with citalopram (Padala et al. 2006). Quinidine and ketoconazole appear to increase serum aripiprazole concentrations (Physicians' Desk Reference 2014).

The most common adverse events with oral aripiprazole in acute mania trials were CNS (headache, agitation/anxiety/akathisia, insomnia, somnolence) and gastrointestinal (nausea, dyspepsia, vomiting, constipation) problems (Keck et al. 2003a; Sachs et al. 2006b; Vieta et al. 2005). The most common adverse events with intramuscular aripiprazole in an acute agitation in mania trial were also CNS (headache, dizziness, insomnia, somnolence) and gastrointestinal (nausea, vomiting) problems. The most common adverse events with oral aripiprazole in a longer-term treatment of bipolar disorder trial were again CNS (anxiety, insomnia, depression, nervousness, tremor, agitation, asthenia, headache, akathisia) and gastrointestinal (nausea) problems, as well as upper respiratory infection, vaginitis, and pain in the extremities. Aripiprazole-related akathisia may respond to aripiprazole dose reduction or the addition of a benzodiazepine, although in some patients it may even be necessary to switch to clozapine (Bratti et al. 2007).

Gastrointestinal adverse effects such as nausea, dyspepsia, constipation, vomiting, and diarrhea may be related to dopamine partial agonist effects and tend to diminish with ongoing exposure. Because of its long half-life, aripiprazole can be dosed once daily; however, during the first few days of treatment, the lower maximum concentrations associated with divided doses may offer enhanced tolerability. Thus, tolerability may be enhanced in patients with gastrointestinal or other adverse effects if aripiprazole is initiated at 7.5 mg twice daily (or lower if necessary) for a few days before being gradually increased to as high as 30 mg/day.

Other noteworthy aripiprazole adverse effects include orthostatic hypotension, syncope (in 0.5% of patients), seizures (in 0.1% of patients), and dysphagia. As of early 2015, aripiprazole had not been associated with congenital malformations in humans (FDA pregnancy category C).

In acute manic and mixed episodes, as monotherapy or as adjunctive (added to lithium or divalproex) treatment, oral aripiprazole is recommended in the USPI to be initiated in adults in a single dose of 15 mg/day, and in children and adolescents at 2 mg/day and titrated to the 10-mg/day recommended dose (Physicians' Desk Reference 2014). The maximum recommended dose is 30 mg/day for both adult and pediatric patients with acute manic or mixed episodes (Table 8–4). In early clinical trials in acute manic and mixed episodes in adults, aripiprazole was started at 30 mg/day, and in approximately 15% of patients the aripiprazole dosage was decreased from 30 to 15 mg/day because of tolerability problems, yielding a mean dose of approximately 28 mg/day (Keck et al. 2003a; Sachs et al. 2006b; Vieta et al. 2005). In monotherapy maintenance treatment for bipolar I disorder, oral aripiprazole final doses averaged approximately 24 mg/day (Keck et al. 2006). In two negative acute bipolar I nonpsychotic depression studies, aripiprazole monotherapy was initiated at 10 mg/day and flexibly dosed within a range of 5–30 mg/day, with a pooled mean dose of 16.5 mg/day (Thase et al. 2008). Citing high discontinuation rates, the authors speculated that this dosing may have been too aggressive for acute bipolar depression. Indeed, in adjunctive (added to antidepressants) treatment of unipolar major depressive disorder, oral aripiprazole is recommended in the USPI to be initiated in adults at 2–5 mg/day and titrated to a recommended dose of only 5–10 mg/day (Physicians' Desk Reference 2014). It may be that the latter more conservative dosing would be better tolerated than higher doses in depressed or euthymic bipolar disorder patients. Intramuscular aripiprazole is recommended to be administered as a 9.75-mg injection, or 5.25-mg injection if clinically indicated, with repeated 9.75-mg (or 5.25-mg) injections as often as every 2 hours as necessary and tolerated, with a maximum of 30 mg/day. The USPI does not recommend 15-mg intramuscular injections, because of concerns regarding adverse effects and the lack of additional benefit with doses over 9.75 mg per injection in clinical trials.

Asenapine

Asenapine is a dibenzo-oxepino pyrrole derivative, which is distinctive because it is an antagonist at multiple serotonin (5-HT$_{1A}$, 5-HT$_{1B}$, 5-HT$_{2A}$, 5-HT$_{2B}$, 5-HT$_{2C}$, 5-HT$_5$, 5-HT$_6$, and 5-HT$_7$), adrenergic (α_1, α_{2A}, α_{2B}, and α_{2C}), dopamine (D$_2$, D$_3$, D$_4$, and D$_1$), and histamine (H$_1$ and H$_2$) receptors, but has low affinity for muscarinic cholinergic receptors (Shahid et al. 2009). Asenapine's complex receptor actions include the SGA "core effects" of serotonin 5-HT$_{2A}$ and dopamine D$_2$ receptor antagonism.

Asenapine's bioavailability using the recommended sublingual route of administration is 35%, whereas its bioavailability using the (not recommended) oral route is less than 2% because of a large first-pass effect (Physicians' Desk Reference 2014). Patients need to be advised to avoid eating or drinking for 10 minutes after taking asenapine. Asenapine is 95% bound to plasma proteins and has a 24-hour half-life. Asenapine is metabolized primarily by UGT1A4 glucuronidation and by CYP1A2 oxidation; it is a weak inhibitor of CYP2D6 so asenapine should be coadministered cautiously with drugs that are either substrates and/or inhibitors of CYP2D6 (Physicians' Desk Reference 2014). Asenapine is not recommended in patients with severe hepatic impairment, which can yield clinically significant increases in serum asenapine concentrations, although asenapine dose adjustment is not routinely necessary in older adults or in patients with renal impairment (Physicians' Desk Reference 2014).

Asenapine does not usually have clinically significant pharmacokinetic interactions with lithium, valproate, or carbamazepine (Physicians' Desk Reference 2014) (Table 8–1), and clinically significant pharmacokinetic interactions with lamotrigine are not anticipated.

However, the CYP1A2 inhibitor fluvoxamine yielded clinically significant increases in asenapine serum concentrations. Because asenapine weakly inhibits CYP2D6, it can increase serum concentrations of CYP2D6 substrates (Physicians' Desk Reference 2014). Tobacco smoking does not alter asenapine pharmacokinetics, in spite of CYP1A2 contributing to asenapine metabolism.

The most common asenapine adverse effects in acute mania trials included somnolence, dizziness, EPS other than akathisia, and weight gain. Weight gain in acute mania trials was greater than with placebo but less than with olanzapine. In addition to the USPI SGA class warnings mentioned above (see introduction to "Second-Generation Antipsychotics"), the asenapine USPI includes warnings of the risks of priapism and QTc prolongation. The asenapine USPI recommendation to avoid combining asenapine with other agents that cause QTc prolongation (e.g., chlorpromazine, thioridazine, ziprasidone) has been criticized as being overly conservative, in view of the modest degree of QTc prolongation observed with asenapine (Preskorn and Flockhart 2009). As of early 2015, asenapine had not been associated with congenital malformations in humans (FDA pregnancy category C).

Patients may complain of a bitter taste or oral hypoesthesia related to the sublingual route of asenapine administration. Use of the black cherry flavor formulation can help mitigate the former problem.

In acute mania monotherapy, asenapine is commonly initiated at 10 mg/day and increased as necessary and tolerated by 5 mg on a daily basis, with final doses ranging between 10 and 20 mg/day (Table 8–4), and averaging 18.2 and 18.4 mg/day in controlled trials (McIntyre 2009, 2010). In acute mania adjunctive therapy, asenapine is commonly initiated at 5–10 mg/day and increased as necessary and tolerated by 5 mg on a daily basis, with final doses ranging between 10 and 20 mg/day, and averaging 11.8 mg/day in a controlled trial (Szegedi et al. 2012). In less acute situations, asenapine is commonly initiated at 5–10 mg/day and increased as necessary and tolerated by 5 mg every 4–7 days, with final doses ranging between 10 and 20 mg/day.

Lurasidone

Lurasidone is a benzoisothiazol derivative, which is distinctive in that it is a serotonin 5-HT$_7$ receptor antagonist (consistent with putative pro-cognitive effects), a serotonin 5-HT$_{1A}$ receptor partial agonist (consistent with putative antidepressant effects), and an α_{2C}-adrenergic receptor antagonist (Ishibashi et al. 2010; Meyer et al. 2009). Like other SGAs, lurasidone is an antagonist at serotonin 5-HT$_{2A}$ and dopamine D$_2$ receptors. Lurasidone has minimal affinities for histamine H$_1$ and muscarinic cholinergic receptors.

Lurasidone has oral bioavailability of 9%–19%, is 99% plasma protein bound, has an 18-hour half-life, and is extensively metabolized, primarily by CYP3A4, but does not have clinically significant effects on CYP isozymes (Meyer et al. 2009). Concurrent ingestion of at least 350 calories of food doubles lurasidone absorption (Meyer et al. 2009). Lower lurasidone doses may be necessary in patients with hepatic or renal impairment but are not routinely necessary in older adults (Physicians' Desk Reference 2014).

The lurasidone USPI states that combinations of lurasidone with carbamazepine (as well as with other robust CYP3A4 inducers) and with robust CYP3A4 inhibitors are not recommended due to the risks of clinically significant changes in lurasidone pharmacokinetics (Table 8–1); lurasidone doses should be reduced by half when used with moderate CYP3A4 inhibitors, and may need to be increased when used with moderate CYP3A4 inducers (Physicians' Desk Reference 2014). There has been a single case report of glossopharyngeal dystonia with lurasidone combined with fluoxetine, hypothesized to be due to fluoxetine's CYP3A4 inhibition, which increases serum lurasidone concentration (Paul et al. 2013).

Ketoconazole and diltiazem increased and rifampin decreased serum lurasidone concentrations (Chiu et al. 2014). In contrast to clozapine (and to a more limited extent olanzapine), no lurasidone dose adjustment is recommended in tobacco smokers (Physicians' Desk Reference 2014).

The most common adverse events with lurasidone in acute bipolar depression studies included nausea, akathisia, EPS, and somnolence. As expected, weight gain and anticholinergic side effects were not commonly encountered with lurasidone. As of early 2015, lurasidone had not been associated with congenital malformations in humans (FDA pregnancy category B).

In acute bipolar depression, lurasidone is commonly initiated at 20 mg/day with dinner, and increased every 4–7 days by 20 mg as necessary and tolerated, with final dosages ranging between 20 and 120 mg/day, and averaging approximately 60 mg/day (Table 8–4). Patients who develop akathisia may tolerate lunchtime dosing better than dinnertime dosing, and may benefit from dosage reduction or addition of a benzodiazepine. The average lurasidone doses in controlled acute bipolar depression trials were 62.7 and 66.3 mg/day as monotherapy and adjunctive (added to lithium or valproate) therapy, respectively (Loebel et al. 2014a, 2014b).

■ Conclusion

Effective pharmacotherapy for patients with bipolar disorder requires familiarity with mood stabilizer and antipsychotic pharmacodynamics, pharmacokinetics, dosing, drug interactions, adverse effects, and their management. In the past, clinicians have relied on observational drug interaction information, but characterization of substrates, inhibitors, and inducers of drug metabolism now allows not only the development of mechanistic models but also enhanced anticipation and avoidance of clinical drug-drug interactions. These developments promise to yield safer and more effective therapeutics when psychotropics are combined with one another in treatment of patients with bipolar disorder.

■ References

Abraham G, Owen J: Topiramate can cause lithium toxicity. J Clin Psychopharmacol 24(5):565–567, 2004 15349023

Adab N, Jacoby A, Smith D, et al: Additional educational needs in children born to mothers with epilepsy. J Neurol Neurosurg Psychiatry 70(1):15–21, 2001 11118242

Adan-Manes J, Novalbos J, López-Rodríguez R, et al: Lithium and venlafaxine interaction: a case of serotonin syndrome. J Clin Pharm Ther 31(4):397–400, 2006 16882112

Adler CM, Fleck DE, Brecher M, et al: Safety and tolerability of quetiapine in the treatment of acute mania in bipolar disorder. J Affect Disord 100(Suppl 1):S15–S22, 2007 17383737

Aichhorn W, Marksteiner J, Walch T, et al: Influence of age, gender, body weight and valproate comedication on quetiapine plasma concentrations. Int Clin Psychopharmacol 21(2):81–85, 2006 16421458

Ali S, Pearlman RL, Upadhyay A, et al: Neuroleptic malignant syndrome with aripiprazole and lithium: a case report. J Clin Psychopharmacol 26(4):434–436, 2006 16855467

Allen MH, Hirschfeld RM, Wozniak PJ, et al: Linear relationship of valproate serum concentration to response and optimal serum levels for acute mania. Am J Psychiatry 163(2):272–275, 2006 16449481

Amdisen A, Gottfries CG, Jacobsson L, et al: Grave lithium intoxication with fatal outcome. Acta Psychiatr Scand Suppl 255:25–33, 1974 4533712

American Diabetes Association; American Psychiatric Association; American Association of Clinical Endocrinologists; North American Association for the Study of Obesity: Consensus development conference on antipsychotic drugs and obesity and diabetes. Diabetes Care 27(2):596–601, 2004 14747245

American Psychiatric Association: Practice guideline for the treatment of patients with bipolar disorder (revision). Am J Psychiatry 159(4)(Suppl):1–50, 2002 11958165

Anderson GD, Yau MK, Gidal BE, et al: Bidirectional interaction of valproate and lamotrigine in healthy subjects. Clin Pharmacol Ther 60(2):145–156, 1996 8823232

Andersson ML, Björkhem-Bergman L, Lindh JD: Possible drug-drug interaction between quetiapine and lamotrigine—evidence from a Swedish TDM database. Br J Clin Pharmacol 72(1):153–156, 2011 21651616

Atherton JC, Green R, Hughes S, et al: Lithium clearance in man: effects of dietary salt intake, acute changes in extracellular fluid volume, amiloride and frusemide. Clin Sci (Lond) 73(6):645–651, 1987 3690979

Baldessarini RJ, Tondo L, Faedda GL, et al: Effects of the rate of discontinuing lithium maintenance treatment in bipolar disorders. J Clin Psychiatry 57(10):441–448, 1996 8909329

Barclay ML, Brownlie BE, Turner JG, et al: Lithium associated thyrotoxicosis: a report of 14 cases, with statistical analysis of incidence. Clin Endocrinol (Oxf) 40(6):759–764, 1994 8033366

Bendz H, Aurell M: Drug-induced diabetes insipidus: incidence, prevention and management. Drug Saf 21(6):449–456, 1999 10612269

Bergemann N, Kress KR, Abu-Tair F, et al: Valproate lowers plasma concentration of olanzapine. J Clin Psychopharmacol 26(4):432–434, 2006 16855466

Besag FM, Berry DJ, Pool F, et al: Carbamazepine toxicity with lamotrigine: pharmacokinetic or pharmacodynamic interaction? Epilepsia 39(2):183–187, 1998 9577998

Bienentreu SD, Kronmüller KT: Increase in risperidone plasma level with lamotrigine. Am J Psychiatry 162(4):811–812, 2005 15800164

Bourgeois BF: Pharmacologic interactions between valproate and other drugs. Am J Med 84(1A):29–33, 1988 3146222

Bourgeois JA, Kahn DR: Neuroleptic malignant syndrome following administration of risperidone and lithium. J Clin Psychopharmacol 23(3):315–317, 2003 12826996

Bowden CL, Janicak PG, Orsulak P, et al: Relation of serum valproate concentration to response in mania. Am J Psychiatry 153(6):765–770, 1996 8633687

Bowden CL, Calabrese JR, McElroy SL, et al; Divalproex Maintenance Study Group: A randomized, placebo-controlled 12-month trial of divalproex and lithium in treatment of outpatients with bipolar I disorder. Arch Gen Psychiatry 57(5):481–489, 2000 10807488

Bowden CL, Grunze H, Mullen J, et al: A randomized, double-blind, placebo-controlled efficacy and safety study of quetiapine or lithium as monotherapy for mania in bipolar disorder. J Clin Psychiatry 66(1):111–121, 2005 15669897

Bowden CL, Calabrese JR, Ketter TA, et al: Impact of lamotrigine and lithium on weight in obese and nonobese patients with bipolar I disorder. Am J Psychiatry 163(7):1199–1201, 2006a 16816224

Bowden CL, Swann AC, Calabrese JR, et al; Depakote ER Mania Study Group: A randomized, placebo-controlled, multicenter study of divalproex sodium extended release in the treatment of acute mania. J Clin Psychiatry 67(10):1501–1510, 2006b 17107240

Bratti IM, Kane JM, Marder SR: Chronic restlessness with antipsychotics. Am J Psychiatry 164(11):1648–1654, 2007 17974927

Bray GA, Hollander P, Klein S, et al: A 6-month randomized, placebo-controlled, dose-ranging trial of topiramate for weight loss in obesity. Obes Res 11(6):722–733, 2003 12805393

Bryant AE3rd, Dreifuss FE: Valproic acid hepatic fatalities. III. U.S. experience since 1986. Neurology 46(2):465–469, 1996 8614514

Burris KD, Molski TF, Xu C, et al: Aripiprazole, a novel antipsychotic, is a high-affinity partial agonist at human dopamine D2 receptors. J Pharmacol Exp Ther 302(1):381–389, 2002 12065741

Byerly MJ, DeVane CL: Pharmacokinetics of clozapine and risperidone: a review of recent literature. J Clin Psychopharmacol 16(2):177–187, 1996 8690833

Bymaster FP, Calligaro DO, Falcone JF, et al: Radioreceptor binding profile of the atypical antipsychotic olanzapine. Neuropsychopharmacology 14(2):87–96, 1996 8822531

Calabrese JR, Bowden CL, Sachs G, et al; Lamictal 605 Study Group: A placebo-controlled 18-month trial of lamotrigine and lithium maintenance treatment in recently depressed patients with bipolar I disorder. J Clin Psychiatry 64(9):1013–1024, 2003 14628976

Calabrese JR, Keck PE Jr, Macfadden W, et al: A randomized, double-blind, placebo-controlled trial of quetiapine in the treatment of bipolar I or II depression. Am J Psychiatry 162(7):1351–1360, 2005 15994719

Callaghan JT, Bergstrom RF, Ptak LR, et al: Olanzapine: pharmacokinetic and pharmacodynamic profile. Clin Pharmacokinet 37(3):177–193, 1999 10511917

Castrogiovanni P: A novel slow-release formulation of lithium carbonate (Carbolithium Once-A-Day) vs. standard Carbolithium: a comparative pharmacokinetic study. Clin Ter 153(2):107–115, 2002 12078335

Chiu YY, Ereshefsky L, Preskorn SH, et al: Lurasidone drug-drug interaction studies: a comprehensive review. Drug Metabol Drug Interact 29(3):191–202, 2014 24825095

Christensen J, Petrenaite V, Atterman J, et al: Oral contraceptives induce lamotrigine metabolism: evidence from a double-blind, placebo-controlled trial. Epilepsia 48(3):484–489, 2007 17346247

Cohen LS, Friedman JM, Jefferson JW, et al: A reevaluation of risk of in utero exposure to lithium. JAMA 271(2):146–150, 1994 8031346

Cohen LS, Sichel DA, Robertson LM, et al: Postpartum prophylaxis for women with bipolar disorder. Am J Psychiatry 152(11):1641–1645, 1995 7485628

Correll CU, Sikich L, Reeves G, et al: Metformin for antipsychotic-related weight gain and metabolic abnormalities: when, for whom, and for how long? Am J Psychiatry 170(9):947–952, 2013 24030606

Cunnington M, Tennis P; International Lamotrigine Pregnancy Registry Scientific Advisory Committee: Lamotrigine and the risk of malformations in pregnancy. Neurology 64(6):955–960, 2005 15781807

De Hert M, Yu W, Detraux J, et al: Body weight and metabolic adverse effects of asenapine, iloperidone, lurasidone and paliperidone in the treatment of schizophrenia and bipolar disorder: a systematic review and exploratory meta-analysis. CNS Drugs 26(9):733–759, 2012 22900950

Denicoff KD, Smith-Jackson EE, Disney ER, et al: Comparative prophylactic efficacy of lithium, carbamazepine, and the combination in bipolar disorder. J Clin Psychiatry 58(11):470–478, 1997 9413412

DeVane CL: Pharmacokinetics, drug interactions, and tolerability of valproate. Psychopharmacol Bull 37(Suppl 2):25–42, 2003 14624231

DeVane CL, Nemeroff CB: Clinical pharmacokinetics of quetiapine: an atypical antipsychotic. Clin Pharmacokinet 40(7):509–522, 2001 11510628

Diav-Citrin O, Shechtman S, Tahover E, et al: Pregnancy outcome following in utero exposure to lithium: a prospective, comparative, observational study. Am J Psychiatry 171(7):785–794, 2014 24781368

Doose DR, Wang SS, Padmanabhan M, et al: Effect of topiramate or carbamazepine on the pharmacokinetics of an oral contraceptive containing norethindrone and ethinyl estradiol in healthy obese and nonobese female subjects. Epilepsia 44(4):540–549, 2003 12681003

Dreifuss FE, Langer DH: Side effects of valproate. Am J Med 84(1A):34–41, 1988 3146224

Duggal HS, Kithas J: Possible neuroleptic malignant syndrome with aripiprazole and fluoxetine. Am J Psychiatry 162(2):397–398, 2005 15677611

Faught E, Morris G, Jacobson M, et al; Postmarketing Antiepileptic Drug Survey (PADS) Group: Adding lamotrigine to valproate: incidence of rash and other adverse effects. Epilepsia 40(8):1135–1140, 1999 10448828

Finley PR, Warner MD, Peabody CA: Clinical relevance of drug interactions with lithium. Clin Pharmacokinet 29(3):172–191, 1995 8521679

Frye MA, Ketter TA, Altshuler LL, et al: Clozapine in bipolar disorder: treatment implications for other atypical antipsychotics. J Affect Disord 48(2–3):91–104, 1998 9543198

Frye MA, Denicoff KD, Bryan AL, et al: Association between lower serum free T4 and greater mood instability and depression in lithium-maintained bipolar patients. Am J Psychiatry 156(12):1909–1914, 1999 10588404

Gadde KM, Franciscy DM, Wagner HR 2nd, et al: Zonisamide for weight loss in obese adults: a randomized controlled trial. JAMA 289(14):1820–1825, 2003 12684361

Gaily E, Kantola-Sorsa E, Hiilesmaa V, et al: Normal intelligence in children with prenatal exposure to carbamazepine. Neurology 62(1):28–32, 2004 14718692

Gelenberg AJ: Lithium efficacy and adverse effects. J Clin Psychiatry 49(Suppl):8–11, 1988 3053673

Gelenberg AJ, Kane JM, Keller MB, et al: Comparison of standard and low serum levels of lithium for maintenance treatment of bipolar disorder. N Engl J Med 321(22):1489–1493, 1989 2811970

Graves NM: Neuropharmacology and drug interactions in clinical practice. Epilepsia 36(Suppl 2):S27–S33, 1995 8784212

Greil W, Ludwig-Mayerhofer W, Erazo N, et al: Lithium versus carbamazepine in the maintenance treatment of bipolar disorders—a randomised study. J Affect Disord 43(2):151–161, 1997 9165384

Hetmar O: The impact of long-term lithium treatment on renal function and structure. Acta Psychiatr Scand Suppl 345:85–89, 1988 3147581

Hirschfeld RM, Keck PE Jr, Kramer M, et al: Rapid antimanic effect of risperidone monotherapy: a 3-week multicenter, double-blind, placebo-controlled trial. Am J Psychiatry 161(6):1057–1065, 2004 15169694

Hung SI, Chung WH, Jee SH, et al: Genetic susceptibility to carbamazepine-induced cutaneous adverse drug reactions. Pharmacogenet Genomics 16(4):297–306, 2006 16538176

Iqbal MM, Rahman A, Husain Z, et al: Clozapine: a clinical review of adverse effects and management. Ann Clin Psychiatry 15(1):33–48, 2003 12839431

Ishibashi T, Horisawa T, Tokuda K, et al: Pharmacological profile of lurasidone, a novel antipsychotic agent with potent 5-hydroxytryptamine 7 (5-HT7) and 5-HT1A receptor activity. J Pharmacol Exp Ther 334(1):171–181, 2010 20404009

Isojärvi JI, Laatikainen TJ, Pakarinen AJ, et al: Polycystic ovaries and hyperandrogenism in women taking valproate for epilepsy. N Engl J Med 329(19):1383–1388, 1993 8413434

Jann MW, Fidone GS, Israel MK, et al: Increased valproate serum concentrations upon carbamazepine cessation. Epilepsia 29(5):578–581, 1988 3137021

Jefferson JW, Greist JH, Clagnaz PJ, et al: Effect of strenuous exercise on serum lithium level in man. Am J Psychiatry 139(12):1593–1595, 1982 6816076

Joffe H, Cohen LS, Suppes T, et al: Valproate is associated with new-onset oligoamenorrhea with hyperandrogenism in women with bipolar disorder. Biol Psychiatry 59(11):1078–1086, 2006 16448626

Junghan U, Albers M, Woggon B: Increased risk of hematological side-effects in psychiatric patients treated with clozapine and carbamazepine? Pharmacopsychiatry 26(6):262, 1993 8127933

Kahn EM, Schulz SC, Perel JM, et al: Change in haloperidol level due to carbamazepine—a complicating factor in combined medication for schizophrenia. J Clin Psychopharmacol 10(1):54–57, 1990 2106534

Kaufman KR, Gerner R: Lamotrigine toxicity secondary to sertraline. Seizure 7(2):163–165, 1998 9627209

Keck PE Jr, Marcus R, Tourkodimitris S, et al; Aripiprazole Study Group: A placebo-controlled, double-blind study of the efficacy and safety of aripiprazole in patients with acute bipolar mania. Am J Psychiatry 160(9):1651–1658, 2003a 12944341

Keck PE Jr, Versiani M, Potkin S, et al; Ziprasidone in Mania Study Group: Ziprasidone in the treatment of acute bipolar mania: a three-week, placebo-controlled, double-blind, randomized trial. Am J Psychiatry 160(4):741–748, 2003b 12668364

Keck PE Jr, Calabrese JR, McQuade RD, et al; Aripiprazole Study Group: A randomized, double-blind, placebo-controlled 26-week trial of aripiprazole in recently manic patients with bipolar I disorder. J Clin Psychiatry 67(4):626–637, 2006 16669728

Kerr BM, Thummel KE, Wurden CJ, et al: Human liver carbamazepine metabolism. Role of CYP3A4 and CYP2C8 in 10,11-epoxide formation. Biochem Pharmacol 47(11):1969–1979, 1994 8010982

Ketter TA: Handbook of Diagnosis and Treatment of Bipolar Disorders. Washington, DC, American Psychiatric Publishing, 2010

Ketter TA, Wang PW: Antidepressants, anxiolytics/hypnotics, and other medications: pharmacokinetics, drug interactions, adverse effects, and administration, in Handbook of Diagnosis and Treatment of Bipolar Disorders. Edited by Ketter TA. Washington, DC, American Psychiatric Publishing, 2010, pp 611–660

Ketter TA, Wang PW: Mood stabilizers and antipsychotics: pharmacokinetics, drug interactions, adverse effects, and administration, in Handbook of Diagnosis and Treatment of Bipolar Disorders. Edited by Ketter TA. Washington, DC, American Psychiatric Publishing, 2010, pp 499–610

Ketter TA, Post RM, Worthington K: Principles of clinically important drug interactions with carbamazepine. Part I. J Clin Psychopharmacol 11(3):198–203, 1991a 2066459

Ketter TA, Post RM, Worthington K: Principles of clinically important drug interactions with carbamazepine. Part II. J Clin Psychopharmacol 11(5):306–313, 1991b 1765573

Ketter TA, Post RM, Parekh PI, et al: Addition of monoamine oxidase inhibitors to carbamazepine: preliminary evidence of safety and antidepressant efficacy in treatment-resistant depression. J Clin Psychiatry 56(10):471–475, 1995 7559374

Ketter TA, Manji HK, Post RM: Potential mechanisms of action of lamotrigine in the treatment of bipolar disorders. J Clin Psychopharmacol 23(5):484–495, 2003 14520126

Ketter TA, Kalali AH, Weisler RH; SPD417 Study Group: A 6-month, multicenter, open-label evaluation of beaded, extended-release carbamazepine capsule monotherapy in bipolar disorder patients with manic or mixed episodes. J Clin Psychiatry 65(5):668–673, 2004 15163253

Ketter TA, Wang PW, Chandler RA, et al: Dermatology precautions and slower titration yield low incidence of lamotrigine treatment-emergent rash. J Clin Psychiatry 66(5):642–645, 2005 15889953

Khanna S, Hirschfeld RMA, Karcher K, et al: Risperidone monotherapy in acute bipolar mania. Paper presented at the 156th Annual Meeting of the American Psychiatric Association, San Francisco, CA, May 17–22, 2003

Kleiner J, Altshuler L, Hendrick V, et al: Lithium-induced subclinical hypothyroidism: review of the literature and guidelines for treatment. J Clin Psychiatry 60(4):249–255, 1999 10221287

Klimke A, Klieser E: Sudden death after intravenous application of lorazepam in a patient treated with clozapine. Am J Psychiatry 151(5):780, 1994 8166326

Koczerginski D, Kennedy SH, Swinson RP: Clonazepam and lithium—a toxic combination in the treatment of mania? Int Clin Psychopharmacol 4(3):195–199, 1989 2794469

Kontaxakis VP, Havaki-Kontaxaki BJ, Stamouli SS, et al: Toxic interaction between risperidone and clozapine: a case report. Prog Neuropsychopharmacol Biol Psychiatry 26(2):407–409, 2002 11817521

Koreen AR, Lieberman JA, Kronig M, et al: Cross-tapering clozapine and risperidone. Am J Psychiatry 152(11):1690, 1995 7485641

Kossen M, Selten JP, Kahn RS: Elevated clozapine plasma level with lamotrigine. Am J Psychiatry 158(11):1930, 2001 11691709

Kukopoulos A, Minnai G, Muller-Oerlinghausen B: The influence of mania and depression on the pharmacokinetics of lithium. A longitudinal single-case study. J Affect Disord 8(2):159–166, 1985 3157725

Lawler CP, Prioleau C, Lewis MM, et al: Interactions of the novel antipsychotic aripiprazole (OPC-14597) with dopamine and serotonin receptor subtypes. Neuropsychopharmacology 20(6):612–627, 1999 10327430

Lee SA, Lee JK, Heo K: Coma probably induced by lorazepam-valproate interaction. Seizure 11(2):124–125, 2002 11945099

Lehman AF, Lieberman JA, Dixon LB, et al: Practice guideline for the treatment of patients with schizophrenia, second edition. Am J Psychiatry 161(2 Suppl):1–56, 2004

Levy RH, Morselli PL, Bianchetti G, et al: Interaction between valproic acid and carbamazepine in epileptic patients, in Metabolism of Antiepileptic Drugs. Edited by Levy RH, Pitlick WH, Eichelbaum M, et al. New York, Raven Press, 1982, pp 45–51

Li X, Ketter TA, Frye MA: Synaptic, intracellular, and neuroprotective mechanisms of anticonvulsants: are they relevant for the treatment and course of bipolar disorders? J Affect Disord 69(1–3):1–14, 2002 12103447

Lima AR, Soares-Weiser K, Bacaltchuk J, et al: Benzodiazepines for neuroleptic-induced acute akathisia. Cochrane Database Syst Rev (1):CD001950, 2002 11869614

Lima WJ, Dopheide JA, Kramer BA, et al: A naturalistic comparison of adverse effects between slow titration and loading of divalproex sodium in psychiatric inpatients. J Affect Disord 52(1–3):261–267, 1999 10357044

Livingstone C, Rampes H: Lithium: a review of its metabolic adverse effects. J Psychopharmacol 20(3):347–355, 2006 16174674

Loebel A, Cucchiaro J, Silva R, et al: Lurasidone as adjunctive therapy with lithium or valproate for the treatment of bipolar I depression: a randomized, double-blind, placebo-controlled study. Am J Psychiatry 171(2):169–177, 2014a 24170221

Loebel A, Cucchiaro J, Silva R, et al: Lurasidone monotherapy in the treatment of bipolar I depression: a randomized, double-blind, placebo-controlled study. Am J Psychiatry 171(2):160–168, 2014b 24170180

Longo LP, Salzman C: Valproic acid effects on serum concentrations of clozapine and norclozapine. Am J Psychiatry 152(4):650, 1995 7694927

López-Muñoz F, Alamo C: Active metabolites as antidepressant drugs: the role of norquetiapine in the mechanism of action of quetiapine in the treatment of mood disorders. Front Psychiatry 4:102, 2013 24062697

Macfadden W, Alphs L, Haskins JT, et al: A randomized, double-blind, placebo-controlled study of maintenance treatment with adjunctive risperidone long-acting therapy in patients with bipolar I disorder who relapse frequently. Bipolar Disord 11(8):827–839, 2009 19922552

Mallikaarjun S, Salazar DE, Bramer SL: Pharmacokinetics, tolerability, and safety of aripiprazole following multiple oral dosing in normal healthy volunteers. J Clin Pharmacol 44(2):179–187, 2004 14747427

Marcus WL: Lithium: a review of its pharmacokinetics, health effects, and toxicology. J Environ Pathol Toxicol Oncol 13(2):73–79, 1994 7884646

May TW, Rambeck B, Jürgens U: Serum concentrations of lamotrigine in epileptic patients: the influence of dose and comedication. Ther Drug Monit 18(5):523–531, 1996 8885114

May TW, Rambeck B, Jürgens U: Influence of oxcarbazepine and methsuximide on lamotrigine concentrations in epileptic patients with and without valproic acid comedication: results of a retrospective study. Ther Drug Monit 21(2):175–181, 1999 10217337

McElroy SL, Keck PE, Stanton SP, et al: A randomized comparison of divalproex oral loading versus haloperidol in the initial treatment of acute psychotic mania. J Clin Psychiatry 57(4):142–146, 1996 8601548

McElroy SL, Guerdjikova A, Kotwal R, et al: Atomoxetine in the treatment of binge-eating disorder: a randomized placebo-controlled trial. J Clin Psychiatry 68(3):390–398, 2007 17388708

McIntyre RS, Brecher M, Paulsson B, et al: Quetiapine or haloperidol as monotherapy for bipolar mania—a 12-week, double-blind, randomised, parallel-group, placebo-controlled trial. Eur Neuropsychopharmacol 15(5):573–585, 2005 16139175

McIntyre RS, Cohen M, Zhao J, et al: A 3-week, randomized, placebo-controlled trial of asenapine in the treatment of acute mania in bipolar mania and mixed states. Bipolar Disord 11(7):673–686, 2009 19839993

McIntyre RS, Cohen M, Zhao J, et al: Asenapine in the treatment of acute mania in bipolar I disorder: a randomized, double-blind, placebo-controlled trial. J Affect Disord 122(1–2):27–38, 2010 20096936

Meltzer HY, Massey BW: The role of serotonin receptors in the action of atypical antipsychotic drugs. Curr Opin Pharmacol 11(1):59–67, 2011 21420906

Meltzer HY, Alphs L, Green AI, et al; International Suicide Prevention Trial Study Group: Clozapine treatment for suicidality in schizophrenia: International Suicide Prevention Trial (InterSePT). Arch Gen Psychiatry 60(1):82–91, 2003 12511175

Meyer JM: Individual changes in clozapine levels after smoking cessation: results and a predictive model. J Clin Psychopharmacol 21(6):569–574, 2001 11763003

Meyer JM, Loebel AD, Schweizer E: Lurasidone: a new drug in development for schizophrenia. Expert Opin Investig Drugs 18(11):1715–1726, 2009 19780705

Mikati MA, Schachter SC, Schomer DL, et al: Long-term tolerability, pharmaco-kinetic and preliminary efficacy study of lamotrigine in patients with resistant partial seizures. Clin Neuropharmacol 12(4):312–321, 1989 2804994

Morrow J, Russell A, Guthrie E, et al: Malformation risks of antiepileptic drugs in pregnancy: a prospective study from the UK Epilepsy and Pregnancy Register. J Neurol Neurosurg Psychiatry 77(2):193–198, 2006 16157661

Murphy DJ, Gannon MA, Hartman ML: Extrapyramidal symptoms with addition of lithium to neuroleptics. J Nerv Ment Dis 177(11):708, 1989 2572677

Nakamura A, Mihara K, Nagai G, et al: Pharmacokinetic and pharmacodynamic interactions between carbamazepine and aripiprazole in patients with schizophrenia. Ther Drug Monit 31(5):575–578, 2009 19701114

Nemeroff CB, Kinkead B, Goldstein J: Quetiapine: preclinical studies, pharmacokinetics, drug interactions, and dosing. J Clin Psychiatry 63(Suppl 13):5–11, 2002 12562141

Nierenberg AA, Friedman ES, Bowden CL, et al: Lithium treatment moderate-dose use study (LiTMUS) for bipolar disorder: a randomized comparative effectiveness trial of optimized personalized treatment with and without lithium. Am J Psychiatry 170(1):102–110, 2013 23288387

Nierenberg AA, Sylvia LG, Leon AC, et al; Bipolar CHOICE Study Group: Clinical and Health Outcomes Initiative in Comparative Effectiveness for Bipolar Disorder (Bipolar CHOICE): a pragmatic trial of complex treatment for a complex disorder. Clin Trials 11(1):114–127, 2014 24346608

Okumura J: Decrease in plasma zonisamide concentrations after coadministration of risperidone in a patient with schizophrenia receiving zonisamide therapy [abstract]. Int Clin Psychopharmacol 14(1):55, 1999

Oral ET, Altinbas K, Demirkiran S: Sudden akathisia after a ziprasidone dose reduction. Am J Psychiatry 163(3):546, 2006 16513883

Padala PR, Sadiq HJ, Padala KP: Urinary obstruction with citalopram and aripiprazole combination in an elderly patient. J Clin Psychopharmacol 26(6):667–668, 2006 17110829

Paul S, Cooke BK, Nguyen M: Glossopharyngeal dystonia secondary to a lurasidone-fluoxetine CYP-3A4 interaction. Case Rep Psychiatry 2013:136194, 2013 23762720

Peano C, Leikin JB, Hanashiro PK: Seizures, ventricular tachycardia, and rhabdomyolysis as a result of ingestion of venlafaxine and lamotrigine. Ann Emerg Med 30(5):704–708, 1997 9360588

Physicians' Desk Reference 2015, 69th Edition. Montvale, NJ, PDR Network, 2014

Pisani F, Caputo M, Fazio A, et al: Interaction of carbamazepine-10,11-epoxide, an active metabolite of carbamazepine, with valproate: a pharmacokinetic study. Epilepsia 31(3):339–342, 1990 2111769

Pope HG Jr, Cole JO, Choras PT, et al: Apparent neuroleptic malignant syndrome with clozapine and lithium. J Nerv Ment Dis 174(8):493–495, 1986 3090198

Potkin SG, Keck PE Jr, Segal S, et al: Ziprasidone in acute bipolar mania: a 21-day randomized, double-blind, placebo-controlled replication trial. J Clin Psychopharmacol 25(4):301–310, 2005 16012271

Potter WZ, Ketter TA: Pharmacological issues in the treatment of bipolar disorder: focus on mood-stabilizing compounds. Can J Psychiatry 38(3) (Suppl 2):S51–S56, 1993 8500079

Poyurovsky M, Pashinian A, Weizman R, et al: Low-dose mirtazapine: a new option in the treatment of antipsychotic-induced akathisia. A randomized, double-blind, placebo- and propranolol-controlled trial. Biol Psychiatry 59(11):1071–1077, 2006 16497273

Preskorn SH, Flockhart DA: 2010 Guide to Psychiatric Drug Interactions. Prim Psychiatry 16(12):45–74, 2009

Quiroz JA, Gould TD, Manji HK: Molecular effects of lithium. Mol Interv 4(5):259–272, 2004 15471909

Raaska K, Raitasuo V, Laitila J, et al: Effect of caffeine-containing versus decaffeinated coffee on serum clozapine concentrations in hospitalised patients. Basic Clin Pharmacol Toxicol 94(1):13–18, 2004 14725610

Rambeck B, Wolf P: Lamotrigine clinical pharmacokinetics. Clin Pharmacokinet 25(6):433–443, 1993 8119045

Rasgon N: The relationship between polycystic ovary syndrome and antiepileptic drugs: a review of the evidence. J Clin Psychopharmacol 24(3):322–334, 2004 15118487

Rasgon NL, Altshuler LL, Fairbanks L, et al: Reproductive function and risk for PCOS in women treated for bipolar disorder. Bipolar Disord 7(3):246–259, 2005 15898962

Rosenhagen MC, Schmidt U, Weber F, et al: Combination therapy of lamotrigine and escitalopram may cause myoclonus. J Clin Psychopharmacol 26(3):346–347, 2006 16702909

Rowland A, Elliot DJ, Williams JA, et al: In vitro characterization of lamotrigine N2-glucuronidation and the lamotrigine-valproic acid interaction. Drug Metab Dispos 34(6):1055–1062, 2006 16565174

Sabers A, Gram L: Newer anticonvulsants: comparative review of drug interactions and adverse effects. Drugs 60(1):23–33, 2000 10929928

Sachs GS, Grossman F, Ghaemi SN, et al: Combination of a mood stabilizer with risperidone or haloperidol for treatment of acute mania: a double-blind, placebo-controlled comparison of efficacy and safety. Am J Psychiatry 159(7):1146–1154, 2002 12091192

Sachs G, Chengappa KN, Suppes T, et al: Quetiapine with lithium or divalproex for the treatment of bipolar mania: a randomized, double-blind, placebo-controlled study. Bipolar Disord 6(3):213–223, 2004 15117400

Sachs G, Bowden C, Calabrese JR, et al: Effects of lamotrigine and lithium on body weight during maintenance treatment of bipolar I disorder. Bipolar Disord 8(2):175–181, 2006a 16542188

Sachs G, Sanchez R, Marcus R, et al; Aripiprazole Study Group: Aripiprazole in the treatment of acute manic or mixed episodes in patients with bipolar I disorder: a 3-week placebo-controlled study. J Psychopharmacol 20(4):536–546, 2006b 16401666

Sattar SP, Ramaswamy S, Bhatia SC, et al: Somnambulism due to probable interaction of valproic acid and zolpidem. Ann Pharmacother 37(10):1429–1433, 2003 14519043

Schou M, Weinstein MR: Problems of lithium maintenance treatment during pregnancy, delivery and lactation. Agressologie 21(A):7–9, 1980

Seeman P: Atypical antipsychotics: mechanism of action. Can J Psychiatry 47(1):27–38, 2002 11873706

Shahid M, Walker GB, Zorn SH, et al: Asenapine: a novel psychopharmacologic agent with a unique human receptor signature. J Psychopharmacol 23(1):65–73, 2009 18308814

Shin JG, Soukhova N, Flockhart DA: Effect of antipsychotic drugs on human liver cytochrome P-450 (CYP) isoforms in vitro: preferential inhibition of CYP2D6. Drug Metab Dispos 27(9):1078–1084, 1999 10460810

Shukla S, Godwin CD, Long LE, et al: Lithium-carbamazepine neurotoxicity and risk factors. Am J Psychiatry 141(12):1604–1606, 1984 6439058

Shulman KI, Mackenzie S, Hardy B: The clinical use of lithium carbonate in old age: a review. Prog Neuropsychopharmacol Biol Psychiatry 11(2–3):159–164, 1987 3114827

Smith MC, Centorrino F, Welge JA, et al: Clinical comparison of extended-release divalproex versus delayed-release divalproex: pooled data analyses from nine trials. Epilepsy Behav 5(5):746–751, 2004 15380129

Smith T, Riskin J: Effect of clozapine on plasma nortriptyline concentration. Pharmacopsychiatry 27(1):41–42, 1994 8159782

Snoeck E, Van Peer A, Sack M, et al: Influence of age, renal and liver impairment on the pharmacokinetics of risperidone in man. Psychopharmacology (Berl) 122(3):223–229, 1995 8748391

Sproule B: Lithium in bipolar disorder: can drug concentrations predict therapeutic effect? Clin Pharmacokinet 41(9):639–660, 2002 12126457

Stahl SM, Shayegan DK: The psychopharmacology of ziprasidone: receptor-binding properties and real-world psychiatric practice. J Clin Psychiatry 64(Suppl 19):6–12, 2003 14728084

Staines AG, Coughtrie MW, Burchell B: N-glucuronidation of carbamazepine in human tissues is mediated by UGT2B7. J Pharmacol Exp Ther 311(3):1131–1137, 2004 15292462

Suppes T, Webb A, Paul B, et al: Clinical outcome in a randomized 1-year trial of clozapine versus treatment as usual for patients with treatment-resistant illness and a history of mania. Am J Psychiatry 156(8):1164–1169, 1999 10450255

Swainston Harrison T, Perry CM: Aripiprazole: a review of its use in schizophrenia and schizoaffective disorder. Drugs 64(15):1715–1736, 2004 15257633

Swann AC, Berman N, Frazer A, et al: Lithium distribution in mania: single-dose pharmacokinetics and sympathoadrenal function. Psychiatry Res 32(1):71–84, 1990 2112261

Szegedi A, Calabrese JR, Stet L, et al; Apollo Study Group: Asenapine as adjunctive treatment for acute mania associated with bipolar disorder: results of a 12-week core study and 40-week extension. J Clin Psychopharmacol 32(1):46–55, 2012 22198448

Terao T, Abe H, Abe K: Irreversible sinus node dysfunction induced by resumption of lithium therapy. Acta Psychiatr Scand 93(5):407–408, 1996 8792913

Thase ME, Macfadden W, Weisler RH, et al; BOLDER II Study Group: Efficacy of quetiapine monotherapy in bipolar I and II depression: a double-blind, placebo-controlled study (the BOLDER II study). J Clin Psychopharmacol 26(6):600–609, 2006 17110817

Thase ME, Jonas A, Khan A, et al: Aripiprazole monotherapy in nonpsychotic bipolar I depression: results of 2 randomized, placebo-controlled studies. J Clin Psychopharmacol 28(1):13–20, 2008 18204335

Tiihonen J, Vartiainen H, Hakola P: Carbamazepine-induced changes in plasma levels of neuroleptics. Pharmacopsychiatry 28(1):26–28, 1995 7746842

Timmer RT, Sands JM: Lithium intoxication. J Am Soc Nephrol 10(3):666–674, 1999 10073618

Tohen M, Castillo J, Baldessarini RJ, et al: Blood dyscrasias with carbamazepine and valproate: a pharmacoepidemiological study of 2,228 patients at risk. Am J Psychiatry 152(3):413–418, 1995 7864268

Tohen M, Sanger TM, McElroy SL, et al; Olanzapine HGEH Study Group: Olanzapine versus placebo in the treatment of acute mania. Am J Psychiatry 156(5):702–709, 1999 10327902

Tohen M, Jacobs TG, Grundy SL, et al; The Olanzipine HGGW Study Group: Efficacy of olanzapine in acute bipolar mania: a double-blind, placebo-controlled study. Arch Gen Psychiatry 57(9):841–849, 2000 10986547

Tohen M, Chengappa KN, Suppes T, et al: Efficacy of olanzapine in combination with valproate or lithium in the treatment of mania in patients partially nonresponsive to valproate or lithium monotherapy. Arch Gen Psychiatry 59(1):62–69, 2002 11779284

Tohen M, Ketter TA, Zarate CA, et al: Olanzapine versus divalproex sodium for the treatment of acute mania and maintenance of remission: a 47-week study. Am J Psychiatry 160(7):1263–1271, 2003a 12832240

Tohen M, Vieta E, Calabrese J, et al: Efficacy of olanzapine and olanzapine-fluoxetine combination in the treatment of bipolar I depression. Arch Gen Psychiatry 60(11):1079–1088, 2003b 14609883

Tohen M, Greil W, Calabrese JR, et al: Olanzapine versus lithium in the maintenance treatment of bipolar disorder: a 12-month, randomized, double-blind, controlled clinical trial. Am J Psychiatry 162(7):1281–1290, 2005 15994710

Tohen M, Calabrese JR, Sachs GS, et al: Randomized, placebo-controlled trial of olanzapine as maintenance therapy in patients with bipolar I disorder responding to acute treatment with olanzapine. Am J Psychiatry 163(2):247–256, 2006 16449478

Vajda FJ, Hitchcock A, Graham J, et al: The Australian Register of Antiepileptic Drugs in Pregnancy: the first 1002 pregnancies. Aust NZ J Obstet Gynaecol 47(6):468–474, 2007 17991111

Verdoux H, Bourgeois ML: A case of lithium neurotoxicity with irreversible cerebellar syndrome. J Nerv Ment Dis 178(12):761–762, 1990 2123235

Vieta E, Bourin M, Sanchez R, et al; Aripoprazole Study Group: Effectiveness of aripiprazole v. haloperidol in acute bipolar mania: double-blind, randomised, comparative 12-week trial. Br J Psychiatry 187:235–242, 2005 16135860

Viguera AC, Newport DJ, Ritchie J, et al: Lithium in breast milk and nursing infants: clinical implications. Am J Psychiatry 164(2):342–345, 2007 17267800

Wang CY, Zhang ZJ, Li WB, et al: The differential effects of steady-state fluvoxamine on the pharmacokinetics of olanzapine and clozapine in healthy volunteers. J Clin Pharmacol 44(7):785–792, 2004 15199083

Watson B: Absence status and the concurrent administration of clonazepam and valproate sodium. Am J Hosp Pharm 36(7):887, 1979 112862

Weisler RH, Kalali AH, Ketter TA; SPD417 Study Group: A multicenter, randomized, double-blind, placebo-controlled trial of extended-release carbamazepine capsules as monotherapy for bipolar disorder patients with manic or mixed episodes. J Clin Psychiatry 65(4):478–484, 2004 15119909

Weisler RH, Keck PE Jr, Swann AC, et al; SPD417 Study Group: Extended-release carbamazepine capsules as monotherapy for acute mania in bipolar disorder: a multicenter, randomized, double-blind, placebo-controlled trial. J Clin Psychiatry 66(3):323–330, 2005 15766298

Wong SL, Cavanaugh J, Shi H, et al: Effects of divalproex sodium on amitriptyline and nortriptyline pharmacokinetics. Clin Pharmacol Ther 60(1):48–53, 1996 8689811

Wyszynski DF, Nambisan M, Surve T, et al; Antiepileptic Drug Pregnancy Registry: Increased rate of major malformations in offspring exposed to valproate during pregnancy. Neurology 64(6):961 965, 2005 15781808

Yasui-Furukori N, Kondo T, Mihara K, et al: Significant dose effect of carbamazepine on reduction of steady-state plasma concentration of haloperidol in schizophrenic patients. J Clin Psychopharmacol 23(5):435–440, 2003 14520118

Yatham LN, Grossman F, Augustyns I, et al: Mood stabilisers plus risperidone or placebo in the treatment of acute mania. International, double-blind, randomised controlled trial. Br J Psychiatry 182:141–147, 2003 12562742

Yatham LN, Paulsson B, Mullen J, et al: Quetiapine versus placebo in combination with lithium or divalproex for the treatment of bipolar mania. J Clin Psychopharmacol 24(6):599–606, 2004 15538120

Yeung CK, Chan HH: Cutaneous adverse effects of lithium: epidemiology and management. Am J Clin Dermatol 5(1):3–8, 2004 14979738

Zarate CA Jr, Tohen M, Narendran R, et al: The adverse effect profile and efficacy of divalproex sodium compared with valproic acid: a pharmacoepidemiology study. J Clin Psychiatry 60(4):232–236, 1999 10221283

Zevin S, Benowitz NL: Drug interactions with tobacco smoking. An update. Clin Pharmacokinet 36(6):425–438, 1999 10427467

Index

*Page numbers printed in **boldface** type refer to tables or figures.*